OXFORD MEDICAL PUBLICATIONS

The Handbook of Alternative and Complementary Medicine

The Handbook of Alternative and Complementary Medicine

Third Edition

STEPHEN FULDER

OXFORD UNIVERSITY PRESS

*This book has been printed digitally and produced in a standard specification
in order to ensure its continuing availability*

OXFORD
UNIVERSITY PRESS

Great Clarendon Street, Oxford OX2 6DP

Oxford University Press is a department of the University of Oxford.
It furthers the University's objective of excellence in research, scholarship,
and education by publishing worldwide in

Oxford New York

Auckland Bangkok Buenos Aires Cape Town Chennai
Dar es Salaam Delhi Hong Kong Istanbul Karachi Kolkata
Kuala Lumpur Madrid Melbourne Mexico City Mumbai Nairobi
Sᴄ o Paulo Shanghai Taipei Tokyo Toronto

Oxford is a registered trade mark of Oxford University Press
in the UK and in certain other countries

Published in the United States
by Oxford University Press Inc., New York

ISBN 0-19-262669-8

Cover illustration: *Mary Evans Picture Library*

Printed in Great Britain by
Antony Rowe Ltd., Eastbourne

Preface to Third Edition

Alternatives to conventional medicine currently command great interest on both sides of the Atlantic. As we shall see, around one-third of the population of the modern world now consult alternative practitioners, and alternative remedies are now on sale in every pharmacy. With the publication of the recent positive report from the British Medical Association, these therapies are set to move into the UK National Health Service. Calls for prior validation of the therapies by clinical studies have been virtually abandoned; the osteopaths are now state-registered without any proper scientific validation of osteopathy. Things are changing very fast. We are moving towards a pluralistic medicine at a pace that is taking everyone by surprise. It is strange, therefore, that there is very little in the way of comprehensive texts for professionals and the interested public on what exactly alternative medicine is, what its practitioners do, how it arrived, what is its status, and what is its future. This is the case as much today as ten years ago. Although many books containing information on individual therapies have been published, hardly any provide a thorough examination of the present state of these alternatives. There is also a considerable need for a comprehensive review of the organizations and training establishments involved with alternative therapies. Nor can one find a summary of the rationale and practice of the therapies which is written with the sceptical conventional medical practitioner as much in mind as the devotees and practitioners of the therapies themselves. I have attempted to rectify the situation with the publication of this book which I hope will fulfil both professional and lay requirements.

Lack of information on the usage and changing role of the therapies has been one reason for the absence of published guides on the therapies, and indeed has prevented an appreciation of their real importance. It was to remedy this that in 1981 the Threshold Foundation provided a generous grant to Robin Monro and myself to gather and compile all available information on the state of the therapies at that time.[1] By means of primary questionnaire-based research, as well as the

[1] Fulder, S. J. and Monro, R. (1981). *The status of complementary medicine in the United Kingdom*, Threshold Foundation, London. Fulder, S. J. and Monro, R. (1985). Complementary medicine in the United Kingdom: patients, practitioners, and consultations. *Lancet*, 2, 542–5. The survey data is referred to frequently in this book. It was collected during 1980/1981, and included a poll which

collection of documents on scientific, social, and legal aspects, a comprehensive classified directory of organizations and their activities, bibliographies, press cuttings, etc., the first full picture of the state of alternative medicine in the UK and Europe was obtained. This resource has made the book possible, is still a useful source of data, and has acted as a foundation upon which more recent studies have built.

My own position within this book is to attempt to be true to both the vast knowledge and experience of scientific medicine, and the equally vast and often contrasting knowledge of the alternative therapies. In principle, after many years as a research scientist in the biomedical field, and more than 20 years' researching, writing, and, most importantly, using alternative medicine, I feel that it should be possible. Yet I also know it to be impossible. For in too many key areas, the two systems of medicine find each other indigestible and in unresolvable conflict. The world views can be incompatable, there are political and commercial interests at stake, the languages used are at times incomprehensible to each other, and the medical systems are in cultural struggle. In many cases I have had to take sides, and it will be clear that I have strong sympathies with some of the vitalistic positions of complementary medicine. If this irritates some medical readers, I can only say in my defence that there are thousand upon thousands of medical books with a very strong bias towards the current biomedical paradigm. Let there be at least a few books with an opposite bias.

The issue of objectivity is very delicate, in part because it has been used as one of the tests by which science has judged non-scientific medicine. Leaving aside the fact that physics today would state that there is no such thing as a totally independent observer, the subjective experiential reality is such an essential component of the healing process and world view of alternative medicine, that it must be honoured in this book, even if this creates conflicts with scientific medicine. To give a personal example, if my family or myself fall ill, I have always gone out into our herb garden, selected the necessary medicinal plants and used them for effective treatments. This experience has no place in a scientific text, but is essential to a portrait of alternative therapies. In the end I include both the position of science, discussing the research issues in general and specific to each therapy, and the subjective position of the alternative therapies and the activities of therapists as they see themselves. I do not aim for reconciliations and integration. Also, no judgements are intended regarding the relative qualities of the therapies. These valuations must be made at a later date by society as a whole.

---

[1] *contd.*
sought information from all the organizations representing therapists (including healers) on various categories of practising membership, growth and estimates as to total number of practising therapists in the UK in that therapy, and other details such as educational programmes. Response was virtually 100 per cent. Another questionnaire was submitted to therapists whose names were obtained from registers, yellow pages, local periodicals, health shops and centres, other therapists, etc. Probably all the therapists practising in Oxfordshire and Cambridge were identified and by means of follow-up interviews 80–90 per cent completed questionnaires. In Cardiff, Exeter, Sheffield, Hereford, and Cumbria detection of therapists was patchy, and only a third of the questionnaires were completed. Only professional therapists who treated members of the public, normally for a fee, were interviewed. A total of 137 completed questionnaires were received.

I must further state at the outset my conviction that complementary medicine has a vital role to play in our future; because of its emphasis on safe and subtle treatment methods and self-care, it will be able to contain many chronic and insidious diseases which conventional medicine has failed to cure. I believe in a pluralistic health system and these views are expressed and supported in this book.

In order to keep this book in manageable proportions some boundaries have had to be drawn. First, the book encompasses therapies that treat the body and the whole being, but I have had to exclude all the purely psychological and psychotherapeutic therapies: encounter, psychosynthesis, meditation, Gestalt, bioenergetics, and the other 140 psychotherapies listed by President Carter's commission on mental health. However, since mental and physical health are interconnected, psychological therapies that are more psychosomatic, such as hypnotherapy, autogenics, and biofeedback, are included. I have also distinguished between healing and general inner development, regretfully omitting such disciplines as yoga, T'ai-Chi, martial arts, or sports. These are primarily designed for the healthy, and although they can also be invaluable in treating the sick, they are rarely tailored specifically to the diagnosed condition of each individual.

Every effort has been made to be accurate and as up to date as possible. Entries for the organizational directory were sent to each establishment for checking; the material is therefore dependent on their willingness to supply accurate information. I hope that organizations will approach the author through the publishers with further information to maintain the accuracy of this handbook.

June 1996   S.F.

Note on terminology. Where the word *medicine* is used, it is distinguished by the adjectives *conventional* or *complementary*. *Practitioner* is used likewise to refer to all professionals with its meaning defined by its context, but of course *doctor* or *physician* are used exclusively in connection with conventional medicine and *therapist* in connection with complementary medicine. *Complementary* and *alternative* are used interchangeably to mean the aggregate of non-conventional healing systems and methods, and *therapy* is used for one of them.

Acknowledgements

First I should like to acknowledge Dr Robin Monro, my friend and partner in the Threshold Project for his extensive and careful work. I thank Ruth West, William Cash, Mr A.J. de Wit of the Dutch Commission on Alternative Medicine, Herta Larive, and the many others who have supplied information to us; the late John Blackwood for his careful reading of the manuscript; Clare Wright whose steady and intelligent assistance is greatly appreciated, and my wife Rachel, for her forbearance and intuition. I would also like to thank Dr Midge Whitelegg and Alison Gould for their careful and insightful research assistance for this third edition.

I am greatly indebted to the following leading practitioners with whom the chapters indicated have been written, and without whom this book would have been impossible: Peter Bartlett LCSP (Applied kinesiology); Robert Davidson R.S. Hom., MCH, (Homeopathy); Colin Dove MRO (Osteopathy); Jonathan Drake MD (Alexander Technique); Michael Endacott (Healing); Michael Evans MD (Anthroposophical medicine); Nicola Hall (Reflexology); Simon Mills MNIMH (Herbalism); Roger Newman-Turner ND, DO, B.Ac. (Naturopathy and nutrition therapy); Iris Oliver (Remedial massage); David Tansley DC (Radionics); Lorraine Taylor, SRN, B.Ac. (Acupuncture and oriental medicine).

I am most grateful to the Threshold Foundation for supporting the national survey which generated a good deal of the data and material on which this book is based, and to Harold Wicks, past General Secretary of the Research Council for Complementary Medicine, for his tireless and continuing support and interest.

Contents

Glossary and classification of therapies   xv

PART 1: GENERAL SURVEY

1 The background   3
Defining complementary medicine, The unique features of
complementary medicine, The art of diagnosis, Holistic
medicine—the new Hippocratism, The history of medicine,
Complementary therapies and the crisis in medicine, Revival of
complementary medicine, The issue of research, References

2 The patient   31
How many people go to complementary practitioners?, Why
do people go to complementary practitioners?, Who are the
patients?, The health problems treated by complementary
practitioners, Patient satisfaction with complementary and
conventional medicine, References

3 The therapist   46
Who are the therapists?, Numbers of therapists practising
in the UK, The cost of complementary medicine, How many
patients do therapists see?, The consultation, Clinics, health
centres, and hospitals, The training of complementary
practitioners, The current state of therapists' education,
Accreditation and standards in complementary medical
training, The biomedical content of complementary
practitioners' education, The complementary content of
medical practitioners' education, Competence and quackery,
The organization of complementary medicine, References

4 **Policy, law, and the National Health Service**   70
The practice of medicine and the law, The lay complementary
practitioner and the law, Approaches to registration
of complementary practitioners, The influence of the
European Union on complementary professions, Advertising
standards, Insurance, Sickness and death certificates,
Homeopathy—medicine's unwelcome bedfellow, Unsuccessful
steps to control hypnotherapy, Acupuncture needles,
Herbs and medicines, Homeopathic remedies, Background,
Breaking the barriers, First steps to integration, Examples
of complementary medicine in primary care, Complementary
medicine in secondary care, References

5 **Complementary medicine internationally**   97
The United States, Western Europe, Germany, France, The
Netherlands, The rest of Europe and Scandinavia, The EEC
and complementary medicine, Russia and Eastern Europe,
Australia, New Zealand, and South Africa, Traditional and
indigenous medicine—its worldwide fate, China, India, References

PART 2: THE THERAPIES

6 **Acupuncture and Oriental medicine**   125
Background, Diagnostic and therapeutic practices,
Applications and contra-indications, Research, New types of
therapy, Obtaining treatment, References

7 **Alexander and Feldenkrais techniques**   143
Alexander Technique, Feldenkrais Technique, Research,
References

8 **Anthroposophical medicine**   147
Background, Fundamental concepts, Health and disease,
Diagnostic and therapeutic practices, Applications, Research
and development, References

9 **Ayurveda**   157
Research, Obtaining treatment, References

10 **Chiropractic**   162
Background, Concepts, Practice, Research, Uses and risks,
References

11 **Creative and sensory therapies**   171
Creative therapies, Colour and sound therapies, References

12 **Healing**   176
Background, Fundamental concepts, Diagnosis and treatment,
Research, Uses and risks, References

13 **Herbalism**   186
Background, Fundamental concepts, Diagnostic and
therapeutic practices, Uses and risks, Research, Types of
therapist, References

14 **Homeopathy**   199
Background, Fundamental concepts, Diagnosis and treatment,
Research, Uses, Risks, Types of therapy, References

15 **Hypnotherapy**   210
Background, Concepts and theory, Method, Research, Uses
and risks, Otaining treatment, References

16 **Manual therapies including reflexology and aromatherapy**   220
Remedial massage, Reflexology, Structural integration—
rolfing, Shiatzu—Japanese pressure point massage, Applied
kinesiology, Spinal touch treatment, Aromatherapy,
References

17 **Mind-body therapies**   232
The mind in disease, The mind in treatment, Relaxation
techniques, Biofeedback, Autogenic therapy, The Bates method
of eyesight training, References

18 **Naturopathy and nutritional medicine**   244
Background, Fundamental concepts, Diagnosis, The treatment,
Fasting and other restricted diets, The dynamics of structure,
The body-mind amalgam, Nutrition therapy, Research, Uses
and risks, References

19 **Osteopathy**   258
Background and fundamental concepts, Diagnosis, Treatment,
Research and development, References

20 **Radionics and psionic medicine**   266
Background, Fundamental concepts, Diagnostic and
therapeutic practices, Applications and contra-indications,
Research and development, Obtaining treatment, Psionic
medicine, References

Bibliography   272
Directory of UK organizations in Complementary Medicine   289
Index   309

Glossary and classification of therapies

Main therapeutic specialities are in **bold** type, therapeutic subspecialities are in *italics*.
Synonyms are in roman type.

Medical systems

Complementary medicine
  Alternative medicine
  Fringe medicine
  Unconventional
  medicine
  Unorthodox medicine
  Natural medicine

The aggregate of diagnostic and therapeutic practices and systems which are separate from conventional scientific medicine. They are usually less interventionist and technical and make more use of self-healing capacities.

Conventional medicine
  Scientific medicine
  Orthodox medicine
  Technical medicine
  Modern medicine

The aggregate of diagnostic and therapeutic concepts and practices which adhere to and employ modern scientific principles, and techniques.

Far Eastern medicine
  Oriental medicine
  Chinese, Korean,
  Japanese, Tibetan,
  etc.

The aggregate of unique diagnostic and therapeutic practices developed in Far Eastern countries, in particular acupuncture, constitutional medicine, Oriental herbalism, movement, massage, and dietary control.

Folk medicine

The aggregate of practices, remedies, and recipes which form a largely unwritten and unsystematic body of knowledge among the lay population.

Holistic medicine	The combined use of conventional medicine, complementary medicine, psychotherapy, and health education by medical and other practitioners and instructors, often within a General Practice setting.
Indian medicine	The unique traditional medicine and remedies of the Indian sub-continent.
Ayurvedic medicine	The aggregate of diagnostic and therapeutic practices, based on the Vedic texts, incorporating a complete life instruction and branches on constitutional medicine, surgery, remedies, longevity practices, etc.
Unani medicine	Ayurvedic medicine joined with ancient Arabic medicine.
Siddha medicine	Ayurvedic medicine joined with the indigenous medicines of the Dravidian people of Southern India.

Traditional medicine
  Primitive medicine
  Indigenous medicine
	The aggregate of indigenous diagnostic and therapeutic practices, which may or may not be formal and systematic, which form an integral part of culture.

Therapies in complementary medicine

Acupuncture	Techniques whereby needles are inserted into specific sites on the body surface to improve the flow of energy around the body, thus preventing and treating disease and disability.
Acupressure Shiatzu	Techniques whereby finger massage is applied to these same points, combined, in shiatzu, with general massage.

Electro-acupuncture	Adaption of acupuncture in which small electrical currents are applied to needles inserted into the acupuncture points.
Ear acupuncture Auricular therapy	Acupuncture solely applied to points in and around the ear in order to affect other parts of the body.
Moxibustion	The burning of rolled cones of dried *Artemisia* (mugwort) over acupuncture points in order to affect the flow of energy at those points to prevent and treat diseases and disabilities.
Anthroposophical medicine	A therapeutic system based on the teachings of Rudolf Steiner in which physical health is achieved through harmony between the various co-existent aspects of man and the environment. Creativity, self-observation, and special (including homeopathic) remedies are used.
Eurythmy	An anthroposophical method using specific rhythmical movements and dance to heal and reintegrate healthy, sick, or disabled people.
Speech therapy	The similar use of sound, speech, and breath.
Art therapy	The similar use of art, colour, and form.
Aromatherapy	External use of concentrated essential oils from plants, often in association with massage, to relieve symptoms and aid well-being.
Breathing therapies	Use of breath for therapeutic purposes.
Pranayama	Indian yogic methods of cultivation of breathing for therapeutic and spiritual purposes.

Diagnosis

Iridology

Diagnosis by observation of the marks, patterns, and colours of the iris, which are reflections of body diseases and experiences.

Auric diagnosis

Psychic diagnosis by analysis of the colours and changes of the aura perceived by sensitives.

Kirlian photography

Diagnostic method which photographs the corona discharge of 'bioenergy' around the body.

Electrical therapies

Use of electromagnetic energy directly for therapeutic purposes.

Magnetic field therapy

Use of a magnetic field to aid repair, regeneration, and healing of tissues.

Diathermy

The use of equipment to send pulses of electromagnetic energy deep into tissues to warm and stimulate them.

Ion generators

Equipment to generate and emit negatively charged ion particles in order to aid mood and concentration.

Healing
  Faith healing
  Spiritual healing
  Magnetic healing
  Mental healing
  Laying on of hands

The direct transmission of psychic energy for therapeutic purposes.

Absent healing

Healing which is given by healer to a patient who is at a distance.

Prayer healing

Healing which is focused, transmitted, and effected by means of prayer.

Spirit healing
  Exorcism

Use of discarnate entities in healing.

Auric healing	Healing directed towards the subtle or etheric aura of the body to cure its susceptibilities and prevent their manifestation in the body as diseases.
Homeopathy	A therapeutic system developed by Samuel Hahnemann, which treats the symptoms of a patient with diluted, microscopic, doses of those remedies which create similar symptoms in the healthy.
Biochemic remedies	Small amounts of salts used on homeopathic principles.
Bach flower remedies	Extracts of flowers diluted according to homeopathic principles which are applied to cure subtle emotional roots of disease.
Hydrotherapy **Balneology**	The use of mineral water, thermal springs, mud, pools, and bathing in therapy.
Spas	Health resorts primarily devoted to hydrotherapy
Manipulative therapies	Treatment by means of manual force or touch or pressure applied to the body.
Chiropractic	A technique in which movement and function of the musculoskeletal system is restored, especially between the vertebrae, by means of massage and short sharp thrusts.
Osteopathy	A technique in which movement and function of the musculoskeletal system is restored by means of leverage and repeated manual articulation.
Cranial osteopathy	Pressure applied to the bones of the cranium to affect musculature and body fluids for the treatment of specific conditions.

Manipulation	Leverage and articulation of the body used pragmatically, usually by medical doctors, without connection to the techniques of osteopathy and chiropractic.
Bonesetting	The restoration of alignment and integrity of limbs after injury.
Massage	Any technique in which pressure and touch are applied to the body to stimulate the circulation and relax the tissues.
Kinesiology	A technique in which muscular strength and balance at distant points is used to determine the site and nature of a local impairment.
Reflexology Reflex zone therapy	Massage of areas of the feet to treat organ systems with which they are in developmental and energetic relationship.
Polarity therapy	Combination of massage and the teaching of awareness of the body and its dimensions and interrelations.
Rolfing	A deep massage technique to make structural alterations in the musculature, to liberate tensions, and to awaken protected, underused areas.
Postural integration	A massage and instructural process which realigns the body, liberating tensions and inhibitions.
Naturopathy Nature cure	Systems which use predominantly the body's own self-healing capacities in a Hippocratic manner, concentrating on diet, self-care, and life habits.
Hygienic systems	Strict nature cure, relying on fasting and purifications, without any recourse to remedies.

Nutritional therapy	Treatment by dietary control and the use of food supplements and components as medicines.
Clinical ecology	Treatment by the detection and elimination of allergenic and irritant foods from the diet.
Dietetics	Planning appropriate diets according to the nutritional principles laid down by conventional medicine.
Monodiets	Diet restricted to one item for a specific period, such as a grape juice diet.
Fasting	A common component of naturopathy in which little or no food is taken for a specific period.
Vegetarianism	A way of life which excludes the consumption of all birds, animals or fish.
Veganism	A way of life which excludes the consumption of all bird, animal or fish products including eggs and milk products.
Macrobiotics	Diets according to the principles established in Zen monasteries in which the grain-, vegetable-, animal-, salt-, heat- or cold-producing and *yin* or *yang* qualities of food are balanced appropriately.
Postural therapies	Treatment of posture by reconditioning mental and physical attitudes to self and habitual patterns of movement.
Alexander Technique	A technique developed by F. M. Alexander for postural improvement by means of constant self-awareness.

Feldenkrais Technique	A technique developed by M. Feldenkrais for restoration of postural balance, relaxation, and ease of movement by learning natural, pleasurable, and harmonious movement.
Radionics **Medical Dowsing** **Radiesthesia**	Use of pendulum and instruments focusing psychic power to diagnose and select appropriate treatments (usually homeopathic), which attack long-term predispositions to diseases, rooted in the subtle body of the patient.
Mind-body therapies	Procedures and therapies which create mental states and behaviour patterns beneficial to general health and recovery from disease.
Autogenic Training Autosuggestion	A technique of implanting positive suggestions into the subconscious by repeated self-instructions, particularly in relation to relaxation and stress diseases.
Hypnotherapy Hypnosis	The use of hypnotic suggestion to treat illness, addictions, and destructive behavioural patterns.
Bioenergetics Biodynamics Reichian therapeutics	Behavioural and psychological encounters with a therapist resulting in an often explosive release of psychological blocks, body tensions, and inhibitions, leading to improved general health and well-being.
Biofeedback	The use of equipment to self-monitor physiological signals from the mind or body and thus to bring involuntary processes under voluntary control.
Relaxation techniques	Techniques for calming the mind and body and releasing muscle tensions so as to induce deep relaxation.

Meditation Visualization	Techniques for calming, concentrating, and purifying the mind by persistent focusing, leading to self-transcendence.

Remedies
  Home remedies
  Natural medicines
	Materials of the natural world, excluding drugs, taken with therapeutic intent. Can be foods.

Herbs	Plant materials so taken.
Health remedies Health products	Remedies or food supplements which are taken for preventive and health promoting purposes.
Mineral remedies	Salts and inorganic materials taken as remedies.
Organic remedies	Tissues, enzymes, extracts, and biological materials, processed or unprocessed, taken as remedies.
Herbalism Phytotherapy	Therapeutic systems based exclusively on the curative power of herbal and mineral remedies.
Sense therapies	Use of specific patterns of sense impressions to heal imbalances and assist in cure.
Colour therapy	Use of specific coloured environments, clothes, and lights for therapeutic purposes.
Sound therapy	Use of patterns of sound for therapeutic purposes.

Part 1
General Survey

1

The background

Defining complementary medicine

It would be unrealistic to attempt an exact definition of those therapies which are found outside mainstream conventional medicine. For they are a diverse assortment, both ancient (e.g. acupuncture) and modern (e.g. biofeedback). Some provide more fundamental curative treatment (e.g. naturopathy), while others can, at times, be highly symptomatic (e.g. chiropractic). Some shun any artificial aid (e.g. nature cure) while others use extensive medicinal intervention (e.g. herbalism). Useful working definitions therefore usually focus on the one aspect that is common to all: the fact that they are separate from conventional scientific medicine. Even here there are no sharp dividing lines: the philosophies of radionics or healing are utterly at odds with conventional medical principles but the bases of osteopathy or herbalism are quasi-scientific and could be incorporated into conventional medicine without stretching its scientific model to breaking point.[1]

It will probably become increasingly difficult to define these therapies by their distinction from conventional medicine. For the 1990s are bringing a convergence of medical and non-conventional systems, and a blurring of boundaries. For the moment we are left with the common currency, and the author and many others who are working in this area have concluded that 'complementary medicine' is the most reasonable general term for, though not much of a description of, the therapies. It depicts them as partners to, though different in nature from, scientific medicine, and is therefore an appropriate definition as we move towards medical pluralism. 'Alternative medicine' is also used, and is the favoured term in the United States, for although the therapies cannot replace conventional medicine as a whole, they do so at times for many people. 'Fringe', 'unorthodox', or 'unconventional' are based on an out-of-date view of the therapies and place them in a rather alienated and embattled light.

'Natural medicine' and 'holistic medicine' are also used very loosely as umbrella terms. However they are approaches to treatment rather than medical systems in their own right. Thus 'natural' applies where the central philosophy is less mechanistic, the techniques are less fabricated and technological, and the goal of health is achieved by harmony with the elemental forces that influence life.[2] For example Oriental medicine and Ayurveda would be 'natural' in their constant reference and use of universal principles such as 'five elements' and 'tridoshas' (see Chapters 6 and 9). A modern naturopath who makes extensive use of purified vitamins and food supplements in pill form, directed by existing scientific evidence, aligns himself less with nature than a German naturopath (Heilpraktiker) who utilizes mostly fasting, diet, and hydrotherapy. Holistic is also an approach, and therapists or doctors can work more or less holistically depending on the breadth and inclusivity of their perspective (see p. 9). Just to make the semantics more difficult, 'traditional medicine' is also sometimes used to describe indigenous alternative medicine, for example by WHO and Third World countries, and sometimes (incorrectly) used by doctors to describe modern medicine!

The unique features of complementary medicine

Despite their diversity, a common bond unites the therapies.[3] They all attempt, in varying degrees, to recruit the self-healing capacities of the body. They amplify natural recuperative processes and augment the energy upon which the patient's health depends, helping him to adapt harmoniously to his surroundings. For example in Western herbal medicine there is very frequent use of a category of herbs called 'alteratives' or 'blood purifiers'. These are herbs such as echinacea (*Echinacea purpurea*), cleavers (*Galium aparine*), burdock (*Arctium lappa*), sage (*Salvia spp*), and myrrh (*Commiphora mol-mol*). They are used during the treatment of most acute and chronic infections and inflammations, along with fasting or special diets and nutrients, and other herbs to promote circulation of lymph and body fluids, all of which is intended to awaken a more powerful immune response and encourage long-term immune function.

The emphasis on restoration of health rather than removal of sickness is a fundamental, and leads to most of those features of complementary medicine which are unique to it and different from conventional medicine. The major themes are summarized below. They may surprise some readers who have imagined that the therapies were just non-conformist techniques that were otherwise quite compatible with modern medicine. This is not so. Even the simplest of therapies, such as reflexology, involves a view of the body unrecognizable to anyone trained in medical school. The real bases of the major therapeutic systems—naturopathy, homeopathy, Chinese medicine, and herbalism—are often radically different from those of modern medicine. They are systems of medicine in their own right, with theoretical bases often grounded in alternative views of nature. Although not all therapists would employ these principles all the time, and more symptomatically oriented therapists hardly at all, they are classical principles inherent in the authentic practice of the main therapies.

1. **Working with, not against, symptoms.** Symptoms are sometimes treated at the outset, or are left to clear up by themselves as the individual progresses towards health, which is usual practise in traditional acupuncture. In all cases, however, the symptoms are used as guides to the origin of the patient's upset or imbalance, and milestones on the journey to a cure. They are therefore managed not suppressed. For example a migraine-type headache might be seen by an acupuncturist as arising from overactive 'liver' metabolism ('liver' fire or 'yang'). The headaches may be relieved, but not removed. Instead the type and location of the headaches (frequency, severity, vertigo, nausea, sharpness, one-sidedness, etc.) is constantly monitored throughout the treatment as a guide to the effectiveness of the deeper treatment of organ function—the draining of the liver's excess. Accompanying symptoms, such as nausea, may be an indication of the energetic state of other organ systems such as the spleen.[4]

2. **Individuality.** Each person's condition is different, has arisen for different reasons, against a different constitutional background, and requires a different path for treatment. Diagnosis seeks to determine the nature of the problem and its causes in that person, and to home in on imbalances or destructive patterns in his or her life. Unlike conventional medicine, it does not rely on statistical norms. Treatment is correspondingly personal. Ten consecutive asthma patients that are treated by an acupuncturist or homeopath may all be treated entirely differently, as the sensitivity and inflammatory condition may have a different source in each case. One of the indications of the richness of the medical system is the development of a typology with which individual differences in health, disease, and response to the environment can be understood. For example the constitutional assessment in Ayurvedic medicine is a highly detailed art, in which hundreds of characteristics of body, skin, personality, habits, etc. are defined and integrated in terms of *Vata* ('airiness'), *Pitta* ('fieriness'), and *Kapha* ('wateriness'). This establishes an individual's susceptibilities, strengths, and weaknesses, and guides both prevention and treatment. Western (Thompsonian) herbalism by contrast does not make extensive use of constitutional differences, and modern medicine generally ignores them unless there are inherited pathologies.

3. **The integrated human being.** Since it is the individual who is treated as well as his symptoms, there are no special reasons to erect or maintain barriers between mind, body, and spirit, or between society and the individual. Lifestyle, caste of mind, vital energy, relationships, posture, and bearing are considered relevant in most of the therapies. In homeopathy and Oriental medicine, emotional, psychological, and behavioural signs are always included in diagnosis. This is rather less so in naturopathy, herbalism, and the manual therapies, but even here holism is often applied as an approach of an individual practitioner. For example naturopaths may encourage relaxation and imagery along with diet and herbs to treat high blood pressure; osteopaths and chiropractors might explore, with the patient, possible psychosocial stresses that may have given rise to a repeated musculoskeletal problem. The therapies are less concerned with anatomy, more

with the flow of energy and life. The patient is encouraged to sense the meaning of the illness within his or her life; the treatment is not only a physical process, but a journey of the soul.

4. No fixed beginning or ending. There is no defined or determined state of illness where treatment must begin or wellness where treatment must end. Such points are defined contextually. One patient may require assistance to reach a state of well-being and accommodation to his cancer. Treatment will finish when this is achieved, although in conventional terms he is still seriously ill. Conversely, another client may be treated so as to improve his energetic balance and condition or vitality. He may seek treatment with Oriental medicine to cope with an addiction, poor vitality and resistance, convalescence, or even to improve *Shen*, i.e. to bring light to his eyes. Treatment in this case, in conventional terms, is of a healthy person. In other words the working definition of health in complementary medicine is in practice more like that defined by the World Health Organization, which stresses states of physical and mental well-being. This is in contrast to modern medicine which in practice defines health as absence of symptoms.

5. Safety is sacred. The therapies are generally harmless when practised competently, and remedies are non-toxic. This arises automatically from the selection of methods that work with, rather than against, normal function, and that seek to promote health rather than attack symptoms. For example in Chinese herbal medicine, the mild, adjustive, health-promoting remedies (such as liquorice) are described as the 'kingly' remedies because of their great safety and general utility, while the more toxic, curative remedies (such as aconite) are described as merely the 'servants'. The opposite is true in conventional medicine which values the more incisive and stronger remedies—'magic bullets'—which inevitably have side-effects. The therapies are minimally interventionist and therefore gentler.[5] There are certain risks with all therapies and these are described in the relevant chapters but they are very small compared with those of conventional medicine.

6. Areas of competence. Alternative therapies are more successful at chronic, psychosomatic, early-stage, musculoskeletal, immunological, 'non-specific/multi-origin', environmental, conditions as opposed to acute, traumatic, infectious, genetic, tropical conditions. This is the opposite, again, of conventional medicine.

7. Patient is partner. The emphasis on self-healing means that the patient must do what he can to help himself. All therapies are partly instructional and some, such as the Alexander or relaxation techniques, are almost entirely so. Virtually all therapists will have something to say about diet and exercise, believing that many current chronic diseases are caused or exacerbated by improper eating habits and superfluous, impure, and unhealthy foods. The patient is encouraged to discover why he is sick and to work for his own cure, with the therapist as a partner whose function is partly catalytic. With most therapies, in particular the Alexander technique, acupuncture, anthroposophy, hypnotherapy, the 'psychosomatic' therapies, and naturopathy, the patient is encouraged to use the changes that happen to him during treatment as part of a learning experience. There is still usually a division into expert and lay roles, but the status difference is less than in conventional medicine, and the tone of the consultation and treatment is more of a dialogue, less of a pronouncement by the dominant professional.

8. **Alternative world views.** Remedies are discovered and employed in conformity to patterns of relationships between all living creatures and their environment. These patterns are often subtle and involve energetic rather than material phenomena. For example *Qi* in Chinese medicine is a tangible but invisible vital force which operates continually as the basis of all function. In Oriental medicine it is sensed and utilized in much the same way that modern man would sense and also utilize gravity. Despite the fact that *Qi* is so universal, it is enormously elaborated as an explanatory principle to describe detailed changes in organ function. For example 'liver' *Qi* might be constrained, stagnant, wild, deficient, excess, rising, etc. This vitalism is in contrast to conventional medicine, which derives from reductionist science, in which body processes are regarded as discrete concrete entities, unconnected to basic forces and elemental qualities.

Modern medicine grew out of Protestant science: the world consists of discrete materials obeying knowable natural laws, which can be used technically to improve life. Alternative medicine, we can see, has a very different philosophical basis which is far less interventionist, reductionist, positivistic, and mechanistic. This affects all aspects of alternative medical practice, but as it confounds research and dialogue with modern medicine, it is often conveniently forgotten by those who unconsciously wish alternative medicine to be just another modern technique, equivalent to physiotherapy. This is to some extent understandable as it is often hard to draw definite boundaries around complementary medicine. There is an overlapping with modern medicine, in the sense that all good medicine is in a way similar. A good doctor will relate to his patients holistically and diagnose intuitively, sometimes employing conservative treatments that rely on self-healing abilities.

There is also an even greater overlapping of complementary medicine with normal cultural daily life habits. A naturopathic diet, for example, may be no different from the usual eating habits of those inclined towards natural unrefined foods. Herbal medicine employs flavourings, spices, and folk remedies as genuine medicines. Anthroposophical methods work through reappraisal of the self so that treatment and self-development become identical. Laying on of hands merges seamlessly with religious faith, prayer, and worship, and points clearly to the connection between healing and spiritual sustenance which has been an essential part of medicine until recently.

The art of diagnosis

Diagnosis in complementary medicine is radically different from that in conventional medicine. The methods invariably consist of very sensitive observation of areas and functions of the body, and detailed questions concerning the patient's feelings, habits, and lifestyle. Diagnosis is not invasive, nor is it intrusive. Just as the conventional medical requirement to probe, assay, biopsy, and X-ray the interior of the body is a necessary product of the anatomical character of conventional pathology, so observational diagnosis is a corollary of the character of complementary pathology.

The diagnostic skills of Oriental medicine are typical of complementary medicine. They are the result of thousands of years of development and refinement, and they contain most of the procedures used by other therapies. The key to Oriental diagnosis is the concept that inner states are projected on to the surface of the body as a film is projected on to a screen. Oriental pathology is highly complex and systematic, classifying diseases by means of qualities of body function (such as hot/cold, watery/dry) and qualities of the various body energies (such as scattered, stuck, and withdrawn). There are no anatomical boundaries to restrict these qualities, which can only be read by a sensitive and trained practitioner. The colour and texture of the tongue and skin, the timbre of the voice, the distribution of hot or cold patches, the responses and actions, the smell or appearance of urine and body secretions, and above all, the textures of the 12 pulses (read like waves on an oscilloscope) are all used as messages. Through them the practitioner gains a type of continuous log of the patient's condition and prognosis, and the alterations produced by treatment or other events. The traditional acupuncturist will use these methods still.

Although the conventional physician will also examine the same parts of the body—the pulse, tongue, skin, and urine—he is looking for very different things and translating his perceptions into a different language. For example he will count pulses to measure heart rate, and will hardly credit that it is even possible to feel their shape and texture, let alone obtain information in this way about the function of various internal organs. Nonetheless, since much of the sensitivity to a patient's condition comes with experience and an open mind, one can find GPs so well versed in their diagnosis that they can tell the condition of some patients as soon as they walk into the surgery.

Other therapies diagnose in a similar manner, although interpretations are again different. Body therapists, including many masseurs, read the postures, actions, balances, and breaths of the body as a language expressing a person's psychophysical make-up. They read character and emotional tone from the patterns of tensions and alignments. Physical therapists, chiropractors, and osteopaths read posture with equal sensitivity, although here it is dimensions, stresses, pressures, and flexions which are invoked to explain the patient's condition. Many naturopaths use a diagnostic technique called iridology, the basic premise of which is that all the parts of the body are specifically reflected in areas of the iris of the eye. An examination of the spots, marks, blemishes, fibres, patterns, and colours of the iris suggests a historical record of the patient's condition.[6] Of course, naturopaths, herbalists, homeopaths, and other therapists will pay very careful attention to the patient's reported symptom picture, often going into details which modern medicine would find irrelevant and essentially untreatable. For example pains might be further analysed: are they dull or sharp, moving or static, continuous or intermittent, diffuse or concentrated, associated with certain activities or certain times of day, etc? A condition of weakness, that a doctor would not regard as a real symptom, might be broken down by a therapist to its subjective experiences such as agitation, nervousness, sleepiness, tiredness, flaccidity, depression, debility, loneliness, boredom, inactivity, etc. These will then be used as a guide to the psychological, post-viral, emotional, nutritional, infective, toxic, or other sources of the imbalance.

All the diagnostic methods described so far use the normal senses as tools. The use of paranormal senses is also common in complementary medicine. The use of paranormal faculties in diagnosis today is not usually expressed in such mystical or sacramental terms as it was before the era of quantum physics. Therapists tend now to regard such faculties as subtle energetic phenomena, below the threshold of normal perception and beyond the threshold of current scientific explanation. Dowsing, for example, has long been used and virtually accepted as a specially developed sense on the physical plane; the pendulum is sometimes used in diagnosis in the same way, to augment minute body responses to the signals that the therapist picks up unconsciously from the patient. The pendulum as amplifier is often used in healing and radionics. Psychic diagnosis can involve visualization of the 'aura' around individuals, or patches of light or shade on their bodies.[7]

Whereas the scientific verification of complementary treatments is fraught with complications and fundamental incongruities, diagnosis should be more easily testable. Indeed, diagnosis of distant pain sites from observation of the ear alone by acupuncturists has been confirmed in a controlled experiment at the University of California. In a further study there, four patients who had lung cancer were correctly picked out from 30 individuals, by measuring the electrical activity of the lung acupuncture points on the hand. The testers saw no other part of the body.[8] Clairvoyant diagnosis of silent patients and even from photographs has been found to be up to 80 per cent accurate, depending on the clairvoyant and the conditions under which he can operate.[9] There are machines available which can detect acupuncture points or measure several pulses on each wrist and record them on a continuous trace. Kirlian photography, a photographic imprint of some kind of bioenergetic corona discharge around the human body, can reveal, when executed properly, patterns which are very sensitive to disease, mood, vitality, drug consumption, and the psychophysical state of the individual. However as the technique is not repeatable between various experimenters using slightly different equipment, it has not been possible to use this technique in routine diagnosis.[10]

Holistic medicine—the new Hippocratism

Holistic medicine is a movement, or an approach to treatment, evolving mostly within the medical profession but also among complementary therapists. It is a response to the need to find new methods of dealing with stress-related and degenerative health problems. It is also a reaction against increasing specialization within medicine. Holistic medicine integrates a variety of potential psychological and physical treatments with preventive instruction. It attempts to give a global treatment to each patient with as much emphasis on psychological and preventive care as on the treatment of pathologies. This is how it is defined by the American Holistic Medical Association: 'Holistic Medicine is a system of health care which emphasises personal responsibility, and fosters a co-operative relationship among all those involved, leading toward optimal attunement of body, mind, emotions and spirit'.[11]

In practice, holistic medicine uses both conventional and complementary methods simultaneously in treatment. There is, however, a more strongly psychotherapeutic approach, including group therapy, sexual guidance, and analysis of important events in the patient's life; and there is an attempt to provide a continuous preventive guide throughout life.[12] For example: 'Holistic practitioners are as interested in the colouring of the mood that preceded an attack of chest pain and the meaning it had for the patient as in the dimensions of the electrocardiographic change that followed it. Their therapeutic approach may include a meditative technique; dietary changes and exercises to improve cardiovascular functioning; psychotherapy to mitigate the depression and rage that predispose an individual to myocardial infarction (heart attack); or pastoral counselling to help someone confront the despair that can be as lethal as any anatomic pathology.'[13]

Holistic practitioners examine minutely the patient's lifestyle, often by means of extensive questionnaires on life habits, attitudes, relationships, and psychological traits, as well as bodily symptoms. In this way they attempt to spot susceptibilities and preconditions for disease. They can then guide the client through his disease towards the discovery of the manner in which his personality and habits influence his physical and psychological health.

Holistic medicine is in consequence concerned with the long-term development of each individual rather than the short-term response to each incidence of disease. It also brings the family, and even the conditions of work into the process of healing since the family is crucial in creating a positive or negative ambience, and may have been instrumental in forming the emotional roots of a disease in the first place. In the same way, since health-promoting or health-destroying habits are carried by society, a holistic health centre will attempt to involve the local community by means of classes, meetings, etc. A good complementary health centre will do likewise, and there may be a great deal of overlap between the two, sometimes making the 'holistic' label redundant.

The history of medicine

A brief examination of the history of medicine may help to place the development of both conventional and complementary medicine in perspective.[14]

The basic principle of modern medicine, that human ill health and incapacity is the result of specific identifiable sets of symptoms (diseases), each of which is curable by specific treatments, has been a constant refrain in history from antiquity. However, it has always been offset against systems of thought which view disharmony with nature as the condition to be treated and physical symptoms as secondary manifestations. In other words the dialogue between 'conventional' and 'alternative' goes back at least as far as the Ancient Greek period (around 500 BC). Aesculapius, the son of Apollo, was the legendary teacher of Greek medicine, and the priests in his temples diagnosed, mixed medicines, and healed diseases by correcting imperfections. However, in the same period, the goddess Hygieia was worshipped by those who believed that good health resulted from man's understanding of how to live. The ascetic Pythagoreans introduced the Hygieian concept of physiological harmony, seeing disease as an imbalance of the constituent elements of man, and treatment as a return to harmony and balance, not so much with medicines, as with life wisdom.

Hippocrates—more correctly the Hippocratics—are interesting because though they are regarded as the fathers of medicine, actually they are the fathers of modern naturopathy, and thus of much of complementary medicine. The Hippocratic corpus generally followed Pythagorean and Hygieian views diametrically opposed to modern medicine. He and his school believed that health was restored by equilibrium (*crasis*) within the fluid essences (*humours*) of man. In their view, the healing process was designed only to aid the body's own self-healing capacities: the *vix medicatrix naturae*. They placed great emphasis on proper diet, natural living and correct habits, and used drugs more to support healing than to cure disease.[15] On the other hand they lost the elemental or sacred view, seeming not to be able to understand how the elements operated, much as a Westerner has trouble understanding the five elements of Chinese medicine: 'Did he who turned wheat into bread remove from it the hot, cold, dry or moist?' The Hippocratics are actually rather materialistic; very busy with details, such as the question of whether the colour of a man's vomit is the primary or secondary essence of the man. There is much about body, and almost nothing about mind or spirit: 'What exists is always visible and recognizable'.

Modern medicine owes more to Galen of Pergamum (AD 130–200), the rationalist and eclectic, than to the earlier Greeks. Galen retained the concepts of humours and the Hippocratic life force, adding to them body functions such as ingestion. He also developed many drugs to restore body functions when they went awry. However, it was the development, during the Renaissance, of anatomy and pathology, which were practised alongside the traditional purgings, leechings, and Galenical remedies, which heralded the rise of scientifically based medicine. Medical theory and diagnosis began to move away from the concept of 'harmony' towards the 'specificity' position, although in practice therapy still mostly involved humour-balancing until about 200 years ago.

The development of new drugs, such as aspirin, digitalis, quinine, and opium (derived, incidentally, mostly from traditional herbal lore), dramatically increased the popularity of scientific medicine. The new drugs had spectacular results, making coughs stop, fevers plummet, and pains disappear; with such symptomatic relief the traditionalists were left with principles but not patients. Humours, secretions, vital energy, balance, and *vix medicatrix naturae* were consigned to dusty books and the herbalist's manuals. With the new drugs as tools, physicians could abandon self-healing in practice as well as in theory. Each disease that arose could be overcome with a specific cure. The patient had become a battlefield on which the war against disease was waged.[16] Modern medicine today is still a theatre of technicality. We may be dazzled by the brilliance of the Intensive Care Unit or the Magnetic Resonance Imagery diagnostic machine, and impressed with the saving of lives. But modern medicine is based on concepts that are recognizable at least since the time of ancient Greece: including reductionism, materialism, and specific treatments for identifiable conditions. The historical perspective counters hubris. It shows that medical systems are transient and that modern medicine has only dominated medical practice for the last 150 years. It may represent no more than a swing of the pendulum from Hygieia to Aesculapius; indeed there are already signs that medicine is beginning to move back from the scientific extreme.[17]

The techniques of complementary medicine have been developed throughout history. Six-thousand-year-old herbal prescriptions still survive from Egypt; the Ebers papyrus is one example. Supposed acupuncture needles made of bone have been unearthed in northern China and are believed to date back to the same period. Bonesetting, shamanism, massage, and dietary control leave less evidence for posterity; however they are practised by the few primitive Stone and Iron Age cultures which survive today. Most of the modern alternative therapies are formalized systems derived from primitive practices. Many were developed in the last century at a time of considerable medical upheaval, when both physicians and traditionalists were exploring new forms of therapy as the inadequacies of blood-lettings and purgations were revealed. For example homeopathy was founded by a Doctor Hahnemann, who was dismayed by the savagery and risk that characterized treatment of disease at the time. His system was a mirror image of medical treatment of the age, using minute doses in contrast to violent medicines and caricaturing symptoms rather than suppressing them.

Complementary medical theory has been intertwined with conventional medicine concepts in a constant discourse throughout history. The debate has heated up in recent times. The development of both branches of medicine, since the Renaissance, has not been at all peaceful, both sides of the medical divide being intolerant and prejudiced. In the middle of the nineteenth century those who held that there were specific drugs for specific diseases were called quacks; a century later the traditionalists were called quacks. In the seventeenth century the early 'Chymists' were harassed by the herbal Galenicists for using poisonous concoctions, yet in this century it is the herbalists who are persecuted by the chemists. 130 years ago scientific medicine was damned as irrational and irresponsible ('out of the false pride of the laboratory . . . has arisen the worst evil of therapeutic nihilism'[16]); yet in modern times, scientific medicine uses precisely the same terms for those practising more traditionally.

During the first half of this century complementary medicine was all but outlawed in this country. The medical profession had a standing regulation that a doctor could be struck off for sending a patient to a practitioner who was not medically qualified. This prevented doctors learning from, or even studying, the methods of complementary practitioners whom they shunned and branded as quacks. Persecution was not as blatant as in America, where osteopaths and chiropractors were harassed in court and out, and where Wilhelm Reich (the founder of bioenergetics) and Ruth Drown (one of the founders of radionics) spent many years in prison for their discoveries; nevertheless it was persistent and effective. Bonesetters were continually accused of harming patients and were starved of resources and respect, hypnotherapists had to run the gauntlet of repeated parliamentary attempts at restriction, and healers were seen as freaks. When acupuncture arrived from the East the medical journals labelled it, too, as witchcraft. In 1975, when I began laboratory research on Oriental tonic herbs, in the hope of finding something useful against senescence, it was very poorly regarded in the two research institutions in which I worked at the time, at best as a joke, and at worst as a kind of brainstorm that would soon pass.

The medical establishment's disapprobation created a very poor public image for the therapies, which persisted until the sudden growth in media reportage on complementary medicine in the 1980s. Even in 1978 a medical public figure felt able to say: 'Jabbering, obscurantist, mysticism . . . most of fringe medicine today is simply survival of techniques used in antiquity because there was nothing better. They're pathological stages in human development, grotesque failures to understand. To go back to them now is like striking flints to light the gas fire'.[18]

Now that a process of accommodation between the various systems is in sight, it would be wise to be positive and encourage a gentlemanly and civilized discourse between world views and systems of medicine that derive from them. It is a historical moment—for the first time in centuries we may be entering a period of pluralistic medicine. There will be much ferment ahead as the systems jostle for position. However it would be foolish to forget that a good deal of the struggle in the past has been vicious and uncompromising, nothing to do with systems of thought, and everything to do with power and the defence of professional boundaries, which is then justified by whatever arguments or phraseology comes to hand at the time.

Complementary therapies and the crisis in medicine

In Chapter 2 we shall see that complementary medicine has not grown because it is good at advertising, because it offers specific cures, because the public cannot get medical treatment (free) from their doctor, or because they are gullible. Rather, the public has turned to complementary medicine as refugees from the inadequacies of conventional medicine. They look for relief from failed treatments, lack of understanding, lack of heart, obsessive technicality, and side-effects. They are turning away from modern medicine just when it is, or is supposed to be (according to the conventional models of progress), better than it has ever been before. Osteopaths and herbalists were there 50 years ago but no-one went to them, even though modern medicine was crude, without penicillin or CAT scans.

At that time surgeons freely pulled out 'unnecessary' body parts like tonsils from an acclaiming public.

What has happened since then is that the magic has worn thin, the birds have come home to roost. Though the professionals seem to be still somewhat intoxicated with the power of science, the illusion doesn't hold, mostly because it is happening within the bodies of people. It does not feel right any more to receive codeine for bad backs, lifelong inhalers for asthma, steroids for skin diseases, chemotherapy for cancers, Valium for psychosomatic disorders, and to know that this is it—nothing more on offer. People *know* that they are basically still in the sickness category. Intuitively, many stop believing in the claims of medicine, and intuitively they drift into the orbit of the alternatives. In essence it is a search for truth, a weariness with the half-truths of unfulfilled claims. Take the example of the most frequent diseases of our times—heart disease and cancer—that constitute major fears for westerners. It is widely known that these are lifestyle problems. Yet apart from smokers, bacon guzzlers, and couch potatoes, for whom there are some easy answers, modern medicine cannot provide real instruction except to wait until it happens, and then roll in the cardiac or oncology juggernaut which, patients know, will not restore them to health. If the public would request from doctors real guidance on how to prevent these diseases, they will be met by a noisy silence, a silence that clearly expresses the unacknowledged limits of medicine: no solutions to stress, no clear answers to cholesterol despite billions of dollars spent on research, no tools for cancer prevention, and such weak dietary advice that it serves only to send patients to naturopaths to find out what is really going on.

Medicine today is in crisis. The critique of medicine has been in process for more than 20 years, since René Dubois and Ivan Illich, and is too well known to repeat here. Readers are referred to the bibliography. It is at last becoming uncomfortably clear that like all other medical systems, modern medicine has areas of excellence and areas of failure. Its tremendous successes are inarguable —the control of acute infection, vaccinations against diphtheria, smallpox, or typhoid; skills in surgery, dentistry, anaesthetics, prosthetics, and parasitology, and the feat of keeping perinatal mortality down to less than 2 children lost per 100 births.[19] Yet the fact remains that the resources ploughed into health are rising steadily, lifespan remains unchanged, and we are getting sicker.

In the last 20 years, there has been a 300 per cent increase in health expenditure, and a 50 per cent increase in the percentage of the Gross Domestic Product spent on health. Yet there has been a third increase, to 34 per cent of the population, in those suffering from long-term illness, and a 64 per cent increase in incapacity, or days of certified sickness.[20] More than one in ten of the UK population now consult their doctor annually for asthma and eczema; 2 million people in the UK now suffer from asthma, from which modern medicine can provide relief, but not cure.[21] More than half a million Americans will die of cancer this year, and cancer death rates continue to rise steadily: the director of the National Cancer Institute confirmed in 1994 that 'death rates for several important cancers are going up'. The US President's Cancer Panel were told, in 1993, that the 'decades of war against cancer have been an unqualified failure'.[22] There has been a 43.5 per cent increase in the incidence of cancer since the 1950s, (adjusted for age), and an almost neglible improvement in the 5-year survival rate after treatment, which raises questions about the real value of current methods which themselves are damaging to health.[23] Though life expectancy has risen, largely because of the drop in infant mortality, US statistics show a steady rise in ill-health: from an average of 0.82 episodes of disabling illness a year in 1920 to 2.12 in 1988.[24] This is the age of 'the vertically ill'. Medical schools today still carry on as if nothing much has changed, as if most of the common diseases of the western world are unpredictable attacks from somewhere else rather than gradual inner deteriorations and disharmonies which are largely the result of behaviour and environment and are therefore adjustable and preventable. Medicine is still shooting magic bullets at them, as at phantom enemies. There is no clear target any more. The medical weaponry is launched against the shifting pattern of life and its shadows, with unpredictable results. The individual is not different from his disease.

A past Director-General of WHO summed up the problem well: 'Most of the world's medical schools prepare doctors, not to take care of the health of the people but instead for a medical practice that is blind to anything but disease and the technology for dealing with it; a technology involving astronomical and ever-increasing prices directed towards fewer and fewer people . . . The medical empire and its closely related aggressive industry of diagnostic and therapeutic weapons sometimes appears more of a threat than a contribution to health . . . the very attempt to diagnose and treat one illness may produce another, be it through side effects or iatrogenesis.'[25]

In a way, complementary medicine can save modern medicine, pull it out of the cul-de-sac into which it has run. It has already given modern medicine most of the ideas it uses in lifestyle and dietary management of chronic diseases, such as the use of fibre, the importance of fresh vegetables and beta-carotene in cancer prevention, or the use of garlic, fish oil, and essential fatty acids in cardiovascular disease. It has provided know-how on stress reduction and other preventive mind – body tools. It has always been, and continues to be, one of the main resources of novel drug concepts, from digitalis to taxol, and so on. It will act as a vast well of knowledge for the future, in the direction of Hygieia rather than Aesculapius. Though scientific medicine responds to these ideas in character, that is, to subject them to the *via dolorosa* of double-blind clinical trials, and if anything is left of their activity, claims to have discovered them, nevertheless the ideas keep coming.

More importantly, patients who go to complementary practitioners do not abandon conventional medicine completely, but use it in addition, often more skillfully than practitioners realize. For example they may obtain treatment for acute or life-threatening conditions, exacerbations or severe symptoms while simultaneously utilizing complementary techniques to gradually effect a total return to health, and ameliorate adverse effects of the medical treatment. The complementarity of the two medical systems are not theoretical—they are being worked out in the present moment within patients' minds and bodies. This is very poignantly expressed with the large number of cancer patients who also use complementary methods. Oncology patients may receive devastating treatment attacking the cancer as if it is a nasty foreign body, and yet add life-affirming, supporting, methods which relate to the cancer as a distorted or unruly part of self, that has to be brought back to line with love rather than aggression.[26] Every patient juggles with these opposite approaches in his treatment plan. Their experimentation is already helping modern medicine to learn a more effective and more gentle way.

Millions of people are now experiencing this complementarity of medical systems within themselves, and there are countless examples, from the simplest use of *Lactobacillus* to avoid antibiotic side-effects, to the complex journey of a treatment of asthma using acupuncture along with steroids. One example that touched me is that of a friend of mine, Dennis, who went blind as a result of diabetic pathology. His kidneys also began to fail. His doctors could only helplessly record the deterioration towards an inevitable kidney transplantation. However 1981 saw a dramatic turnaround in Dennis's fortunes. He went to a traditional acupuncturist. His kidneys began to improve. The clinic found this phenomenon inexplicable but refused to consider the possibility that acupuncture might be responsible. Dennis's health continued to improve through the use of acupuncture and herbal and dietary treatment, although he must also take insulin. It seems that only the subtle methods of complementary medicine can help Dennis to adjust to his disturbed glands. Conventional medicine (insulin) is keeping him alive. Complementary medicine is helping him live.

Dennis's case illustrates the potential of pluralistic medicine, if it avoids the professional territorialism of conventional medicine that looks on all alternatives as humbug, and the naturalistic extremism of alternative medicine that views all technical interventions as dangerous symptomatic meddling. All it requires is that both doctors and therapists wisely appreciate the limitations of their own systems.

Revival of complementary medicine

The 1960s witnessed the birth of a strong grass roots health movement. It was especially popular with young people, who saw in complementary medicine tools for self-care and autonomy, ways to avoid the degenerative diseases of the age, and a response to the increasing environmental deterioration, particularly in relation to impure and unnatural foods, and the sterility that characterized much of modern life. Complementary medical knowledge was welcomed as part of a search for new values.[27]

The alternative health movement is no longer a movement; it is now an accepted part of modern life. Its focus has changed from the negative—disquiet with modern medicine—to the positive—the quest for a reliable, practical, universal cultural knowledge on natural medicine, both for self-care and professional care. A public opinion poll carried out in 1984 found that 10 per cent of the population 'believed strongly' in alternative medicine.[28] By 1989, three quarters of the British public stated that they wanted alternative medicine available on the health service,[29] and a 1993 survey by the British Market Research Bureau found that only 11 per cent of the population would not use complementary medicine, and did not believe in it.[30] Other European countries are showing the same trend—only more so. For example, even by 1979, 75 per cent of the Dutch population wanted complementary medicine included in the national health insurance scheme, and 80 per cent said that there should be freedom of choice in medicine with all systems of equal status.[31]

GPs have found themselves caught between their obligation to cater for the health needs of their patients and their adherence to scientific medicine. Some did refer patients, albeit quietly. The Threshold Survey found that in 1981, 10 per cent of the patients of lay therapists arrived through a recommendation from their GP despite discouragement from the British Medical Association (BMA). In 1995, Baroness Cumberlege, the Minister in the Department of Health responsible for complementary medicine, reported that 40 per cent of registered medical practitioners delegate patients to complementary medicine.[32] The majority of GPs no longer make a secret of the fact that they are relieved to have somewhere to send their difficult cases. A survey of GPs in the county of Avon found that no less than three-quarters referred patients to therapists. Above half of the 145 doctors wanted complementary medicine available on the NHS.[33] Other GP surveys have confirmed these figures in other regions, but derive from the 1980s.[34] However the most recent and methodologically careful study is of great interest because it compared the views of GPs, hospital doctors, and medical students. Generally, all the respondents were interested in alternative medicine, medical students more than doctors. 85 per cent of the medical students, 76 per cent of the GPs, and 69 per cent of the hospital doctors felt that the therapies should be available on the National Health Service, and 79–91 per cent of the respondents felt that therapists should be formally qualified and registered. 70 per cent of the hospital doctors and no less than 93 per cent of the GPs had referred patients to alternative practitioners, many at the first consultation. Still, the number of consultations in which referral happens is small—one third of the GPs estimated that they referred during 1–5 per cent of the consultations. Twenty per cent of the GPs and 12 per cent of the hospital doctors practise some form of complementary medicine.[35] The Threshold Survey found, in 1983, that 2000 doctors in the UK, around 4 per cent, practised some kind of alternative therapy.[36] Today it is four times that number. Times have truly changed!

More doctors than ever wish to learn about complementary medicine, although all too often their resulting knowledge is superficial. A 1983 survey of doctors training to be GPs showed that 70 out of 86 wanted such training.[37] In 1994 the proportion of medical students who felt that alternative medicine should be a topic course in medical schools was 84 per cent. Three quarters of GPs want training in alternative medicine.[35] 'Medical education . . . must recognise that there is a growing demand for treatments that do not conform to conventional orthodoxies' stated the General Medical Council in its 1993 report entitled '*Tomorrow's Doctors: recommendations on undergraduate medical education*'.

As we shall see in Chapter 3, there is still very little opportunity for medical undergraduates to learn about complementary medicine in medical school, and most teaching is postgraduate. In addition, the courses available to doctors to train them in complementary medicine are often perfunctory, in some cases no more than two or three weekends compared with the several years' training required for lay therapists in the major therapies to gain the appropriate qualification. However the British Medical Association is now aware of the problem, and this could make a big difference in the future.

In 1983, the Prince of Wales was elected president of the BMA. Much to the chagrin of that august body, Prince Charles, in a careful yet forceful manner, exhorted doctors to re-examine the basic assumptions of technical medicine and to be more open-minded about alternatives: 'Sophistication is only skin deep, and it seems to me that account has to be taken of those sometimes long-neglected complementary methods of medicine which in the right hands can bring considerable relief, if not hope, to an increasing number of people.'[38] Encouraged by Prince Charles the BMA had no choice but to launch an inquiry into complementary medicine. After three years work the team of eminent specialists, which failed to include anyone who knew anything about the subject, scored a much publicized own goal. Their report is a defensive polemic in support of scientific medicine, charging the natural therapies with being primitive, untested, ineffective, and, absurdly, 'inconsistent with natural laws'.[39] It was like the last gasp of the dinosaurs. Things had already moved on. The report only served to create a powerful backlash, and gave complementary medicine a new boost. It gave ammunition to the All Party Parliamentary Group on Alternative and Complementary Therapies, who requested the Department of Health to define their position. In response, the Health Minister, made a statement on December 3 1991, which reiterated the stated position of the General Medical Council, that doctors could refer patients to non-registered therapists, provided they retained clinical responsibility and accountability. But he went further: 'It is open to any family doctor to employ a complementary therapist to offer NHS treatment within his practice.' This was a previously unthinkable invitation to alternative medicine to come in out of the cold into the National Health Service, the state medical structure, and work with doctors there.

The British Medical Association itself quickly put together another team in 1990, directed by Dr Fleur Fisher, to revise the disastrous previous attempt, and now it was much more conciliatory. This time, it did not set out to judge complementary medicine, but to assume that it was here to stay and examine how to accommodate to it. It saw it as a public health issue, and endorsed the freedom of choice of the consumer. In the new 1993 report the BMA set out information to the medical profession on complementary medicine, its use, its nature, its standards and ethics, and so on, and recommended principles of good medical practice.[40] The report's recommendations took into account the views collected from the various complementary therapy organizations. It recommended that each therapy organize itself into a single regulating body which should be capable of enforcing codes of conduct and professional practice, and also supervising educational standards. It recommended statutory registration of the main therapies, and since it was medical opposition that has basically stopped registration of alternative therapists for more than a century, osteopaths and chiropractors became state registered as soon as it was clear that the medical opposition had collapsed (see Chapter 4).

The BMA's educational recommendations are also groundbreaking. They agree that all doctors must become sufficiently familiar with alternative medicine in order to know what to expect from it, who might benefit, and how and to whom to refer. They recommend accredited postgraduate courses, and also 'a familiarization course on non-conventional therapies within the medical undergraduate curriculum.' Learning how to refer could be quite a project in itself. For the therapies are not mechanical techniques that if carried out properly will produce a predictable result. And certainly there is no specific therapy that is best for a specific disease. Rather, there are best combinations of individual therapist, appropriate methods, and individual patient. It takes experience, knowledge, and intuition to make rational choices when referring patients. Still, if a start is made in educating doctors about what to expect from alternative medicine, it would be a big step. But the BMA goes further. It has woken up to the fact that 'serious professional misconduct may arise by "a doctor persisting in unsupervised practice of a branch of medicine without having acquired the experience which is necessary"'. It therefore recommends that doctors wishing to learn a therapy must take 'recognised training in that field approved by the appropriate regulatory body, and should only practice the therapy after registration.'[40] The importance of this statement is that the BMA, representing the medical profession, at last acknowledges that the therapies are full systems in their own right, substantial bodies of knowledge and skills, that cannot be learnt by anyone overnight.

The medical profession has all but accepted complementary medicine and seeks accommodation with it. About one third of the population of Europe now use it at some time (see Chapter 2). Most people, as well as medical professionals, want it state registered, incorporated into the National Health Service, and more freely available. Indeed more and more complementary medicine is becoming available under the aegis of the Health Authorities. It is not hard to see that within a relatively short time, even hospitals will be unrecognizable: mothers will be giving birth in hospital holistic birthing units with the help of acupuncture, massage will be provided to all long-stay patients, the chemical smell of Intensive Care Units will give way to the sweet vapours of aromatherapy oils, and, more important, many beds will be empty because patients will have been treated by alternative therapists in the community at a stage when they can avoid the surgeon's knife. Medicine will never be the same again. 'Medicine everywhere is in the middle of a profound structural change.' states a recent editorial in the *British Medical Journal*. The editorial sees a brighter future for medicine in which doctors have less power but work with other specialists in a wider health-promoting effort, serving more powerful and sophisticated consumers.[41] Complementary medicine will be part of this revolution.

As we shall see in subsequent chapters, the development of a pluralistic medical system necessitates a rapid development of organization and teaching in complementary medicine. Therapists will need to become more professional, and more accountable and supervised. Many therapists will think that the price of a standardized education is not worth the prize of acceptability. They will have to let go, painfully, of some extreme and unrealistic attitudes, especially that their therapy is good for everything. Above all, the concepts used in the therapies may need to be updated. Previously, therapists were reluctant to tamper with the purity of their systems for fear of losing them altogether. Therapists now find themselves burdened by some outmoded concepts which they find hard to adapt to the modern age, such as the innate intelligence in chiropractic, the physicomedicalism of herbalism, or the tubercular miasms of homeopathy.

The issue of research

At a time when as many Westerners with back trouble are going to chiropractors and osteopaths as to doctors, the basis of vertebral manipulation remains uninvestigated. This doesn't matter so much in itself, since a large part of complementary medicine, and a great deal of conventional medicine too, has not been scientifically assessed or understood, and may never be. But what is interesting is that osteopaths became state registered by the UK parliament, without any scientific proof of the effectiveness of osteopathy. The chiropractors too won state recognition after only a single recognized trial of chiropractic, supported reluctantly by the Medical Research Council, only on pressure from the Cochrane committee on back pain, after they had turned down two requests to do so from Parliament itself. What has happened is that scientific medicine's demand that the non-scientific alternatives should prove themselves scientifically has collapsed. With it has gone any pretence that this call was about science or about proof. It was about preservation of existing professional boundaries.

Therapists found it irksome that for decades the medical world called for controlled clinical trials while at the same time refusing to fund them or carry them out. The 1986 BMA Working Party clearly stated that it would be 'for practitioners of alternative therapies to mount any trial'. The Medical Research Council consistently refused to fund any research. Heads of departments squeezed out embryonic ventures from their laboratories. Neither the pharmaceutical industry nor the large medical charities such as the British Heart Foundation or the Imperial Cancer Research Fund would have anything to do with such research.[42] Not only were the billions of dollars in research funding denied to complementary medicine, but even when the tiny resources of therapists' time and money were spent on research, it was almost impossible to get it into the major medical literature because of publication bias. Editors and peer-reviewers gave the thumbs down, research was shunted out to the fringe publications, which gave further ammunition to medical professionals—and peer reviewers—to exclude it. When two high-quality acupuncture papers finally made it to The *Lancet* in 1986, they were accompanied by a patronizing editorial which said: 'In this issue we take courage into our hands (and trust in the seasonal goodwill of our readers) and offer two contributions on acupuncture treatment of lung disease.'[43] When *Nature* finally published Professor Benveniste's impeccable research on high dilution phenomena *in vitro* involving 13 researchers and six separate laboratories (see Chapter 14) it was accompanied by a similar dismissive editorial: '. . . prudent readers should, for the time being, suspend judgment.'[44] *Nature* called for its repetition, sent over a fraud-busting squad, and when the trial was successfully repeated, refused to publish it. All of this is like Goliath challenging David to a contest in which Goliath makes up all the rules while David pays the costs. It is cynical to call out, in these circumstances, as *The Lancet* has done, 'Let the best man win'.[45]

A closer examination confirms that the issues are not about proof but about power and competition between opposing systems of thought. For example, all herbs were dropped from the official pharmacopoeias during the first half of the century, without any testing to see if indeed they were ineffective as was claimed. They were accused of being 'grandmother's remedies' and peremptorily kicked out. A recent study has examined the reporting of acupuncture in the medical literature over the last two centuries, and found that the changing number of papers published follow the alternate waves of public interest and ridicule. Whatever this literature showed, it was anyway never admitted that acupuncture might have advantages over conventional medicine in certain areas of health care. The medical reports were 'marked more by the closed nature of professional thinking . . . than the kind of open-minded, impartial inquiry which is held within the profession to be associated with the rise of scientific medicine.'[46]

All over Europe, it was the same 'dog-in-the-manger' attitude towards the rise in consumer interest in alternatives: 'No we will not recognise them without scientific proof; No we will not invest in scientific testing'. It is little wonder that the Dutch Minister of Health, exasperated with this situation, stated that she could not wait for scientific verification of the therapies, and would consider legalizing complementary medicine purely on the basis of public demand. The Dutch Government's Commission for Alternative Systems of Medicine put it clearly: '. . .the division between alternative and orthodox medicine is not—or is not principally—of a scientific nature . . . The demand that alternative practitioners must demonstrate the effectiveness of their treatments before they can be granted any form of recognition thus seems to the Commission to be indefensible.'[47]

Alternative medicine practitioners too shunned research as it did not seem to help them, either with the authorities or with their patients. Many therapists felt closed, convinced that the call to research was a cultural ethnocentricity of modern medicine that did not touch them. In other words, it was modern medicine's problem if it believed more in the efficacy of the randomized double-blind clinical trial than in the therapeutic process. It was modern medicine's problem if it isolated itself from the rich ancient healing arts which utilized a more experiential and direct way of knowing, assuming a frozen technical superiority, like being alone on a cold mountain top. However other therapists took a much more open and pragmatic approach. Research was the language of modern civilization within which all must live and work. It was a way of explaining oneself to others, not necessarily a way of proving that one was right. From this arose the Research Council for Complementary Medicine (RCCM), an attempt to co-ordinate research so as to make best use of limited resources, and so, at least, to introduce the therapies as rational systems.

This pragmatic approach has now won. The RCCM, therapy organizations, and the British Medical Association, all encourage a research attitude within complementary medicine. The RCCM not only supports research but has also set up a Centralised Information Service on Complementary Medicine (CISCOM). Research is now seen as not only about proof. It also helps the clarification, development, and professionalization of the therapies. Research is no longer an entrance ticket but a form of discourse with conventional medicine, a way of moving closer to the mainstream. Most therapists are happy to oblige if it is felt that research is not a 'trial by ordeal', for it can help the therapies themselves to assess, audit, and improve their practice, and also to promote it to the wider public in conventional language. A survey of all UK acupuncturists in 1993 found that only around 30 per cent committed a half a day a week to research and development activities, but that 80 per cent would do so if they received more support, such as financial support, training in research methods, and collaboration.[48] At the same time the Medical Research Council is much more ready to support studies, especially on usage; the European Community is investing in research and has set up the Committee for Science and Technology project on Complementary medicine (COST B4); and charities are slowly coming round to looking at alternative methods for hard to treat diseases.

But even where there is the will to research the therapies there may be no way. It is so difficult to scientifically explore systems of treatment that do not obey scientific principles, that many in the conventional and complementary camps do not know how to begin. With which experimental tools, for example, can the relationships between acupuncture meridians and health, the actual results of chiropractic manipulation, or the use and effect of homeopathic potencies be investigated? This is a complex question, which cannot be deeply explored in this brief review. However some general comments follow.

Modern research is reductionist and objective, an attempt to break down reality into manageable bits and know whether each one of them is actually happening 'out there'. It is singularly inappropriate for the examination of a holistic alternative clinical situation in which a therapist, in close alliance with a patient, provides a therapeutic environment, unique to just this patient, in which he can find his way back to health. If no therapy is involved, and science is applied to, for example, *in vitro* cell culture dishes in the laboratory, some useful objective information can be obtained, for example that healing energies can affect plant cell growth and enzyme activity, or that certain ultra-high dilutions of poisons, when potentized by shaking in the homeopathic manner, can detoxify cells or laboratory animals. But this does not demonstrate therapy, and indeed tens of thousands of such studies exist in the scientific literature without apparent effect on the practice or the status of complementary medicine.

In clinical research the 'gold standard' is the randomized double-blind clinical trial (although it must be said that they constitute only 16 per cent of published articles in leading medical journals[49]). The investigator attempts to gain maximum control over the conditions of the study by stripping therapy down to a single isolated intervention (a drug compared with a placebo or another drug) on a single target (a homogeneous group of patients with a single diagnosed symptom or condition). Objectivity is obtained by removing the healing potential inherent in the therapeutic interaction by double-blind conditions. Besides the huge expense, difficulty and slowness of such trials, they represent an unreal world that hides the effects and side-effects of the treatment on each individual. When the treatment is used in practice on individual patients all kinds of new problems and inadequacies come to light. And the less powerful the treatment, the more difficult it is to obtain clear knowledge of anything. For example, billions of dollars have been spent on trials with hundreds of thousands of people to ask the following simple question: is it a good idea to lower blood cholesterol by drugs for those with raised blood cholesterol? For those whose hypercholesterolaemia is not extreme, the answer is still not clear.[50]

An example of how such methods fail when applied to complementary medicine is the current research on Chinese herbal remedies for eczema being carried out by teams from certain London hospitals. Patients with long-standing eczema unresponsive to modern treatments were cured by a Chinese herbalist. Researchers became aware of this but ignored the principles in the rush for the product: 'Once you've heard the theory you can't really believe that a treatment based on it could work—but this is the big mistake, because it does.'[51] Though researchers do know that different patients need different herbal mixtures, in order to study this success they set up a series of classical double-blind controlled studies.[52] For this purpose they standardized the precise herbal mixture used (lost: the entire theoretical and practical basis of Oriental medicine), are using it under double-blind conditions (lost: the therapist), with a restricted group of eczema cases (lost: the applicability of Oriental medicine for all kinds of diseases, conditions, and individuals), and are attempting to isolate the single active ingredient from the mixture so as to test it (lost: much of the effectiveness and safety). There will be left a single powerful and toxic new Western drug 'discovery', probably merely symptomatic, with a very narrow field of use. It would be exactly equivalent to primitive people hunting for modern medicine, entering a hospital to search for its essence, finding it and emerging triumphantly with 'the scalpel'. Shorn of its conceptual background it will be of little help and can do much harm.

Some of the problems inherent in applying controlled trial methodology to complementary medicine are obvious. How does one get a homogeneous group when each patient should be treated differently? For example, each member of a group of mildly hypertensive patients may need radically different treatments according to complementary diagnosis. The opposite is also true, a 'kidney-yin' deficient group can manifest a wide variety of symptoms, each of which could be diagnosed as having a different disease according to Western medicine.[53] It would be absurd to test one treatment in complementary medicine as the treatment is always complex and changing, and instructions as to the patients' lifestyle are often of the essence in therapy. So what should be tested: a single herb? a series of herbs? a series of herbs plus instructions as to diet? or all that plus ancillary treatments by one or more practitioners of different kinds? If the trial is to be double-blind neither patient nor researcher must know whether they are actually being treated. But the psychological dimension in most complementary therapies is part of the therapy, and to attempt to cancel it out invalidates the treatment. In addition in many cases it is simply impossible. Either the patient will always know whether he is receiving real or placebo treatment, such as in chiropractic where the results are felt immediately. Or, a real placebo cannot be constructed, because, as in acupuncture, almost everything the therapist does will affect the patient energetically. Finally, since complementary treatments are often undertaken over a considerable period of time, such studies cut some arbitrary slice out of a lengthy return to health. It will be a mere snapshot.

The entire field is ridden with fundamental methodological problems that arise from the attempt to employ observational methods based on one culture and world view to practices that are based on radically different world views. The methodological problems have been well reviewed in a recent book by Lewith and Aldridge,[53] who nevertheless believe the attempt to be worth it. Randomized double-blind controlled trials can, of course, be carried out, and some researchers strongly support them to address the effectiveness and safety of complementary medicine.[54] However most researchers agree that the kind of answers that emerge are of uncertain value and applicability.

A series of homeopathic clinical studies illustrate these points in practice. In the mid-1970s, a team in Glasgow explored the effect of homeopathy on 54 rheumatoid arthritis patients compared with the effect of conventional aspirin on 41 similar patients. A further control group were given a placebo. Homeopathic treatment was given by the homeopathic doctors, conventional treatment by the conventional doctors, and an independent assessor reviewed progress. It turned out that both doctors and patients agreed that progress was much better with homeopathy than salicylates (aspirin), and homeopathy produced substantially less side-effects. Both groups did better than the placebo group.[55]

However, this trial engendered a bitter debate, with some justification.[56] How can a single conventional treatment be compared with a whole system of homeopathic treatments in which a total of 200 remedies were used? There was also the problem that the homeopathic, salicylate, and placebo groups could not be exactly matched. It was also argued that the trial was not controlled as the homeopathic doctor would have a vested interest in the success of his treatment and would communicate this to the patients. There is the question of the wisdom of giving a placebo to arthritis patients in pain. There is the complex problem of whether to allow the homeopathic patients to continue their previous conventional treatment. Finally, there is the question of assessment. In this, trial factors such as joint mobility were used. However, many other signs of health or sickness which are read by the homeopathic practitioner were ignored. The controversy raised by this trial was discouraging for research and researchers. However it was repeated in a truly double-blinded fashion with all patients maintaining their previous therapy but receiving in addition homeopathy or placebo, and again homeopathy was highly significantly better.[57]

Now the researchers went one step further and attempted to move from *one disease/any medicine* to the more conventional *one disease/one medicine* clinical trial. The first attempt found no difference between placebo and Rhus tox in osteoarthritis.[58] But now it was the homeopath's turn to complain that the full prescribing criteria for Rhus tox were not applied. Again, the study was repeated, but this time using selected fibrositis patients for whom Rhus tox was indicated. The trial was double-blind and now homeopathy was clearly better than placebo.[59]

Another instructive example is the clinical testing of acupuncture. Many double-blind clinical trials have been confounded by the failure to find a true placebo. Years of such trials used acupuncture at incorrect (sham) or inert points, or at a very shallow depth.[60] But it has been demonstrated that such insertion produces non-specific physiological effects, sometimes providing actual therapeutic benefits, i.e. that acupuncture at true points and at sham points both produce results, such as relief of asthma, which are better than baseline.[61] No placebo has been found that is truly comparable to acupuncture and yet inert. The best is probably the use of electroacupuncture equipment with the current switched off or at inappropriate settings. Yet this may be an inadequate placebo if it is used as a placebo against real acupuncture.[62] There are further severe problems in trial design, that have been elegantly described in a recent review,[63] such as the fact that double-blinding of needle acupuncture is impossible, because, like surgery, it needs the full awareness of the practitioner, and patients too may easily intuit the difference between real and sham treatments. In addition, trials have to be assessed from the perspective of Oriental medicine, not just conventional methodology: how authentic was the diagnosis, how were points selected, how were patients followed-up, what was the effect of any concomitant conventional drugs on the treatment, etc.[63]

There is a growing movement within the research community to look for appropriate research methods. In particular, to adopt the 'comparative outcomes approach' and examine the outcome in selected groups of patients of the entire therapy performed authentically by the therapist, compared with conventional treatment by doctors, with the protocol agreed by both. In these studies the crucial importance of the intangible in medicine is acknowledged, and the fruitless attempt to dissect it out of medicine as 'the placebo effect' is abandoned. The therapist is not 'blind', so his intention to heal is recruited, as in real life. Assessors can be used, and they can be 'blind'. The use of such outcome studies has been strongly supported in a recent authoritative *Lancet* paper.[64] Even here though, there are problems. Since the basic notions of health and disease are different between medical systems, it is often hard to come to an agreement on whether a therapy has produced an improvement in health, let alone the nature of this improvement. For example, a symptom, such as a cough, may be seen by the therapist as the result of deeper vulnerabilities which if left untreated would eventually erupt into a life-threatening disease. In this case the presenting symptom is the main one in Western terms but a minor one to the therapist. On which basis does one judge success? It is very common too, that alternative medicine produces a major improvement in patient symptoms, but when it is judged by conventional physical diagnostic criteria, such as the degree of airway obstruction in asthma, or ESR sedimentation in rheumatic conditions, the disease is still present. There has been intensive discussion of these issues.[65] One of the ideas to emerge is to make more use of health indices, validated questionnaires which assess the patient's state of health before and after the treatment, such as the Nottingham Health Profile or 'SF 36', adapted from the American Medical Outcomes Trust measures.[66] The advantage of using these tools is that they include assessment of physical, mental, and social function and well-being. Instead of trying to eliminate the patient's subjective universe, the patient is recruited into the research team.

There are new methods under development which may be more appropriate for the study of the therapeutic process, giving more importance to the entire healing relationship rather than stripping therapy to bare technique. Co-operative inquiry is a method in which researchers, therapists, and patients can form a group which inquires together about the process in which they are all partaking.[67] There is a strong case for using qualitative methods derived from the social sciences in order to assess and evaluate treatment. For example, biographic methodology involves in-depth structured interviews, to probe deep into the subjective experience of treatment. It can obtain valued insights into effects and side-effects that would be hard to obtain any other way.[68] The way of the anthropologist has been proposed as a model for research tools to cross systems of thought.[69] Anthropologists examine existing records, observe human interactions in detail by taking part in them, use open interviews without predetermined questions, and use maps, games, or other tools for revealing subjects' knowledge. The validity of the information is constantly improved by cross checking for internal consistency. These methods can give us a real insight into what happens during the therapeutic process.[70] Cassidy, in proposing such methods for the study of alternative medicine, reminds us that science itself, in researching new subjects, usually goes through stages of qualitative research for the purposes of exploration, description, and correlation.[69]

Yet investigation is always needed. Without it neither conventional nor complementary medicine would exist beyond the folk remedy level. Society would not know which therapy would do what, and conventional medicine would not understand in what way other therapies could be complementary to it. The problem lies not with the need for research but with the methods. Modern medical research is highly standardized and rigorously controlled; only certain ways of observing the world are admitted as knowledge. This arises from professionalization. The imposition of these methods on alternative medicine could be a form of 'epistemological aggression'. Alternative medicine is a loose and non-professionalized body of knowledge which flexibly adapts to observations drawn from practice. In other words, there always has been alternative research, in which therapists study the potentials of their remedies on patients and on themselves. Its epistemological basis is not standardized; but is more like a 'conversational field'.[71] If this approach was respected, complementary medicine could provide to modern society not only new practical approaches and radical new concepts, but also a refreshing and powerful new methodology of looking at the body, at health and disease, and at life itself.

References

1. Pietroni, P. (1990). *The greening of medicine*. Gollancz, London. Stanway, A. (1994). *Alternative medicine: guide to natural therapies*. Penguin, Harmondsworth. Hill, R. and Gould, A. (1996). *Complementary medicine: its practice in the health service*. Blackwell Scientific, Oxford. Lewith, G. T. (ed.) (1985). *Alternative therapies. A guide to complementary medicine for the health professional*. Heinemann, London. Weil, A. (1991). *Health and healing: understanding conventional and alternative medicine*. Houghton Mifflin, Los Angeles.
2. Fulder, S. J. (1995). Natural health and healthy nature: the neo-Hippocratic revolution in alternative medicine. In *Studies in alternative medicine II. Bodies and nature in alternative medicine*, Johanessen, H., Olesen, S. G. and Andersen, O. (eds.). Odense University Press, Odense.
3. For good summaries of the conceptual basis of complementary and holistic medicine see: Bannerman, R. H., Burton, J., and Wen-Chieh, C. (1983). *Traditional medicine and health care coverage*. World Health Organization, Geneva. Pietroni, P. (1990). *The greening of medicine*. Gollancz, London. Weil, A. (1990). *Natural health, natural medicine*. Houghton Mifflin, Boston.
4. Siegel, B. (1986). *Love, medicine and miracles*. Rider, London. Farquhar, J. (1994). *Knowing practice: the clinical encounter in Chinese medicine*. Westview, Oxford and Boulder.
5. Vickers, A. J. (1994). Complementary medicine, intermediate medicine and the degree of intervention. *Complementary Therapies in Medicine*, 2, 123–7.
6. Kriege, T. (1969). *The fundamental basis of iridiagnosis*. Fowler, London. Jensen, B. (1978). Iridology: Its origin, development and meaning. In *Wholistic dimensions in healing*, (ed. L. Kaslov). Doubleday, New York. (See Chapter 18.)
7. Shealy, N. (1988). *The creation of health. Merging traditional medicine with intuitive diagnosis*. Stillpoint, U.S. Regush, N. M. (ed.) (1974). *The human aura*. Berkeley Medallion, New York.
8. Bresler, D. E., Oleson, T. D., and Kroenig, R. J. (1978). *Ear acupuncture diagnosis in musculoskeletal plain: Final report of a preliminary investigation*. Institute of Noetic Sciences, San Francisco. Sullivan, S. G. (1985). Evoked electrical conductance on lung acupuncture points in healthy individuals and confirmed lung cancer patients. *American Journal of Acupuncture*, 3, 261–6.
9. Karagulla, S. (1967). *Breakthrough to creativity*. Scarecrow Press, New Jersey. Benor, D. (1990). Survey of spiritual healing research. *Complementary Medical Research*, 4, 9–33.
10. Moss, T. (1981). *The body electric*. Granada, St Albans. Gennaro, L., Guzzon, F., and Marsigli, P. (1987). *Kirlian photography*, East West Publications, London.
11. Lowenberg, J. S. (1989). *Caring and responsibility: crossroads of holistic practice and traditional medicine*. University of Pennsylvania Press, Philadelphia. Pelletier, K.

(1979). Holistic medicine: From pathology to prevention. *Western Journal of Medicine*, 131, 481–2. Power, R. (1991). Ideologies of holism in health care, *Complementary Medical Research*, 5, 151–9.

12. Pelletier, K. (1994). *Sound body, sound mind*. Simon & Schuster, New York. Borysenko, J. (1988). *Minding the body, mending the mind*. Bantam, New York.

13. Hastings, A. C. (ed.) (1981). *Health for the whole person*. Westview Press, Boulder, Colorado.

14. Inglis, B. (1979). *Natural medicine*. Collins, London. Inglis, B. (1979). *A history of medicine*. Fontana/Collins, London.

15. Brock, A. J. (1921). *Greek medicine*. Dent and Sons, New York. Bynum, W.F. and Porter, R. (eds.) (1993). *Companion encyclopaedia of the history of medicine*. Routledge, London. Lloyd, G. E. R. (1978). *Hippocratic writings*. Pelican, Harmondsworth.

16. Rosenberg, C. E. (1977). The therapeutic revolution: medicine, meaning and social change in the nineteenth century. *Perspectives in Biology and Medicine*, 20, 485–506.

17. Dubos, René (1968). *Man, medicine and environment*. Praeger, New York.

18. Miller, Jonathan (1978). Interview. *Vogue*, November, London.

19. Office of Population Census and Surveys. (1974). *Morbidity statistics from general practice: second national study 1970–71*. HMSO, London. Howe, G.M. (1976). *Man, environment and disease in Britain*. Pelican, Harmondsworth, Middlesex.

20. Department of Health (1992). *Compendium of health statistics*. HMSO, London.

21. Office of Population Census and Surveys. (1995). *Social trends*. HMSO, London.

22. Beardsley, T. (1994). Trends in cancer epidemiology. A war not won. *Scientific American*, January, 118–26.

23. National Cancer Institute (1991). *Statistics review. 1973–1988*. NIH Publication No. 91–2789. NIH, Bethesda, Maryland. Bailar, J. C. (1986). Progress against cancer? *New England Journal of Medicine*, 314, 1226–32.

24. Barsky, A. (1988). The paradox of health. *New England Journal of Medicine*, February 18, 414–18.

25. Mahler, H. (1977). Editorial. *WHO Chronicle*, 31, 60–2.

26. Downer, S. M., Cody, M. M., McCluskey, P., Wilson, P. D., Arnott, S. J., Lister, T. A., and Slevin, M. L. (1994). Pusuit and practice of complementary therapies by cancer patients receiving conventional treatment. *British Medical Journal*, 309, 86–9. Sikora, K. (1990). Complementary medicine in cancer. *Cancer Care*, 7, 9–11.

27. Seminal books that helped to initiate the resurgence were: Clark, L.A. (1968). *Get well naturally*. Arco, New York. Forbes, A. (1976). *Try being healthy*. Health Science Press. Holsworthy, Essex.

28. Taylor Nelson Ltd (1985). *The monitor programme*. Epson, Surrey. Annual survey of social trends using a base of 2135 adults throughout the UK.

29. MORI Poll (1989). *The Times*, 13 November 1989.

30. Mintel (1993). *Alternative medicines, market intelligence report*. Mintel, 18–19 Long Lane, London EC1A 9HE.

31. Opinion Research (1980). *Opinions about natural therapists*. Opinion Research, Lagendijk, Foundation Central Bureau NWP, The Netherlands. The survey which led to this report was carried out in November 1979 among 1030 Dutch males aged over 18 years.

32. Editorial (1995). *Journal of Alternative and Complementary Medicine*, 13, 3

33. Wharton, R. and Lewith, G. (1986). Complementary medicine and the general practitioner. *British Medical Journal*, 292, 1498–500.

34. Anderson, E. and Anderson, P. (1987). General practitioners and alternative medicine. *Journal of the Royal College of General Practitioners*, 37, 52–5. Schachter, L., Weingarten, M. A., and Kahan, E. E. (1993). Attitudes of family physicians to

nonconventional therapies. *Archives of Family Medicine*, 2, 1268–9. Hadley, C. M. (1988). Complementary medicine and the General Practitioner: a survey of General Practitioners in the Wellington area. *New Zealand Medical Journal*, 101, 766–8.

35. Perkin, M. R., Pearcy, R. M., and Fraser, J. S. (1994). A comparison of the attitudes shown by General Practitioners, hospital doctors and medical students towards alternative medicine. *Journal of the Royal Society of Medicine*, 87, 523–5.

36. Fulder, S. J. and Monro, R. (1985). Complementary medicine in the United Kingdom: patients, practitioners and consultations, *Lancet*, 2, 542–45.

37. Reilly, D. T. (1983), Young doctors' views on alternative medicine. *British Medical Journal*, 287, 337–9.

38. *The Times*. 30 June 1983.

39. Board of Science and Education (1986). *Alternative therapies*. British Medical Association, London.

40. British Medical Association (1993). *Complementary medicine. New approaches to good practice*. Oxford University Press, Oxford.

41. Morrison, I. and Smith, R. (1994). The future of medicine. *British Medical Journal*, 309, 1109–10.

42. Tonkin, R. (1987). Research into complementary medicine. *Complementary Medical Research*, 2, 5–9.

43. Anon. (1986). Editorial. *Lancet*, 2, 1427–8.

44. Maddox, J. (1988). When to believe the unbelievable. *Nature*, 333, 787.

45. Editorial (1981). At the centre and on the fringes. *Lancet*, 2, 1209.

46. Saks, M. (1991). The flight from science? The reporting of acupuncture in mainstream British medical journals from 1800 to 1990. *Complementary Medical Research*, 5, 178–82.

47. Commission for Alternative Systems of Medicine (1981). *Alternative medicine in the Netherlands*. Ministerie Van Volks Gezondheid en Milieuhygiene. Staatsuirgeverij, C., The Netherlands.

48. Fitter, M. and Blackwell, R. (1993). Are acupuncturists interested in research? *The European Journal of Oriental Medicine*, 2, 44–50.

49. St. George, D. (1994). Research into complementary medicine: going beyond the limits of clinical trials. *Advances*, 10, 59–61.

50. Davey Smith, G. and Pekkanen, J. (1992). Should there be a moratorium on the use of cholesterol-lowering drugs? *British Medical Journal*, 304, 431–484. Muldoon, M. F., Manuck, S. B., and Matthews, K. A. (1990). Lowering cholesterol concentrations and mortality: a quantitative review of primary prevention trials. *British Medical Journal*, 301, 309–14.

51. Wroe, M. (1992). Treatment that is more than skin deep. *The Independent on Sunday*, 28 June 1992, p.55.

52. Sheehan, M. P., Rustin, M. H. A., Atherton, D. J., Buckley, C., Harris, D. J. Brostoff, J. *et al.* (1992). Efficacy of traditional Chinese herbal therapy in adult atopic dermatitis, *Lancet*, 340, 13–7. Atherton, D. J. (1994). *Eczema in childhood: the facts*. Oxford University Press, Oxford.

53. Lewith, G. T. and Aldridge, D.(eds.) (1993). *Clinical research methodology for complementary therapies*. Hodder & Stoughton, London. Vickers, A. (1994). Special problems of clinical research in complementary medicine. *Journal of Alternative and Complementary Medicine*, 12, 47–51. Heron. J. (1986). Critique of conventional research methodology. *Complementary Medical Research*, 1, 12–22.

54. Ernst, E. (1995). Complementary medicine. Common misconceptions. *Journal of the Royal Society of Medicine*, 88, 244–7.

55. Gibson, R. G., Gibson, S. L. M., MacNeill, A. D., Dick, W. C., and Buchanan, W. W.

(1978). Salicylates and homeopathy in rheumatoid arthritis: Preliminary observations. *British Journal of Clinical Pharmacology*, **6**, 391–5.

56. Huston, G. (1979). Salicylates in homeopathy. *British Journal of Clinical Pharmacology*, **7**, 529–30. Dick, W. C., Gibson, R., Gray, G. I. L., and Buchanan, W. W. (1979). *British Journal of Clinical Pharmacology*, **7**, 530.

57. Gibson, R. G., Gibson, S. L. M., MacNeill, D. A., and Buchanan, W. (1980). Homeopathic therapy in rheumatoid arthritis: evaluation by double blind clinical trial. *British Journal of Clinical Pharmacology*, **9**, 453–9.

58. Shipley, M., Berry, H., Broster, G., Jenkins, M., Clover, A., and Williams, I. (1983). Controlled trial of homeopathic treatment of osteoarthritis. *Lancet*, **1**, 482.

59. Fisher, P., Greenwood, A., Huskisson, E. C., Turner, P., and Belon, P. (1989). Effect of homeopathic treatment on fibrositis (primary fibromyalgia). *British Medical Journal*, **299**, 365–6.

60. Vincent, C. A. and Richardson, P. H. (1987). Acupuncture for some common disorders: a review of evaluative research. *Journal of the Royal Society of Medicine*, **37**, 77–81.

61. Lewith, G. T. and Machin, D. (1983). On the evaluation of the clinical effects of acupuncture: concepts and methods. *Pain*, **16**, 111–27.

62. Jobst, K. A., Chen, J. H., and Hext, A. (1992). Review of acupuncture for bronchial asthma; a double blind cross-over study. *Complementary Medical Research*, **6**, 57–8.

63. Jobst, K. A. (1995). A critical analysis of acupuncture in pulmonary disease: efficacy and safety of the acupuncture needle. *Journal of Alternative and Complementary Medicine. Research on Paradigm, Practice and Policy*, **1**, 57–85.

64. Joyce, C. R. B. (1994). Placebo and complementary medicine. *The Lancet*, **344**, 1279–81.

65. RCCM Methodology Conference 1987 (1988). How do we know it works?—measures of outcome. *Complementary Medical Research*, **2**, No. 3. 1–106.

66. Bowling, A. (1991). *Measuring health*. Open University Press, Milton Keynes.

67. Reason, P. (1994). Three approaches to co-operative inquiry. In *Handbook of qualitative research*, (eds. Denzin, N. K. and Lincoln, Y. S.). Sage, London. Reason, P. and Rowan, J. (eds.) (1981). *Human inquiry: A sourcebook of new paradigm research*. Wiley, Chichester.

68. Lafaille, R. and Fulder, S. (eds.) (1993). *Towards a new science of health*. Routledge, London.

69. Cassidy, C. (1995). Social science theory and methods in the study of alternative and complementary medicine. *Journal of Alternative and Complementary Medicine. Research on Paradigm, Practice and Policy*, **1**, 19–40.

70. Mitchin, A. (1995). Modelling the therapeutic process. *Journal of Interprofessional Care*, **9**, 1.

71. Schied, V. (1993). Orientalism revisited. Reflections on scholarship, research and professionalisation. *European Journal of Oriental Medicine*, **1**, 23–33. Leslie, C. and Young, A. (eds.) (1992). *Paths to Asian medical knowledge*. University of California Press, Berkeley.

2

The patient

How many people go to complementary practitioners?

This is a question upon which future health policy decisions will turn. It is therefore unfortunate that in contrast to other countries such as The Netherlands or Australia, such a simple question has not been asked by official medical or sociological research bodies in the UK. It may well be that the failure to spend a tiny fraction of the total medical expenditure to find out what proportion of the population have embraced alternatives to modern medicine expresses an unconscious hope that the whole uncomfortable phenomenon will eventually go away. In fact, the preliminary data shows that usage is increasing as rapidly as ever.

The most recent study is a pilot population survey carried out by a team at the University of Sheffield on behalf of the Research Council for Complementary Medicine. Postal questionnaires were sent to 921 voters; 78 per cent were returned. These showed that roughly 10 per cent of the population had visited a professional complementary practitioner in the previous year.[1] Estimates of the numbers of people who have consulted complementary medicine at some time, vary from one-fifth[1] to around one-third of the population.[2] A 1991 Consumers Association survey of some 1000 readers of *Which?*, the consumer magazine, found that a quarter had visited a non-conventional practitioner in the previous year.[3] This level of annual consultation is close to the extent of consultations with GPs which stood at 16 per cent of the population per year in 1990.[4] This is despite GP consultations being essentially free. This astonishing fact seems to have gone largely unnoticed. Indeed, one cannot avoid the impression that official medical institutions including the Department of Health, the National Health Service, and the local Health Authorities, are continually and needlessly caught unawares by the extent of usage of alternatives, and the strength of feeling of adherents.

This scale of usage is transnational. In Europe as a whole, 20–50 per cent of the European population consult complementary practitioners.[5] In Holland, which has the best statistics, 5.9 per cent of the population consulted a lay complementary practitioner during 1990, while 15.7 per cent of the population consulted a practitioner with medical qualifications, making 20.6 per cent in total.[6] Even in the United States, the bastion of modern medicine, no less than 1 in 3 of the population use alternative medicine.[7] Despite alternative medicine being defined in this case as everything beyond the pale of orthodoxy, even megadose vitamins, this statistic shocked the US medical community there and led to the immediate establishment of the Office of Alternative Medicine. Whichever way you look at it, the extent of use is massive, despite most of these consultations being paid for out of pocket, and the numbers do not even include all those who purchase and use alternative remedies.

Obviously, the usage of complementary medicine has been growing rapidly. The Consumers Association study mentioned above found that usage had almost doubled in the years from 1986 to 1991. Larger national polls give the same picture. Two commercial surveys found that 13 per cent of the UK population had sought such treatments in 1983.[8] This means that usage has more than doubled in the intervening 13 years until today. The same kind of growth has happened in Europe. An influential national survey carried out by The Netherlands Institute of Preventive Medicine found that 6.4 per cent of the Dutch population had visited a complementary practitioner in 1981.[9] Ten years later, as we saw above, the numbers had more than doubled. The use of homeopathy in France also more than doubled, from 16 per cent of the population to 36 per cent in the ten years from 1982 to 1992.[5]

Another way of gauging how much complementary medicine is used is to assess the total numbers of consultations. This tends to give an understimate as it is virtually impossible to find and to canvass those therapists who keep a low profile. The Threshold Survey found that in 1981 there were from 11.7 to 15.4 million consultations in the UK.[10] These figures excluded healers, who often provide therapy without personal face-to-face consultations. If they were included the numbers would be much higher. Acupuncture, chiropractic, and osteopathy were the therapies most commonly consulted with two million annual consultations for each. This is followed by naturopathy with 1.2 million, then hypnotherapy, herbalism, homeopathy, and the others. Healing is frequently used but hard to quantify. The number of consultations today is unknown. However if we assume a very approximate 3-fold increase in the number of lay practitioners since then (see Chapter 3), there could now be between 33 and 45 million consultations in the UK per year. In the USA there are even more *pro rata*. The Harvard Medical School study found that there were 425 million consultations with alternative therapists in 1990, exceeding by a considerable margin all visits to primary care physicians in that year.[7]

The total number of UK alternative medical consultations demonstrates again that an entire medical system, distinct from conventional medicine, now exists. The number of consultations is similar to the number of GP consultations which are now running at about 42 million per year.[4] However, it should be remembered that consultations with GPs are free and are used for treatment, enquiry, and vaccination. Therefore, it may be more appropriate to compare complementary medical consultations with those of conventional medical specialists, as in both cases patients are likely to have a history of illness, and have often already seen a GP for their health problem. This is the point made by the Dutch survey, which only used specialist consultations as a comparison.[9] Consultation rates for specialists are not published in the UK.

The giant of modern medicine has indeed been caught napping. Available statistics indicate a much heavier use of medical alternatives than has previously been suspected. As a result a profound re-orientation is already occurring in the culture of medicine, the choices of consumers, the economy of health, the pharmaceutical and natural medicines industries. The future is sure to be full of even more dramatic change and opportunity.

Why do people go to complementary practitioners?

Everyone involved in the caring professions has an intention to relieve human suffering, and most have patients' well-being at heart. It is therefore of great importance to understand what people are saying in their drive to seek and pay for alternatives. In searching for these reasons, we are no longer in the realm of objective and verifiable facts, or of health issues. The question is about people's subjective experience and their inner motivations, their cultural assumptions, and world view. Those who look for new ways of thinking may be going to complementary practitioners because of ideological identification with the alternative health subculture. Others who need to be heard will go to seek a deeper kind of listening, others may be simply shopping around for a cure, or maybe they have encountered suffering and failure at the hands of conventional doctors. Others may be beginning to feel that different medical systems are each suitable for different kinds of health problems. Should medical professionals regard such patients simply as medical rejects, incurable chronic cases which the medical world is glad to pass on? Or are they the complete reverse—seekers, on a quest for a more healthy, fulfilling, and meaningful life? And it is not a question of either/or, since any or all of these reasons may be working together in different individuals at different times.

In particular, some questionnaire-based studies have attempted to assess the attitudes and expectations of patients of complementary practitioners compared with GPs. Like all such research, the subject is constrained by the questions to give an artificial summary in the present moment of a long personal story, so the results are limited. For example, patients also often express a distrust in medical professionals. But it is unclear if such a view caused or resulted from a commitment to self-responsibility in health, unsatisfactory experiences with medical professionals, or other reasons. As Ursula Sharma has pointed out in her book on the subject, patients of complementary medicine have moved steadily towards it as a result of chains of experiences, shifts in attitude, and decisions:

Evidently many people are in the process of changing their approach to medical authority and to family healthcare, and the decision to consult a non-orthodox practitioner may represent only one moment in a series of connected shifts in practice.[10]

In other words, we are in the midst of a cultural transformation in medicine, in which attitudes, beliefs, practices, choices, habits, and knowledge are shifting gradually across a broad front which includes lay and professional people. In such a situation only longitudinal, long term, biographical, and qualitative research can tease out causes and consequences; the way of the anthropologist.[11]

In any event, whenever people are asked why they are going to an alternative practitioner, two answers stand out: people are usually driven to seek alternatives after disappointing experiences with conventional doctors, or are advised by a successfully treated friend or colleague. Thirty-nine per cent of Dutch complementary patients gave the former as their main reason while somewhat less had been motivated by the success of complementary treatment with someone known to them.[9] The three-city study in Australia, carried out by a team from the University of Queensland, found that disappointment with other forms of treatment and personal recommendation of a friend or relative were the two main reasons for consulting therapists. Only a relatively small proportion gave belief in complementary medicine as their motive.[12] Recently, a series of studies by Adrian Furnham, of University College, London, investigated beliefs and attitudes of homeopath and GP patients. Patients of homeopaths confirm that they went to them because of dissatisfaction with previous medical treatment rather than belief in alternative medicine.[13] It is evidently necessity, not ideology, which draws people to the complementary consulting rooms, although it doesn't rule out cultural and belief systems as distant, rather than proximal causes.

Studies in both America[14] and the UK[15] have also put paid to the notion that alternative practitioners flourish in medically under-served areas. Indeed, both studies point to the opposite conclusion—that where conventional medicine increases its coverage, complementary medicine follows suit. In addition, the evidence described in the next section shows that complementary medical patients are not ignorant, gullible, and underprivileged. Indeed, studies have shown that they seem to be less trusting of professional care providers, less willing to leave things in the hands of their therapist, and less confident about the outcome of the treatment than the patients of modern medicine.[16] In other words, contrary to commonly expressed views, blind faith or the placebo effect may be stronger within a modern medical treatment than a complementary medical treatment.

Surveys show that there are differences in the beliefs expressed by patients of complementary therapists and of GPs. In particular, those using complementary medicine have a more internal locus of control: they believe that they are more responsible for their health, that disease is not just a matter of chance, and that the threat of disease is overstated. They also seem more knowledgeable about the body and more conscious about health. Besides, they represent the holistic position, believing that treatment should involve the whole person and not just the symptoms.[13,16] These beliefs are expected, and represent the current shifts in world-view.[17] However, one cannot know if the person felt like that in the first place and therefore sought a complementary consultation, or whether the views developed as a result of contact with alternatives, during which, the belief system is inevitably swallowed along with the pill.

So, a patient, often frustrated with medical care, is ready to try something new. How does he first hear of a complementary practitioner? Is he attracted by advertising and enticing health magazines? How often does a doctor actually suggest a visit to his erstwhile rival? The Dutch survey found that 71 per cent of the patients had first heard of a complementary practitioner from friends or relatives. Only 14 per cent first thought about it as a result of books or media coverage, while for 12 per cent of the patients it was their medical practitioner who put the idea forward.[9] A recent public survey by the Daily Telegraph and the Open University found that five times more users of complementary medicine went as a result of recommendation from a friend or relative than because of professional recommendation.[18] These figures demonstrate that patients arrive largely as a result of a groundswell of opinion and shared experience. The flight to medical alternatives is a grass roots phenomenon, solidly based on personal experience. It is not a temporary media-enhanced fashion.

In my experience, people find it hard to articulate the deeper reasons for change. But behind their frustration with modern medicine is a strong and intuitively held sense that what is lacking in modern medicine is respect. Patients may feel that the totality of their life brought them to this disease at this time. Yet the reductionist basis of modern medicine can hardly do more than fix a problem and send the patient on his way, without connection to his feelings, questions, vulnerabilities, biography, and life experience. In that sense, however nice the medical staff, reductionism reduces the human being and takes its toll. Biographical research would be able to draw out these feelings, and would be of great help in understanding where the social movement towards alternatives is heading.

Who are the patients?

There are a number of myths about the types of people who go to complementary therapists and the kind of relationships that result. For example, some doctors of the author's acquaintance assume that complementary therapy patients are either neurotic or hypochondriacal, or that they go to therapists for sympathy rather than treatment.

The Threshold Survey's data on therapists' patients indicates that they tend to be predominantly young to middle-aged, an impression confirmed by the Dutch and Australian studies, and recent surveys of patients in the USA and UK.[2,7,9,19] There are few infants and few elderly patients nationally, although there may be regional differences. This is in contrast to conventional medicine, where more patients are derived from the two ends of the lifespan than the middle. Possibly the aged are less willing to experiment with complementary medicine and have less money with which to do so, while the very young tend to have acute rather than chronic diseases.

Patients appear to come from all social classes. However, there are more patients from socio-economic grades A and B (professional, managerial, technical, business, academic, etc.) than the others. They are also likely to be more highly educated than doctors' patients.[7,9,19] For example, 16 per cent had higher education as opposed to 12 per cent of doctors' patients in Australia.[20] Healing (often free) is weighted towards the less well off, as is herbalism and to some extent hypnotherapy. Nearly two-thirds of the patients are women, much the same distribution as doctors' patients.[2,19]

Complementary medicine is more widely practised in the more prosperous areas of the UK. Oxford, for example, with its students and proximity to a large acupuncture college, and Exeter, with many retired people, both have considerable numbers of acupuncturists. Exeter and Hereford have a high proportion of naturopaths and osteopaths, and few hypnotherapists. In industrial areas there is less complementary medicine, though the North is traditionally strong in hypnotherapy and healing.[19]

There are certainly no grounds for believing that the alternative health system battens on the less educated, elderly, or poorer people who are somehow enmeshed in its promises. If anything, the reverse is true, for patients are generally sufficiently knowledgeable to make discriminating choices, old enough to act on them, and rich enough to pay for them.

The health problems treated by complementary practitioners

Since the major proportion of complementary practitioners' patients come for consultation following unsuccessful treatment elsewhere, we might expect that most of the conditions with which they arrive are those which conventional medicine finds hard to cure. There are several such areas:

1. Musculoskeletal, including chronic backache, rheumatic, arthritic and structural problems, slipped discs, etc.
2. Chronic pain, including headaches, migraine, sciatica, and neuralgia.
3. Chronic infections, such as cystitis and bronchitis, which are only manageable by constant use of antibiotics.
4. Allergic conditions.
5. Cardiovascular problems such as hypertension and arteriosclerosis.
6. Neurological diseases such as multiple sclerosis.
7. Sleep disorders, fatigue, and debility.
8. Stress-related and psychosomatic disorders.
9. Chronic diseases related to inadequate immunity, such as AIDS, ME.
10. Non-specific conditions that are hard to diagnose conventionally.

These are health problems which conventional medicine cannot easily cure. The symptoms may be successfully managed. But despite continual medical care, it may become clear to the patient, sooner or later, that he or she still has the condition. Complementary therapists present an almost irresistible opportunity to tackle the disease at its root. The patient with a persistent ailment will also be more likely to be prepared to make the curative alterations to his lifestyle demanded by complementary medicine, and more attracted to therapies which do not themselves gradually undermine health. One would therefore expect almost all complementary medical clients to have chronic ailments of the type described above, apart from the healthy who go for preventive purposes.

Checking this supposition is not so easy to do accurately. It has been carried out by querying complementary practitioners. However they usually diagnose patients in their own terms (such as 'blood impurities', 'yin-yang', 'vertebral adhesions') and, if pressed for a medical diagnosis, often simply quote what the patient has told them concerning some previous medical contact, so the diagnostic categories are somewhat general and vague. Nevertheless, the general picture is clear. The University of Queensland research team carried out a poll of no less than 17 258 new patients of chiropractors and other practitioners throughout Australia.[20] Their list of major symptoms seen is given in Table 2.1. This is compared with data from a survey by the Department of Public Health Medicine at the University of Sheffield, of 2473 patients of various complementary practitioners, giving the main problems that the patients reported.[2]

Looking at the main diagnostic areas it is obvious that the majority of patients arrive with musculoskeletal problems. In the UK these problems are the major causes of physical impairment, with 26 per cent of the population reporting long-term musculoskeletal problems.[4] Two million people go to their GP complaining of back pain every year. It seems as if complementary practitioners take on a very large number of the chronic and potentially crippling musculoskeletal cases that conventional medicine, by its own admission, is poorly equipped to help. Of the other conditions seen, headaches and migraines are common and the rest fall into the groups of chronic medically intractable conditions discussed earlier.

Though these surveys seem straightforward, they contain major uncertainties that themselves illustrate the alternative nature of complementary consultations.

Table 2.1 Health problems presented to complementary practitioners (%)

Sheffield study		*Australian study*	
Musculoskeletal	78.2	Aches, strains, in back, limbs	42
Neurological	5.6	Neuralgia, sciatica	11
Psychological	4.6	Postural and joint problems	10
General, including checkup	3.7	Migraines, headaches	8
Respiratory	1.9	Respiratory, digestive	7
Urogenital, obstetric	1.7	Muscular problems	5
Digestive	1.6	Arthritis, bone problems	5
Skin	0.9	Nervous and mental disorders	2
Metabolic	0.9	Skin conditions	1
Circulation	0.6	Others	9
Others	0.3		

For patients arrive complaining of a set of symptoms, not just one, and the one recorded here may not be medically the most significant. Nor can the therapist be relied upon to define the health problem as a known medical diagnostic condition. For example, according to complementary medicine, most health problems have a psychosomatic basis, so very few problems are reported as purely psychosomatic, giving an underestimate of this category. Moreover these studies polled only the established complementary professions in the UK, which are dominated by osteopaths and chiropractors, so exaggerating the extent of musculoskeletal problems. A poll of healers or reflexologists might give rather different results, again emphasizing the mind – body dimension. The picture also looks a bit different if one asks patients for what health problems they use all of complementary medicine, including remedies that they bought and folk medicine, rather than just professional consultations. This was done in the recent US study which ascertained that 52 per cent of the problems that people brought to therapists were musculoskeletal, whereas they were only 37 per cent of the problems that they sought treatment with all complementary methods, including alternative self-care. Instead, 33 per cent reported using alternative methods for insomnia, anxiety, and depression and 13 per cent for headache.[7]

The Australian Study also addressed the issue of how diseases were distributed among the different kinds of practitioner.[20] Table 2.2 confirms the preponderance of chronic musculoskeletal problems, and that these are mostly treated by the chiropractors. Acupuncturists see a much wider spread of conditions, similar to that seen in general practice, but again, more chronic in nature. This evidence confirms the position of chiropractic as more of a supplement to conventional medicine, seeing a limited range of health problems, while acupuncture and naturopathy are more of a substitute. Doctors see far fewer musculoskeletal

Table 2.2   Distribution of patients' diseases among complementary Practitioners in Australia 1977 (%)[12]

Diagnostic classification	Therapy			General practice
	Chiropractic	Naturopathy	Acupuncture	
Respiratory	3	8	8	26
Musculoskeletal	77	47	31	10
Cardiovascular	1	–	2	11
Genito-urinary	1	–	4	5
Central nervous system	12	16	11	12
Gastro-intestinal	1	5	4	5
Psychological	1	11	19	2
Other	4	13	21	29

patients but several times as many patients with respiratory problems than therapists, reflecting the fact that these infections—particularly bronchitis, pneumonia, influenza, and tuberculosis—are still very much a medical preserve. Naturopaths and acupuncturists take several times as many patients with psychologically based problems than either doctors or chiropractors. This indicates, perhaps, a growing realization of the psychogenic component of illness, and a desire to seek treatment involving both mind and body.

Complementary medicine is thus gradually moving into those areas, particularly chronic musculoskeletal, psychosomatic, neurological, digestive, and preventive areas, where modern medicine is weak. This is clearly the beginning of a differentiation of roles of therapist and doctor according to the strengths of each system. This process can only continue in the future as complementary medicine works more and more closely with modern medicine. However it will not be easy. For different professions will no doubt fight over therapeutic territories. For example, after a long struggle, modern medicine has conceded back problems to the chiropractors providing they agree to remain within that therapeutic boundary. The major traditional medical systems of naturopathy, Oriental medicine, herbalism, and homeopathy will continue to state their claim to be full alternatives, able to be first-call therapists treating the whole person whatever his symptoms. The public is unfortunately caught in the middle of this conflict, and finds it very hard at the present time to know to which therapy or medical system to go to for which problem. They are, in a sense, caught between the two systems. However this may well be because of the relative immaturity of complementary medicine in the modern world. As time goes by, one might expect the public to be better informed on what can do what. It would be a return to a cultural knowledge of how to use the competing skills on offer that used to be there in history, and may well be a sign of the coming of age of complementary medicine.

Patient satisfaction with complementary and conventional medicine

It would be interesting to obtain some indication of patients' opinions of their treatment by various kinds of practitioners. This would take account of the patient as medical consumer, a point of view rapidly gaining in importance today. Naturally, patient reports are subjective interpretations, not objective evaluations on outcomes or on the quality of health care. Research on outcomes is just beginning, and is discussed elsewhere in this book. Here we look at the patients' experience, an evaluation that should be given no less prominence than evaluation by detached professionals, but which has been sadly lacking until recently. There are indications of an awakening of interest in the subjective experience of medicine, and new research tools such as SF 36 (Short Form 36, a validated questionnaire on patient satisfaction) are beginning to be used, but results using this research tool have not been published to date.

According to a random poll of nearly 2000 members of the UK Consumers

Association who had been to a complementary practitioner, 82 per cent said they were cured or improved, and 74 per cent would use the same method again.[21] Most had been to a GP previously for the same problem, and 81 per cent of these said that they were dissatisfied with conventional medicine because it could not help them. A similar result emerged from the more sophisticated Australian studies, which found that 93 per cent of those using complementary therapy stated that they were satisfied with their current treatment.[12] Of those who had switched from medical practitioners, only 8 per cent were very satisfied with the treatment they had previously received, while of those who had switched from a different complementary practitioner, 51 per cent were very satisfied with the treatment they had previously received.

A recent study examined the use of complementary medicine by 415 cancer patients who were receiving medical treatment. Sixteen per cent of them also made use of complementary medicine. Four out of five of those who used complementary medicine stated that they were satisfied or very satisfied with the treatment they were getting, even if it did not amount to a cure of the disease. There were distinct psychological benefits. They felt calmer and emotionally stronger, and they felt more optimistic and hopeful about the future. Physically, there were also benefits including more strength and energy, less nausea and easier breathing. These patients were using conventional medicine as well, with which they were also satisfied, although they complained that it left them in a no-hope situation.[22]

It is somewhat misleading to compare the degree of satisfaction that patients experience with conventional and complementary therapists by asking only those patients who had been converted to complementary medicine. Naturally, they give overwhelming support to their current therapy. In fact, when the University of Queensland team compared the satisfaction of patients seeing complementary therapists with that of patients seeing medical practitioners, they were both equally satisfied with their current practitioner, even though many more of the doctors' patients had reservations about the treatment. Those people who were not happy with their complementary practitioner were found to be uncured, but unharmed, while those dissatisfied with their doctor were not necessarily unharmed.[12] It is at least possible to conclude that although all patients have a strong loyalty to their current practitioner, complementary therapy patients are generally more satisfied with their overall treatment than doctors' patients.

Does this satisfaction with treatment stand the test of time? The Australian team evaluated the response of patients both straight after their treatment and 10 weeks later. Eighty-eight per cent still experienced improvement after 10 weeks, which not only indicates a high degree of improvement, but that the therapists' treatments are also long term, although it should be pointed out that the less chronic cases might have returned to health during this period whether or not they saw a practitioner.[12] Also, the satisfaction depends on expectations. A recent study of osteopathic patients found that their degree of expectation from treatment was so high that after 4 months the improvement was not as great as expected.[23] This ought to strike a warning note to complementary medicine not to get too excited about its successes so as not to unduly raise patient expectations. In any event, such research does suggest that patients are pleased with complementary therapists because of their actual results, not simply because they enjoyed the treatment.

In a recent study, Professor Furnham pointed out that satisfaction is also a belief in competence, and so subject to all kinds of influence such as advertising and the media. One cannot then ask about such perceptions in general, as people feel differently about the treatability of different health problems. When asked about competence, patients of complementary practitioners rated them more competent than GPs to deal with symptoms such as allergies, anxiety, musculoskeletal problems, colds, headaches, insomnia, menstrual problems, and migraine. However there were some more serious conditions for which even those consulting complementary practitioners would first consult a GP, including cancer, angina, kidney problems, and pneumonia.[13]

The Dutch study also related the types of complaints that people had experienced and their view of the success of their treatment. The results are given in Table 2.3. Like other studies before this the major symptoms reported particularly by the complementary therapy patients, were musculoskeletal, tiredness, non-specific sickness, pain, tension/depression, and insomnia. There were only minor differences between the complementary practitioners and the specialist. For example, the complementary practitioner was better than the specialist in relieving insomnia, dizziness/fainting, and shortness of breath, while the specialist did better in relieving poor vision and hearing.[9] One could conclude that complementary patients feel at least as successfully treated as patients of medical specialists, if not more so, but it depends on the health problem. This is important because the delineation of therapeutic boundaries between modern medicine and therapies depend on the perceptions of consumers about what conditions are more successfully treated by each system.

This raises the important question whether patients are so satisfied with their complementary treatment that they abandon their conventional doctor. According to the above studies, one might surmise that patients would by and large not abandon conventional medicine, but rather pick and choose depending on their health problem. This is indeed what is found. In Australia the government-sponsored survey found that 33 per cent of all complementary patients would not use conventional medicine. These patients stated that they would go to a complementary therapist first for any kind of symptom, including cancer, chest pain, internal bleeding, or influenza. This group tended to be young, female, and health conscious and saw complementary medicine as a true alternative primary health care system. However, the majority still appear not to be so converted, but to be attempting to get the best of both systems.[24]

Similar results emerged from a recent UK study: one third of complementary medicine patients will have come there first, one half will have received conventional medicine for the main complaint and then switched, and the remaining 15 per cent will be receiving both concurrently.[2] The dual use is still not easy for the patient to handle. The majority of cancer patients who are receiving

Table 2.3 *Comparison of the success rate in the treatment of symptoms by complementary practitioners and medical specialists in the Netherlands, 1980*[2]

Symptom	Patients of complementary practitioner		Patients of medical specialist	
	% reporting symptom	% improved	% reporting symptom	% improved
Palpitations	19	12	17	10
Stiffness	39	26	24	13
Feeling very ill	36	27	27	21
Itching or burning sensation	14	10	10	5
Tiredness and lethargy	57	40	47	28
Fever	7	6	9	9
Pain	64	45	55	32
Tension and depression	48	33	43	28
Coughing and chestiness	17	13	14	7
Blood loss	3	3	10	10
Tingling, numbness	27	16	20	8
Shortness of breath	26	20	19	10
Nausea and vomiting	14	10	12	8
Diarrhoea and constipation	12	8	10	5
Poor vision and hearing	13	4	19	9
Paralysis	5	4	3	2
Insomnia	40	23	31	14
Dizziness and fainting	20	16	17	9
Anxiety	26	17	28	18
Rash	12	7	8	4
Emotional instability	16	9	16	10
Sexual problems	7	4	7	4
Other	12	9	9	5

complementary medicine concurrently, cannot bring themselves to tell their doctor.[22] In the United States the climate seems more polarized, since only 4 per cent of those seeing providers of non-orthodox healthcare were seeing doctors concurrently, and here too, most people using therapies did not tell their doctor.[7] In other words patients today generally pick and choose their medical system according to their current needs, without burning their boats, and without strong loyalties or beliefs. Medical and complementary professionals may be irked by this apparent public capriciousness. However it surely is the expected pattern of pluralistic use in a consumer-oriented society. Indeed, medical professionals with a caring attitude might encourage this experimentation and learning so as to reveal the true benefit of the therapies. Only time will tell whether this shopping around represents an end-point, or a transitional moment, catching in mid-stream a major shift in healthcare systems.

In either case, if complementary therapies are indeed being used as complements rather than substitutes it augurs well for both systems. The individuals concerned are ceasing to be mindless consumers of drugs and services, becoming more discriminating and aware in their choices. They are also bringing their new options back home to their family physicians, and contributing to an awareness among doctors of the existence and potential of natural therapies. It is the patients, rather than organized lobbies, who will bring about the co-existence and mutual respect between the various medical systems which is as obvious as it is inevitable. It is the patients who are breaking down the walls around medical fiefdoms, and the professionals, both conventional and complementary, are peeping a little nervously through the gaps.

It is a welcome wind of change, that also sweeps away some excessive professional pride that is the ever-present shadow of doctors and therapists. Indeed professionals and academics are finding it hard to keep on top of the game; they constantly wake up to find it has already moved on somewhere else. One of the many reasons for this is that the consultation with a practitioner or doctor is the end result of a long inner dialogue between the person and his or her health problem. Included in this dialogue, consciously or unconsciously, may be the extent of his own competence to cope with the situation, his beliefs about the causes and prognoses, his fears, knowledge, freedoms, views, habits, rituals etc. The issue of to whom he would most entrust his body-mind is only one of the considerations. Even in the case of alternative medicine as such, much of the healing work is also out of the hands of professionals, and in the realm of self-help groups, counselling, spiritual movements, religious circles, family and folk traditions, and the health shops. Seventy-five per cent of health problems are never seen by a professional, but are dealt with by self-care (63 per cent) or doing nothing at all.[25] This is somewhat patronizingly called 'the Hidden Healthcare System'; it is only hidden because inadequate objective research methods fail to approach the subjective world from which healthcare choices emerge. For this reason, the patterns of consultations described in this chapter are the tip of the iceberg. The rest is a powerful and unpredictable force for change.

References

1. Vickers, A. (1994). Use of complementary medicine. *British Medical Journal*, **390**, 1161.
2. Thomas, K. J., Carr, J., Westlake, L., and Williams, B. T. (1991). Use of non-orthodox and conventional health care in Great Britain. *British Medical Journal*, **302**, 207–9.
3. The Consumers Association (1992). Alternative medicine. *Which?* November 1992, 45–9.
4. Department of Health (1992). *Compendium of health statistics*. HMSO, London.

5. Fisher, P. and Ward, A. (1994). Complementary medicine in Europe. *British Medical Journal*, **309**, 107–11.
6. Menges, L. J. (1994). Regular and alternative medicine: the state of affairs in the Netherlands. *Social Science and Medicine*, **39**, 871–3.
7. Eisenberg, D., Kessler, R., Foster, C., Norlock, F., Calkins, D., and Delbanco, T. (1993). Unconventional medicine in the United States. *New England Journal of Medicine*, **328**, 246–52.
8. Research Surveys of Great Britain Ltd. (1984). Survey reported in *Journal of Alternative Medicine* (July 1984). Taylor Nelson Ltd (1985). *The monitor programme*. Epsom, Surrey.
9. Oojendijk, W. T. M., Mackenbach, J. P., and Limberger, H. H. B. (1980). *What is better? An investigation into the use of, and satisfaction with, complementary and official medicine in The Netherlands*. The Netherlands Institute of Preventive Medicine and the Technical Industrial Organization. The survey took place at the beginning of 1980 among 3782 Dutchmen aged 18 and over; 300 people were followed-up later.
10. Sharma, U. (1995). *Complementary medicine today: practitioners and patients*. Tavistock/ Routledge, London.
11. Cassidy, C. (1994). Social Science theory and methods in the study of alternative and complementary medicine. *Journal of Alternative and Complementary Medicine (US)*, **1**, 19–40.
12. This is the third study of a series of four carried out by Professor Western, Professor of Sociology at the University of Queensland, and his colleagues. A total of 484 patients derived from complementary practitioners in Perth, Brisbane, and Melbourne were interviewed at length. The study forms Appendix 8 of the *Report of the Committee of Inquiry into Chiropractic, Osteopathy, Homeopathy and Naturopathy*, Parliamentary Paper No. 102 (1977). Its title is: Current patients of alternative health care—A three city study, by Boven, R., Lupton, G., Najman, J., Payne, S., Sheehan, M., and Western, J.
13. Furnham, A. and Forey, J. (1994). The attitudes, behaviours and beliefs of patients of conventional vs complementary (alternative) medicine. *Journal of Clinical Psychology* **50**, 458–62.
14. Yesalis, C. E., Wallace, R. B., Fisher, W. P., and Tokheim, R. (1980). Does chiropratic utilisation substitute for less available medical services? *American Journal of Public Health*, **70**, 415–17.
15. Hewitt, O. and Wood, P. H. N. (1975). Heterodox practitioners and the availability of specialist advice. *Rheumatology and Rehabilitation*, **14**, 191–9.
16. Furnham, A. and Smith, C. (1988). Choosing alternative medicine: a comparison of the beliefs of patients visiting a General Practitioner and a homeopath. *Social science and medicine*, **26**, 685–9.
17. Capra, F. (1982). *The turning point: science, society and the rising culture*. Bantam, New York.
18. *Daily Telegraph*, 6 April 1993.
19. Fulder, S. J. and Monro, R. (1985). Complementary medicine in the United Kingdom: Patients, practitioners and consultations. *Lancet*, **2**, 542–5.
20. Boven, R., Genn, C., Lupton, G., Payne, S., Sheehan, M., and Western J. (1977). *New patients to alternative care*. Western Report No. 1 published as Appendix 6 to the Report of the Committee of Inquiry on Chiropractic, Osteopathy, Homeopathy and Naturopathy, Parliamentary Paper No. 102 (1977). This study concentrates on questionnaires sent out to new patients.
21. The Consumers Association (1986). Magic or medicine? *Which?* October, 1986, 443–7.

22. Downer, S. M., Cody, M. M., McCluskey, P., Wilson, P. D., Arnott, S. J., Lister, T. A., and Slevin, M. L. (1994). Pursuit and practice of complementary therapies by cancer patients receiving conventional treatment. *British Medical Journal*, **309**, 86–9.
23. Pringle, M. and Tyreman, S. (1993). Study of 500 patients attending an osteopathic practice. *British Journal of General Practice*, **43**, 15–18.
24. Parker, G. and Tupling, H. (1977). *Consumer evaluation of natural therapies*. Parker Report No. 2, Appendix 11 of the Report of the Committee of Inquiry into Chiropractic, Osteopathy, Homeopathy and Naturopathy. Australian Government Publishers. The survey was based on 144 completed questionnaires from complementary therapy patients.
25. Helman, C. G. (1987). General practice and the hidden health care system. *Journal of the Royal Society of Medicine*, **80**, 738–40.

3

The therapist

Who are the therapists?

The public image of a complementary practitioner has been at a nadir for over a century. However, there has been a considerable change in recent years. The public is now more ready to see therapists as true professionals. The therapists themselves, especially if recently qualified, are more confident, more forthcoming, and more politically and socially active in the furtherance of their profession. It is my impression that their older colleagues are somewhat exhausted after the years of struggle with mainstream medicine, and tend today to retire from the arena to devote themselves instead to practice and teaching. Complementary practitioners are mostly male, a disappointing fact to many who hoped that the new broom would sweep away the old inequitable social distinctions.

About 20 years ago, a survey of UK osteopaths put their average age at 37 years. They had been in practice for an average of 13 years.[1] Today, as the therapies are growing so rapidly, these therapists' average time in practice would be less than 10 years.[2] The characteristics of therapists would seem to be similar to those of any other set of healthcare professionals although they might tend to come from more diverse backgrounds than the average professional, who tends to come from a middle-class home. No less than 80 per cent of Australian therapists have had previous occupations of one kind or another.[3] One can understand why, for the profession of complementary practitioner is marginal, holding an uncertain status. Entrants are usually motivated more by the calling itself than by any of the ancillary social benefits that may result. A study of the motivation that draws people to study and work in the therapies found that 'there was a high level of expressed interest in people, a satisfaction in treating patients as individual persons, and in seeing them healed and well'.[2] Along with this there was a desire for independence and autonomy, for work outside hierarchical and institutional structures. These motives mirror those of patients who also turn to alternative therapies seeking for more conviction and autonomy, to be seen as 'a whole person'. This is quite different from the motives that draw young people to become doctors, for entrance to medical school, by contrast, usually occurs immediately after completion of secondary education, at an age when social and parental pressures are still determining factors on careers, and status is an important goal.

Numbers of therapists practising in the UK

In 1981 the Threshold Survey made a serious attempt to estimate the total number of therapists in the UK.[4] All organizations representing or training complementary practitioners were contacted. Steps were taken to weed out therapists appearing on more than one register and those retired, honorary, or abroad. The figures are given in column 1 of Table 3.1. In addition many therapists chose not to join professional bodies, and there are always some who are untrained or very part-time. Their numbers were obtained by combining rough estimates from the various organizations, and they are added to those in professional bodies to give a total number of UK therapists in column 2.

Today there is little concrete information on the numbers of therapists practising in the UK. The Research Council for Complementary Medicine and the BMA committee studying complementary medicine both made an informal attempt to log numbers of therapists in professional bodies in 1993, but as they only included certain professional bodies, their numbers are underestimated by at least 50 per cent. The author carried out a rough survey in 1995 by contacting all the main organizations and umbrella bodies. The figures are given in column 3. They include both members of the main professional bodies, medically qualified and lay, and an estimate of those in practice who do not belong to professional bodies. Because of rapid professionalization, it can be safely assumed that today far fewer therapists practise outside professional bodies than in 1981.

There are about 50 000 alternative practitioners in the UK, including a very large number of healers and manual therapists, which is around 60 per cent more than the number of GPs. There are around 8000 professional therapists who practise the main therapeutic modalities of complementary medicine: acupuncture, osteopathy, etc. These could be regarded as primary care practitioners who, in market terms, compete with GPs, and sometimes with medical specialists. They are about one third the number of GPs.

The 1981 Threshold Survey found that over 2000 doctors, or 8 per cent of the number of GPs belonged to complementary medical professional bodies. This figure seems to be underestimated, however, as three studies between 1986 and 1988 reported that from 16 to 38 per cent of GPs in different areas of the UK and New Zealand practised some kind of complementary medicine[6-8]. There are certain to be more medical doctors doing so today, but the numbers are not known. These GPs, however many there are, play an highly important role in the spread of complementary medical services, providing it with legitimacy, though, as we have seen, at the cost of dilution.

There is a very large number of healers in the UK. Every country seems to have

Table 3.1   Complementary practitioners in the UK

Therapy	Nos. in professional bodies (1981)	Estimated total (1981)	Estimated total (1995)
Acupuncture	708	958	3000
Alexander Technique	175	225	850
Chiropractic	157	357	900
Hakims, Chinese doctors	40	80	100
Healers	6300	19 300	20 000?
Herbalists	238	438	600
Homeopaths	461	696	1200
Hypnotherapists	1507	1670	?
Manual therapies	1650	4000	20 000?
Creative therapies	815	905	?
Naturopathy	210	400	750
Osteopathy	989	1139	3039
Radionics	119	219	219
Total	13 369	30 137	Approx. 50 000

Notes.

* All columns include both medically qualified and lay complementary practitioners.
* Manual therapists excludes beauty therapists, and includes massage therapists, aromatherapists, reflexologists, practitioners of Applied Kinesiology, Polarity therapists, etc. The current figure in column 3 is very rough. It is obtained from the membership of the British Complementary Medicine Association (includes massage therapists, reflexologists, aromatherapists, miscellaneous physical therapists and some healers) which now stands at 22 000. In addition, massage therapists who are affiliated to the Independent Therapists Examining Council (ITEC) stands at around 10 000. This gives a total of 32 000 from which healers have to be subtracted.
* There are 11 000 healers associated with the Confederation of Healing Organizations (CHO) and another 3500 church-connected healers, associated with the Spiritualist National Union (SNU), plus others. The estimate of 20 000 today is rough, but likely to be more accurate than the estimate of 1981 which is an over-estimate.
* Other therapies may not have been specifically included, but are incorporated into these categories, such as iridology into naturopathy.
* Osteopathy figures are based on reference.[5] The figures for acupuncturists, Alexander teachers, chiropractors, herbalists, homeopaths, naturopaths, osteopaths, and radionics practitioners are based on figures the author obtained from organizations in July 1995. They are reasonably accurate.

its favourite therapies; for Germany it is Heilpraktikers (who use homeopathy and naturopathy) and anthroposophical therapists, for Switzerland herbalists, for France homeopaths, so for England it is spiritual healers. This is a tradition that goes back into history, some say to the time of the Hyperboreans who were said to come from the British Isles! Healing organizations in the field guess there may be around 20 000 healers, including healing circles in churches. The largest complementary profession in the UK is osteopathy, which has always been regarded as the most senior and respected of the therapies. It now has more than 3000 practitioners. However acupuncture is rapidly catching up and is now in close second place.

Numbers of therapists have been increasing rapidly. The annual trends in numbers of practising UK therapists were calculated from membership organizations for 1978–81 and show an average increase of 11 per cent per year.[4] This is nearly six times the annual increase in the total number of UK general practitioners. The growth since 1981 until today has continued at more or less the same rate, increasing from two and a half to three and a half times since then, or between 8 to 10 per cent annually. (The uncertainty arises because of changes in the proportion of therapists within and without professional bodies since 1981.) The numbers of osteopaths, according to good evidence, is increasing currently at around 10 per cent a year.[5]

The cost of complementary medicine

A Consumers Association survey in 1992 found that an initial diagnosis and consultation with an osteopath, chiropractor, herbalist, homeopath, or acupuncturist is likely to cost £30, with subsequent consultations costing £15–20.[9] These fees are less than those of a medical specialist and roughly equivalent to the total cost per consultation of providing general practitioner services (including drugs). If we assume that 33–45 million complementary consultations are given annually (excluding healers – see Chapter 2) then £825–1125 million are spent annually on consulting complementary practitioners. With the UK herbal market alone now at £100 million,[10] the additional cost of vitamins, supplements, herbs, X-rays, and mechanical aids could bring the figure to roughly £1250 million per year. This is equivalent to only 2 per cent of the total health services bill, despite serving some 16 million people annually.

Europeans as a whole spent over £1200 million on complementary medicine in 1986, 60 per cent of which was for consultations and physical therapies and the rest for remedies and supplements.[11] It could be at least £3 billion today. In the United States there is a comparable total cost on a population basis of some $13.7 billion in 1990, which is actually more than the total spent by the US population on all hospitalizations in that year.[12]

How many patients do therapists see?

The demand for therapists is an indication of the popularity of the practices, the popularity of the practitioners, and the room for future expansion. The Threshold Survey's statistics are given in Table 3.2 together with those from the University of Queensland alternative practitioner study.[3,4] In the UK, a surprising number of practitioners, 16 per cent, saw hardly any patients. This reflects a large group of part-time therapists who obtain their livelihood by other means. In the UK, more than half the total consultations are accounted for by less than a quarter of the practitioners. Chiropractors and osteopaths see the greatest number of

Table 3.2   Numbers of patients seen by complementary practitioners per week in the UK[4] and Australia[3]

No of patients seen	UK practitioners (%)	No of patients seen	Australian practitioners (%)
<5	16	<20	22
6–20	24	21–60	38
21–50	31	61–100	16
51–100	19	101–200	14
101–200	10	<201	1
>201	0		

patients. This is both because treatment takes less time than other therapies and because the therapists themselves tend to be more organized. Acupuncture and naturopathy follow, then hypnotherapy, and finally, healing. Many healers see very few clients. The average number of weekly consultations overall was 43 in 1981. A more recent study based on 1987 data found a very similar average workload of 44 patients/week.[13] This is between one third and one half of that of GPs, who see 21 patients per day.

The consultation

At a first consultation with a complementary practitioner, the patient will usually be required to give a full personal history. The practitioner will go much deeper than symptoms, trying to decode the origin of disease from the cipher of constitution, vulnerabilities, energetic conditions, psychological disposition, and lifestyle. The diagnosis also generally involves non-invasive and subtle reading of the signs of internal function projected onto the exterior, for example patterns of colour, heat, and pulses on the outside of the body in Oriental medicine; the feel and tone of muscles, joints, and ligaments in osteopathy; the texture of skin and appearance of irises and nails in naturopathy, etc. Laboratory tests are sometimes ordered by herbalists and modern naturopaths.

First consultations in traditional acupuncture and homeopathy can take up to two hours. The Threshold Survey found that most first consultations take between 30 and 60 minutes and average time for all consultations is 36 minutes. This is six times that of a GP. We need look no further for one of the reasons for the popularity of complementary medicine. Although it is not just a question of time, as is often erroneously portrayed. It is also a question of what happens in this time, and new patients who arrive at complementary practitioners mostly get a pleasant shock at the depth to which the therapists investigate their individual selves, and the real origins of their condition. Although GPs rightly claim that they are too overworked to give sufficient time to patients, *if doctors were given 36 minutes per patient per visit would they know what to do with it?* Because a complementary practitioner sees one-third to one-half of the number of patients as a GP, but for six times as long, he or she may have, on average, two to three times as much total patient contact as a GP. Even allowing for the house calls and administrative duties of the latter, we can conclude that complementary practitioners are as busy as GPs and that demand is still outstripping supply.

The once-only visit to a complementary practitioner is a rarity. The practitioner is involved in a programme which with the active participation of the patient, will steer him to a state of maximal health. Often the patient will be suffering from chronic or deeply rooted conditions which require lengthy management and gradual change to life habits. Generally, acute cases need a linked series of 3–4 visits, chronic cases 10–12. Some healers, hypnotherapists, and radionicists gave up to and over 30 treatments in a course: the average was 9.7 overall.[4] The Dutch study found that an average patient made 7.5 visits to his complementary practitioner per year.[14]

Clinics, health centres, and hospitals

Many professional therapists practise from private houses, with simple treatment rooms that would remind one of a family doctor with a small practice, minus receptionist. In fact, it would be quite difficult to tell therapists apart, were it not for their equipment. Osteopaths have a padded raised table and simple medical diagnostic instruments; chiropractors usually have a much more complex hinged, spring-loaded table, and sometimes an X-ray room; herbalists their tinctures and bottles; naturopaths their charts; homeopaths their bottles of little pills, repertoire books, and a nearby computer; and acupuncturists, packets of sterilized needles and perhaps electro-acupuncture apparatus.

There is a growing trend for therapists to share their treatment facilities rather than work in isolation. Two or more therapists of the same or different disciplines may work together in a shared clinic at which they are likely to be able to employ a secretary and provide a more efficient service. At least half of all therapists now work in a group practice of this kind.[4] It is worth remembering that complementary therapists do not have any general administrative infrastructure to channel patients to them and their code of ethics does not permit advertising more than their name in the Yellow Pages or local newspapers. So they are, like GPs, dependent on patients' recommendation. When therapists pool resources their influence increases. For example, an acupuncture clinic at Farmoor near Oxford existed for a number of years, building up sufficient clientele to be able to support no less than nine acupuncturists. The existence of this centre was instrumental in the growth of an awareness of acupuncture itself throughout Oxfordshire.

A growing number of therapists feel that a shared clinic is only a prelude to a much more powerful establishment: the natural or holistic health care centre. The Nature Cure Clinic or the Hale Clinic in London are perhaps the best known examples of this kind of polyclinic, but there are now many dotted throughout the country. Such a centre (which under a legal ruling cannot be called a 'health centre' to avoid confusion with NHS health centres) employs the services of several therapists practising different disciplines. There are sometimes classes in yoga, relaxation, diet, or other self-care methods. It is an attractive arrangement to both therapist and patient as it can deal with a wider range of problems more effectively. For example, acupuncturists and osteopaths both treat a large number of back pain cases. However, while the osteopath can provide relief and the opportunity for repair of the physical frame, the acupuncturist can deal with underlying metabolic or energetic disturbances. A mixed treatment of this kind is better than the sum of its parts. For the patient, this kind of centre is a boon. It drastically reduces the confusing search for the right therapist for a specific health problem, which understandably discourages so many potential patients. The patient can instead put himself in the hands of a group of natural therapists whose skills complement each other, enabling them to guide the patient to the most appropriate therapy for his condition. Though it is very attractive in theory, in practise the actual degree to which therapists of different kinds can work together to shunt patients intelligently to different therapies sometimes falls far short of their dreams. For it is no easy matter to decide which therapy would be best for which condition, at least without a substantial prior diagnosis. And anyway, it is often not a particular therapy that is suitable for a patient but a particular therapist, irrespective of his or her basket of techniques. There is also the inevitable question of power relations and personalities within centres, and the time and effort needed to discuss and co-operate on cases. Therefore despite the best intentions such centres sometimes end up doing little more than renting space to different therapists that come and go.

A centre that is solely a group practice of professionals is still to some extent a sickness centre. A health centre that is true to its name should play a preventive, health-promoting role in the community, and there are a growing number that do this. Like the US Holistic Health Centres, these places become a focus where workshops and classes are held on relaxation, diet, yoga, T'ai-chi, natural childbirth, and other self-care techniques. To this may be added the more consciously social goal of the spread of natural health attitudes among the public. Examples include the Wellbeing Centre in Cornwall and the Bristol Natural Health Centre.

There is as yet not a great deal to offer in the way of natural therapy hospitals or residential clinics. This is a sad state of affairs, for many people with chronic conditions, such as high blood pressure, could be substantially cured by intensive residential natural treatment combined with a drastic alteration in their lifestyle. The best-known and most successful natural hospital is the Tyringham Clinic near Newport Pagnell in Buckinghamshire, set up as a charity in the mid-1960s. When someone books in to this stately manor house, he or she is seen by a multidisciplinary consultant and therapies are assigned according to individual need. A large number of therapies are available and careful attention is given to a patient's diet. The Kingston Clinic in Edinburgh is noted for its purificatory procedures and emphasis on nature cure. Other clinics include Shrubland Hall in Ipswich, Enton Hall in Godalming, and Grayshott Hall in Hindhead. A new natural health hospital is planned in Devon, the Ottery St Mary's Hospital, to be run both by doctors with experience in complementary medicine and therapists. Besides complementary medicine, there will be health instruction and counselling, i.e. it will be a 'Teaching Hospital' in a new sense of the word—to teach patients not medical students. There are, also, of course, health resorts too, the best-known being Champneys at Tring. Here relatively healthy people can clean out the residues of their indulgences in an amenable but expensive environment.

The training of complementary practitioners

There are basically two ways to learn the healing arts. At one extreme is the apprenticeship in which a student learns his skills through a gradual process of osmosis from long periods of working with accomplished therapists. At the other extreme is the highly formal and standardized training, as in modern medicine today. At one time complementary therapies, such as traditional medicine, were all taught by apprenticeship. Private instruction by charismatic and innovative teachers was how acupuncture arrived in the West, homeopathy was taught to lay people, and chiropractic and osteopathy were initiated by Palmer and Stills. The knowledge was passed down as a semisecret art from master to disciples, whose entrance requirements were aptitude, enthusiasm, and endurance. Under these circumstances, there was every opportunity to be very good or very bad. Such experiential training is still the main method for the intuitional healing arts which involve special sensitivities, for example healing, radionics, Alexander Technique, or reflexology. However for the main therapeutic systems, the last 30 years saw the establishment of small formal colleges which varied widely in quality of training, depending on the competence and ability of their founders. They often taught different interpretations of each therapy, fragmenting the knowledge and preserving the fragments with professional rivalries. Attempts in the past to set up common standards were fruitless, and possibly unnecessary as therapists could practise anyway under common law. There was no chance of formal recognition, and the medical profession successfully marginalized complementary medicine. Therapists therefore arrived at the end of the 1980s as a mixture of the highly competent and less competent, highly trained and untrained, and with widely differing interpretations of each therapeutic modality.

Today, as we have seen, the new position of government and the medical institutions, characterized by the 1993 BMA report, concentrates on accreditation and standards, not on scientific verification. The response of the therapies has generally been a scramble towards professionalization and establishment of standards of education and training. For example, the lay homeopaths who used to regard themselves as a radical populist health alternative, now teach a previously unthinkable content of anatomy, physiology, and modern biomedical subjects. Therapists who are so trained and join the official registers, now attempt to distance themselves from untrained and non-professional lay therapists who can still practise under common law. All the therapies are attempting to close the profession by agreeing minimum educational standards and the permitted courses by which they are obtained. Different schools with previously conflicting and antagonistic interpretations of what constitutes acupuncture, osteopathy, or chiropractic have been going through a painful process of dialogue in order to set common standards of what it means to be an acupuncturist, osteopath, or chiropractor. Interestingly, they have unwittingly followed the track of modern medicine, which began to be taught by apprenticeship, continued during the early part of the last century with different colleges of widely varying standards and conflicting approaches, and ended up today at the other extreme: precisely delineated teaching sequences, producing similarly trained practitioners, of reasonable competence and deep-seated conservatism.

Undoubtedly this process weeds out the grossly incompetent and untrained, and protects the public to a degree. But insofar as it is intended to defend the profession rather than the patient, it bears a serious cost. There are indeed dissenters within the complementary movement who are deeply worried about the trend. There is an obvious loss of educational freedom to teach novel, derivative, or indeed ancient forms that are outside the standard syllabuses. For example the chiropractors have accepted a standardized education and a greatly reduced therapeutic role, much like opticians, in return for increased status for their profession. Besides, to use education as a test of acceptability produces a subtle shift in the way a therapist is judged by society at large. Instead of being judged by results, as in the pre-professional era, a therapist will be judged on qualifications. The fluid world of alternative medicine requires great flexibility and authenticity in matters of training and assessment. Otherwise the very strengths of these systems—their adaptive and unconventional healing strategies—will be crushed. Then alternatives to the alternatives will be needed and will no doubt arise. Admittedly, there is no substitute for therapists who are selected as to ability, who are carefully and intensively trained, and who have built up a resource of experience, sensitivity, and understanding. Even spiritual healing can be, and is, taught so that healers learn to amplify their energy and channel it into the required therapeutic form. However, training should be true to the unfathomable and ancient wellspring of knowledge and experience from which modern complementary medicine draws its skills.

The current state of therapists' education

The author's first contact with a complementary therapy college was in 1970 as a young student seeking cheap osteopathic treatment. The college used a large and rather gloomy Victorian house. The secretary who made the appointments also seemed to rule the entire establishment, from a glass partitioned office on the ground floor. Nearby were classrooms with ancient books in glass-fronted cases, old wooden desks, and a skeleton or two dangling quietly in the corners. Apart from the secretary, the place had a rather lethargic air, with an occasional student in a crisp white jacket calling patients for treatment. The course there was a full-time, four-year course, which students might enter straight after school, with certain minimum O- and A-level entrance requirements. The students were mostly in their late-teens or early-twenties. They gave a pleasing impression of devotion and dedication to their therapy. But they were a world on their own with a private therapeutic tradition; an interpretation of the respected founding fathers. My concerns about the relationship between their method and other complementary and conventional techniques, including drugs, for my problem, were met with vague and defensive answers. The hidden message was: if you want to be treated by us, believe as we believe.

It turned out that this first impression was rather typical of the full-time colleges at the time. They were autonomous, inward-looking, idiosyncratic, and sometimes slack. However they compensated by being authentic and true to their tradition, and provided a fascinating alternative world view to students. Today the courses are of similar length, the buildings may be the same, but everything else has changed. Chiropractic, now state registered, is mostly taught in a modern college, the Anglo-European College of Chiropractic, with a medical-school type course, leading to a 4-year B.Sc. Honours degree in Human Sciences (Chiropractic), awarded by the University of Portsmouth. To join the register and practise as a licensed chiropractor, students need to complete a fifth postgraduate year, and do a further year of supervised clinical practice. There is also another smaller college offering a somewhat more holistic interpretation, the McTimoney Chiropractic School, which is on the path to accredition, and it is expected that this college will also be accredited in a year or two and its graduates will then also be able to join the official register. Osteopathy is taught in several colleges in four-year full-time courses. These courses are validated by the accreditation body, the General Council and Register of Osteopaths and also have degree status. Previously they received degrees from the Council for National and Academic Awards. Now B.Sc. (Honours) Osteopathy degrees are awarded to graduates of the British School of Osteopathy by the Open University Validation Service, B.Sc. (Honours) Osteopathic Medicine degrees are awarded by the University of Westminster to graduates of the British College of Naturopathy and Osteopathy, and B.Sc. (Osteopathy) General Degree with Honours is awarded to graduates of the European School of Osteopathy by the University of Wales.[14] Herbalism has also succeeded in obtaining degree status for its main course, which is now taught at Middlesex University, leading to a four-year full time B.Sc. Honours in Herbal Medicine (Phytotherapy). Herbalists can practice as members of the National Institute of Medical Herbalists after the four years training, which includes clinical experience, plus a further year of supervised practice. Students at these University courses are eligible for mandatory grants from their local authority which pay something towards the fees.

Although the process has not been easy, chiropractic, osteopathy, and herbalism have been more or less wholehearted about joining the conventional tertiary education system, because they are more comfortable with the language, concepts, and world-view of modern scientific medicine. However acupuncture and homeopathy are not quite so ready, for both are complete alternative therapeutic systems that fear that their unique alternative theoretical and practical basis will be subverted by the dominant biomedical model of health and disease. This is especially true in the field of education where students already come from school systems and from a life dominated by the same model. There has been a good deal of heart searching on the issue. Homeopathy is now taught to non-medical students in some 20 colleges in the UK as a three years full-time, and four years part-time course. The course core curriculum is being formulated by the Homeopathic Training Forum, representing all homeopaths.

Acupuncture is taught in three or four years part-time courses at a number of colleges, which with supervised clinical practice, leads to membership of the acupuncture register and permission to practise. The British Acupuncture Accreditation Board now oversees the five main acupuncture colleges and provides a voluntary self-validation system for the colleges. It has not, as was first feared, imposed a straightjacket of a standardized acupuncture system on the colleges, but has allowed the colleges to preserve their unique interpretations while ensuring basic standards of education. The British Acupuncture Accreditation Board claims that acupuncture courses are already quasi-postgraduate courses, as most of their students are mature students, and many already have degrees or equivalent qualifications. Therefore the Northern College of Acupuncture has recently obtained validation of a three-year part time course, leading to a postgraduate diploma, rather than B.Sc., at the University of Wales which permits practice. A fourth year leads to an M.Sc. This postgraduate route has allowed the college to maintain the traditional nature and content of their course without imposing extensive mandatory biomedical teaching on their students which would have been necessary at B.Sc. level. It is a route which other acupuncture colleges are studying.

Besides chiropractic and osteopathy, the therapies can be taught freely under common law by anyone in any way. This still stands despite an European directive that recommends that all the therapies be taught in courses equivalent to three years tertiary education.[15] Therefore one can still find superficial and even correspondence courses which provide their students with a fancy-looking but relatively worthless diploma to hang on the wall. But these days, with the current pressure for standards and self-validation such courses are disappearing. It is a general rule that if courses of several years' duration exist in a therapy, this is an indication that that subject needs it, and colleges offering only minimal training in the same subject should be looked at with suspicion.

Some subjects however do not require extensive courses—a four-year, full-time course in reflexology, for example, would be a ridiculous idea. These subjects can be described as the accessory or limited techniques, and not full first-call alternative medical systems. They would include the various types of massage, aromatherapy, healing, relaxation, biofeedback, and so on. In addition, anthroposophy, autogenic training and Alexander technique, are as much teachings as therapies, and the therapist and client need to develop new sensitivities rather than knowledge. Here too a full-time course would be inappropriate; training happens gradually over a considerable period. Short courses are available even in the main therapies, especially homeopathy, herbal medicine, and nutrition therapy, for the public to acquaint themselves with the rudiments of the therapy for first-aid or self-care purposes. These short courses are an important facet of complementary medicine. They help to bring the wisdom of the therapies into the lives of ordinary people so as to improve their health awareness, and prevent the therapies from becoming distant professional preserves.

Another recent development is the training of therapists and students in research. After a generation, the medical world has given up the requirement of scientific proof of the non-scientific therapies. It has requested that therapists think like scientists instead. The British Medical Association expects:

'the student of non-conventional therapy must be trained to be a competent practitioner and also be given the skills to carry out audit and research . . . it is important that students should acquire the basic principles of research methodology at undergraduate level so that a research culture is inculcated at an early stage.'[16]

As we have seen in Chapter 1, research here is a loaded word. It implies developing a biomedical view. It is paying dues to science. But it is also relatively painless, and when carried out sympathetically, can be useful in the development of the professions and sorting the wheat from the chaff. Research has, consequently, been taken up by all the therapies without exception and encouraged and taught in the colleges. Postgraduate courses in complementary medical studies started at the University of Exeter which has been taking M.Phil. and Ph.D. students for some years, and are now available at the University of Westminster and at other centres.

The BMA report also insisted that practitioners take part in continuing education, and postgraduate education is a compulsory part of maintaining registration as an osteopath or chiropractic. In other words, in theory, an osteopath can be 'struck off' the register for not taking part in postgraduate education. This is stricter than the rules for doctors which encourage but do not insist on postgraduate education. Postgraduate education has in fact been popular and very useful to practitioners, who find that they can broaden their practice and extend their therapeutic skills. For example, acupuncturists and herbalists have been keen to study Oriental or Ayurvedic herbal medicine.

Accreditation and standards in complementary medical training

In recent years the therapies have finally come to realize that the main obstacle to acceptance was teaching standards. Standards began to be set by therapist organizations who also give the right to join the professional register. This still fell short of full accreditation of courses by a body that had the blessing of government, and the government in turn kept pressing for the formation of such accrediting bodies before registration could be contemplated. At first the Council for Complementary and Alternative Medicine (CCAM) attempted to become an accrediting body representing the main therapies. However there was so much dispute that it became clear that, as Baroness Hooper, the Undersecretary of State for Health stated:

'the Government's stance on umbrella organisations has changed in recent years . . . we now firmly believe that it must be up to each therapy group to determine its own future development.'[17]

CCAM suggested a programme of accreditation of educational establishments by a process of self-validation. That means that each teaching body would articulate its goals and the goals of competency of its graduates, and demonstrate to a controlling board for each therapy how those goals were being met. This would force a minimum standard, yet retain the individual nature of each therapy.

The acupuncturists were keen to get going on this process, partly because they were concerned at possible heavy-handed control of their education in the future by authorities that did not understand the nature of Chinese medicine. In 1990 the Council of Acupuncture, a working group of the main lay colleges and professional bodies in Chinese medicine, swallowed their differences and set up the British Acupuncture Accreditation Board. They were followed at the end of 1994 by the British College of Acupuncture which teaches acupuncture to medically qualified students. The Board established the core teaching syllabus that was agreed as the minimum for safe and effective practice of acupuncture. The Board guides the colleges in their self-evaluation process, helping them to define acceptable criteria and goals, and then assess compliance to those standards. The colleges can, in addition, seek university degree validation as an 'optional extra.' The BAAB accreditation process takes at least three years, and the first colleges were eligible for accreditation in 1995. The Board consists of members from the profession, as well as representation from education, medicine, and the public.

This structure is being watched by the other non-registered therapies and could be an excellent model, for it has apparently succeeded in retaining the unique and independent character of acupuncture teaching in the various streams of Chinese medicine, while making sure that basic standards are maintained. Acupuncture requires a world view of elements and energies, yin and yang, radically different from that in which the students have grown up. It needs elegant and sensitive teaching, and special methods to develop subtle skills like pulse diagnosis. There is no sign that the accreditation process has hindered this. The acupuncture colleges are still very different from each other. It may be instructive to review some acupuncture colleges here in more detail to provide some insight into the educational structure of an alternative therapy which is far away from modern medicine yet constrained to co-exist with it.

The British College of Acupuncture was founded in 1964 as a postgraduate college that requires students to have some prior qualification in another healing area, either conventional or complementary, a knowledge of basic medical sciences. The course lasts three years at the end of which students receive the licence to practise. In the first year, the students learn western medicine and the rudiments of the Chinese view of the body, the acupuncture points, and basic principles of diagnosis and treatment. They then move on to explore diagnosis of diseases in western terms, and the rules and approaches of treatment. This is combined with clinical work. Attendance is on weekends and there is an examination at the end of each year. Practitioners tend towards a modern and scientifically acceptable adaptation of acupuncture, including the use of electrical equipment. The College trains some 250 students a year in large new premises in Hunter Street, in the centre of London.

The College of Traditional Acupuncture, in Leamington Spa and Glasgow is very different. Around 100 students a year are taken through a full three-year course, assuming no prior knowledge of acupuncture or any other therapy. In this college, acupuncture is taught as a complete therapy with a full traditional grounding in Chinese concepts and therapeutic practices, especially the practical philosophy of the Five Elements. It also concentrates on the development of natural diagnostic abilities in the sensitive reading of pulse, skin colour, tongue, voice, and so on. The college expresses a commitment to

'educating caring, independent practitioners who are instruments of Nature, rather than mere acupuncture technicians.' (CTA Prospectus).

During the first two years the students attend at the college for 14 weekend sessions per year, together with extensive home study. They receive teaching in the theory and laws of traditional medicine, the five element system, the meridians, the basis of traditional (not western) diagnosis, and courses in conventional surface anatomy and physiology, which aim to be of a standard equivalent to nurses and physiotherapists. The third year has weekly attendances for clinical training for six months, after which the students set up in supervised practice for a further six months. Basic conventional medical pathology and diagnosis is also taught at this time, as well as the rudiments of conventional drug treatment. The students find the course profound and exciting. It is felt that the part-time nature of the course is not a disadvantage, since the student has time to absorb what he has learnt, relating the initially outlandish concepts to his or her own experience.

The International College of Oriental Medicine, was founded in 1972. It is located in a large old house in a quiet cul-de-sac in East Grinstead. Students need at least two 'A' levels and some basic human biology, but mature students can study if they show inclination and ability, particularly qualities such as sensitivity, care, perceptiveness, and flexibility in thinking. As the College of Traditional Acupuncture, the college teaches authentic traditional acupuncture without compromise to western principles. However it differs in a number of respects. Its emphasis in traditional philosophy is towards the 'eight principles' system; teaching is more intensive, involving three days per week as well as extensive home study, over three years. A full range of approaches within Oriental medicine are taught including oriental massage, T'ai chi, herbalism, and even Chinese language. Traditional Chinese acupuncture is explored more fully and in a more traditional manner than in any other college. There is also a thorough grounding in Western medical pathology in which, interestingly, diseases are examined simultaneously from conventional and Oriental medical positions. Clinical practice is carried out during the second and third years and requires the most hours of any UK acupuncture college. There are only around 75 undergraduates as well as postgraduates, and the stated intention of the college is to produce an élite, well grounded in the rich and complex basis of Oriental medicine.

The Northern College of Acupuncture is a second generation college attempting to offer high quality teaching and not wedded to any of the traditional lineages of Chinese medicine. It is perhaps midway between all the other colleges offering a traditional yet eclectic and empirical interpretation, similar to the Traditional Chinese Medicine as practised currently in Chinese hospitals and clinics. They aim to produce well-rounded acupuncturists who are

'able to engage with the subtleties of the therapeutic relationship and the richness and diversity encompassed by a holistic medical approach.' (NCA prospectus, 1995).

There is probably more emphasis on particular disease conditions, and the interface with modern medicine, including research, than at the two more traditional colleges. This summary of the teaching of acupuncture must in fairness state that there are one or two establishments that are outside the accreditation process and offer wholly inadequate weekend-type courses.

Herbalists have also set up an accreditation board, and an educational board, and they are following a similar track to the acupuncturists, although they are some time behind. They wish to organize themselves so that state registration is possible if it would be seen in their best interest in the future. The full-time course at the main college, the School of Phytotherapy, is validated by the University of Wales, and as we have seen they have a course at Middlesex University.

Homeopathy too is considering self-validation and accreditation. Currently non-classical medical homeopathy is taught to doctors by the Faculty of Homeopathy, in a six-months course, while lay students learn more classical homeopathy in three- to four-year part-time courses, which entitle them to join the registers of the Society of Homeopaths or the UK Homeopathic Medical Association. Though it began as an exciting alternative social movement, a way of self-treatment and empowerment that was freely taught in the community, homeopathy has gradually professionalized over the last 20 years. The insistence on the long courses is partly intended to close the profession. However the distinction between 'expert' and unqualified lay homeopaths is still not entirely clear. Even today many go to these courses as a learning experience rather than a preparation for practice.[18]

The Society of Homeopaths has begun to accredit courses, set standards, and insist on a core curriculum. However the accreditation process is behind that of the acupuncturists and there is no formal Board as yet representing the whole profession. Homeopathy, because of its historical and conceptual opposition to modern medicine, is finding it difficult to develop an appropriate model which will be acceptable both to classical homeopaths and to the conventional tertiary education system. There is a great deal of debate on these issues, and an atmosphere of 'reluctant professionalism'.[18] The London College of Classical Homeopathy is perhaps a good example of a recently set up college. It offers a four-year full-time course for students who can join with little or no formal entry requirements. The course covers homeopathic philosophy extensively, especially at the beginning, and then moves on to materia medica, human sciences, psychology and psychotherapy, history of medicine, and computer studies. There is a good deal of guided clinical work. There are also shorter courses for doctors and other health professionals, introductory courses for the public, and postgraduate courses for homeopaths. It rents its premises from Morley College in London.

Other therapies which are not full primary contact therapeutic systems are also on the track towards more accreditation and approval of their courses. This is especially after both the BMA report and the NAHAT report acknowledged the demand for, and importance of, these accessory therapies, yet at the same time voiced concern over the issues of competence and called for educational standards. Reflexology, massage, aromatherapy, and hypnotherapy have been working towards validation of their courses as training courses under the National Vocational Qualifications scheme. The rewards of such a process are great—a stable future, and acceptance and employment within the National Health Service. In addition the chances of legislation and regulation of these professions would recede. The National Vocational Qualifications scheme focuses on occupational standards rather than academic success, that is they are oriented towards skills and the quality of performance or outcome. This would favour a strong clinical and practical emphasis in these therapies. The development of standards is under the aegis of the Occupational Standards Councils (OSCs), the one relevant to complementary medicine being the OSC for Health and Social Care. Complementary therapists' organizations have obtained support, information, and resources from the OSC for Health and Social Care and the Employment Department of the government to begin defining educational standards and the road to them. This would lead in the end to accreditation of the training in these complementary professions, yet the standards would be set essentially by the therapists themselves.[19]

The biomedical content of complementary practitioners' education

How much medical science should be taught? This is a thorny question. All but the most extreme natural medicine zealots now accept that there are some diseases or body repairs that are best left to doctors and surgeons, although naturally there is a continuing contention about how much. Some degree of daily accommodation with the medical world is essential. If a diabetic comes to a naturopath for treatment the therapist cannot ignore the patient's dependence on insulin. A traditional acupuncturist needs to know the effect of medical drugs on the pulses and Oriental diagnostic signs. A therapist needs to know what cortisone does, how it changes the symptom picture, and what will happen if the patient stops taking it. Therapists who are unable to diagnose certain serious conditions, such as venereal disease, tuberculosis, cancer, or multiple sclerosis, imperil the patient and themselves. If complementary professionals are to care for the public they must have sufficient medical knowledge at least to diagnose those conditions which require referral elsewhere. And in order to communicate with GPs all therapists ought to know what the doctor's diagnosis means.

These are the obvious minimum requirements for the safety and benefit of patients. But beyond this are requirements which modern medicine would wish on therapists: they are not for talking to doctors, they are for being like doctors. They are to protect the biomedical paradigm as much as the patients. For example, the BMA report states that graduates in the therapies should have the ability

'to use currently accepted clinical testing procedures as well as the ability to interpret any ancillary tests. In reaching a diagnosis, a practitioner must be able to show that he or she has thought differentially using a rationale based upon current knowledge of anatomy, physiology, and pathology.'[21]

This is a political request; differential diagnosis is the essential core of modern medicine but it is unnecessary and disturbing to the good practice of therapies such as Oriental medicine or classical homeopathy. A homeopath does not need it to talk to a patient's GP just as a GP does not need to learn pulse diagnosis before talking to a patient's acupuncturist.

There are wide variations in the extent to which colleges fulfill this responsibility. The larger ones are all able to provide extensive teaching and laboratory study of preclinical medically oriented subjects. The smaller ones sometimes also do very well, depending on the teaching staff, and teach anatomy, physiology, pathology, and pharmacology to a reasonable standard, in some cases equivalent to that of physiotherapists. Others have found the new requirements for basic medical sciences beyond them, and farm out the biomedical teaching to local colleges and universities. But there are still colleges that do little more than pay lip service to the new call for minimal biomedical content, and pad the curriculum; for example, the study of anatomy and physiology might be included in the prospectus, but in reality the students are flung a couple of weighty tomes and told to get on with it. The pressure for standards and accreditation of courses is being felt throughout complementary medicine, and there is no doubt that the quantity and quality of biomedical teaching, even in therapies such as shiatsu, aromatherapy, and healing, is at a level unthinkable even 5 years ago.

A full tertiary medical preclinical course is only necessary if the therapist intends to use those principles in his or her practice. This applies to some of the more scientifically oriented therapies, such as chiropractic, osteopathy, and herbalism, which actually use modern medical terminology and concepts in treatment. For example, in the teaching of chiropractic all of the first year, and more than half of the courses in years 2, 3, and 4, are biomedical not chiropractic courses. The director of studies is an experienced university teacher and academic. There is no dissection, but histology, biochemistry, and physiology are well covered by laboratory studies. Clinical subjects include orthopaedics, obstetrics and gynaecology, dermatology, geriatrics, paediatrics, and neurology.

The complementary content of medical practitioners' education

It is worth remembering that there is nothing inherently second-rate about the major alternative medical systems; it is only the cultural fact that modern medicine happens to be the dominant system today that requires therapists to learn the principles of medicine but does not require doctors to learn the principles of natural therapies. Despite a clear interest in alternative medicine expressed by the majority of young doctors and undergraduates, described in Chapter 1, there is still virtually no teaching of the therapies to medical undergraduates. Every few years for the last 20 years, the author has tested the temperature by writing to the Deans of the local medical schools, offering to teach courses. Deans have come and gone but the answer is the same: sorry, the syllabus is packed. No room on the bus. But with around one quarter of patients now using alternative medicine, at the very least trainee doctors ought to know what all the fuss is about. More than that, doctors should know how and when to refer patients to alternative medicine, what alternative medicine is and what to expect from it, and how to interface with its therapists. Most of the problems that arise when doctors work with alternative practitioners under the NHS or otherwise, arise from the lack of education of doctors and administrators in alternative medicine rather than the other way round.

In fact this call for the education of doctors is backed both by the British Medical Association which states that

'doctors need to know more about different therapies in order to delegate care appropriately, and to advise patients as to the benefits and likely hazards of treatment.'[20]

and also by the General Medical Council which says:

'Medical education must . . . also recognise that there is a growing demand for treatments that do not conform to the conventional orthodoxies'.[21]

But the medical schools are inherently conservative, and reluctant to take up the call. At an undergraduate level there is a little experimental teaching of the therapies, as student projects or lectures by local therapists, for example at Oxford University's Department of Public Health and Primary Care, at King's College, and at the City and East London Confederation for Medicine and Dentistry. At the Department of Medicine of the University of Glasgow, Dr Taylor Reilly polled nearly 600 undergraduates, and found that three-quarters regarded complementary medicine as useful and 69 per cent wanted it in their curriculum. They expressed their concern that they would be placed at a disadvantage if their patients knew more about these areas than they did. It was consequently taught to undergraduates as a series of seminars, which did not delve into the therapeutics, but raised issues for discussion such as self-healing and the placebo effect, the rise of complementary medicine, lay versus medically qualified therapists, and the question of integration of the therapies within the NHS, and so on.[22]

Postgraduate courses on complementary medicine are more widespread and are eligible for medical credits. They are available at the University of Westminster, University of Exeter, and other centres. However, doctors go to established colleges of complementary medicine, such as the British School of Osteopathy or the Faculty of Homeopathy, to actually learn to practise the therapies. An interesting scheme at the University of Glasgow has trained some 20 per cent of Scottish GPs in homeopathy to date. The teaching is modular, so that the medically qualified participants can learn a basic introduction to homeopathy, with the understanding that this allows only a limited use of homeopathy in practice, such as for first aid. A Primary Health Care Certificate is offered. About one-third move on to a further two years training to become full homeopaths. This kind of model would entirely answer the criticism that doctors usually receive skimpy training in the therapies, and then go on to practise a diluted version believing it to be the real thing. Interestingly, a two-year follow-up found that not only did 78 per cent still use homeopathy two years later, but it also helped practitioners to listen more, be more aware of natural healing, and be more holistic in their medical practice.[23]

Competence and quackery

There are no laws that prevent incompetence in medicine, complementary or conventional. Legal registration only ensures a proper standard of training, which is merely partial protection against incompetence. If a licensed practitioner becomes incompetent after training, he can usually plod along for years doing mild damage, only risking dismissal if something goes spectacularly wrong. The public does have redress against incompetent practitioners by suing for negligence in the civil courts (see Chapter 4).

The absence of formal registration of most of the therapies leaves them without any legal requirement for proper training. It might be thought that this is an open invitation to snake oil salesmen. In actual fact, quackery, the practise of medicine for profit by the untrained and incompetent, is relatively rare. In 1981, well before the current wave of educational renovation, the Threshold Survey found only 4 untrained practitioners out of 137, and these claimed to have been in practice for some time and to have been taught by apprenticeship.[3] The Australian studies have come up with a similar analysis. They found that 80 per cent of the 600 active therapists who returned their questionnaires had a formal diploma or doctorate. Most of the others were older therapists who had miscellaneous kinds of training and qualifications. The average number of years in practice of the therapists who were not formally trained was 15. Out-and-out quacks are unlikely to last that long.[4]

So the fear of incompetence in complementary medicine may be over-rated. But there certainly have been many superficially trained therapists who belong to impressive-sounding organizations and provide utterly inadequate treatment. For example, there was one hypnotherapy organization in the UK which trained practitioners in a brief correspondence course, after which it gave them recorded tapes and a franchise on an area of the UK. The practitioners advertised hypnotism as a cure for smoking or obesity, and the public paid dearly. However this kind of thing is disappearing, as therapy organizations today are much more concerned about the standards of those on their register, and the registers themselves are becoming centralized. A more benign form of incompetence arises when a member of the public who has received some introductory or self-help instruction, is tempted to take on patients. The author has witnessed one comical episode of therapeutic theatre in which a middle-aged lady chased a visitor around her house with bottles of Bach Flower Remedies, to which she had been recently converted. Since complementary medicine gives so much responsibility to the patient, there is always the risk that the patient grabs more. This probably does little harm, and may even be helpful in raising interest in health promotion and self-care, providing it is kept to a domestic scale.

Competence has become a hot word recently. Since the BMA report it has usurped 'proof of efficacy' as the passport to legitimacy. Competence is tied in with the drive for education and standards. But it is hard to define and is also a loaded word: competent to do what, to whom? and who is to decide? There will be little problem with the demand to be accountable, to provide truthful information, to refer cases which would be better dealt with elsewhere, to work within codes of ethics and disciplinary procedures, and to be generally professional. However competence is usually defined according to the responsibility for outcome, and here it gets difficult. Invisible qualities are much more important in alternative medicine, technical qualities in conventional medicine. The British Acupuncture Accreditation Board encourages:

'a reflective, research-minded practitioner with qualities of integrity, humanity, caring, trust, responsibility, respect and confidentiality'.[24]

These are immeasurable, but essential to the patient's and the practitioner's estimation of competence. Modern medicine would judge competence entirely differently, as if talking another language. Competence would be described in terms of full-time accredited courses, or as sensitivity to the risk/benefit ratio of a treatment.[25] This is fine, but it alters the role model for a 'good practitioner'. Since this model is defined by peers, practitioners are likely to adopt a new self-image accordingly.

But who is to judge competence: the patient, the GP, the therapist? The conventional medical argument that alternative medicine is 'mild' and the benefit less clear, so that risks should be less acceptable,[25] is specious: is it really more risky to be less interventionist? To reduce competence to the tangible and the measurable is what has happened to conventional medicine and is why there are alternatives in the first place. Competence of alternative therapists is also being defined today as knowing limits, that is knowing when to refer patients to doctors. This awareness of limits is indeed an important wisdom for all professionals who otherwise betray the trust of patients. But such an obligation must apply to medical practitioners too otherwise the issue of competence is simply another political weapon used to keep therapists 'knowing their place'—in the servants' quarters. The British Medical Association's call that

'therapists should be aware of which conditions and individuals they are not able to treat and when patients should be directed to medically qualified practitioners'[20]

should be symmetrical. In the end competence can only be judged from within not without each therapeutic tradition.

The organization of complementary medicine

Professional associations of therapists have usually borrowed a structure from medical associations. They have an elected council, a management committee, a code of ethics, a register to which only suitably qualified practitioners will be admitted, and often a research co-ordinator. Some are charities, others companies limited by guarantee. There are perhaps 100 professional bodies in the UK, with members ranging from half a dozen to several thousand. The larger and more established bodies are stricter in relation to membership and will normally only draw their membership from specific approved colleges. This is true with all therapies except osteopathy, chiropractic, and acupuncture, which have transcended the college based system, and control standards across the profession by means of a single council. Most organizations require candidates to practise for a period as a licensed associate, becoming a full member at the end of their candidacy.

The umbrella bodies representing complementary medical practitioners have played a key role in encouragement, information, facilitation, and the inevitable fire-fighting when things have become too hot between various organizations and factions. Their history has been truly Byzantine, and requires a book on its own. Today, the Council for Complementary and Alternative Medicine represents the central professional therapies, including herbalism, acupuncture, naturopathy, and osteopathy, as a discussion forum, representative, and spokesman where necessary, such as on the European legislative stage. The Institute for Complementary Medicine after failing in the attempt to represent all of complementary medicine, and to set standards, now assists various other groups of therapists to improve their education and political profile. The British Complementary Medicine Association represents therapists in the supplementary therapies, such as reflexology, in issues such as vocational training, and working with the National Health Service. They accept a secondary role for their therapists. These therapies are now also represented by the new Guild of Complementary Practitioners, a professional body set up to represent the graduates of the Independent Therapists Examining Council.

Complementary medicine has been beset by divisiveness. Many parallel organizations, often having little to choose between them as far as standards are concerned, have been at loggerheads for years. For example, among the eight osteopathic organizations, the half-century of bickering, splits, reconciliations, camps, associations, and disassociations would beggar belief. It is often because of a perceived difference in standards, or a more or less naturopathic or medical or classical orientation, or no reason at all.

'Perhaps this is not surprising', commented one osteopath, 'for practitioners brought up in an age of small 'training' units where the apprentice-master model was prevalent, followed by years of independent private practice, largely divorced from peer evaluation'.[26]

However all this has changed now. For the last few years, the mantra has been: 'get your act together'. The promise of legitimation in return for professionalization has dragged previous enemies into the meeting rooms. Now each of the therapies is developing co-ordinating bodies, councils, research offices, educational committees and merging their registers. Old colleges have adapted or closed. New, broader, second-generation colleges have begun. Younger, less xenophobic, more professional therapists are now in charge.

For example, the General Council and Register of Osteopaths has become the accrediting body for the osteopaths, somehow roping together five osteopathic colleges in the process. This body represents osteopaths and will be in charge of the register. Only because the therapy became sufficiently united, was legal registration possible. Registration also involves the setting up of a General Osteopathic Council (GOC) to regulate the profession in the same way that the General Medical Council regulates conventional medicine. This body has 24 members, including 12 elected osteopaths, 8 lay members appointed by the Privy Council, 3 members of the osteopath's education committee, and one adviser appointed by the Secretary of State for Education. Though the osteopaths are still contentious, continuing with struggles for positioning between the colleges, gradually the emphasis is moving away from separate associations, into one profession representing individuals who may practise a little differently from each other.

Acupuncture has gone through a similar process, with the five main associations amalgamating into the new British Acupuncture Council which holds a combined register of individual therapists, supervises ethics, and is the governing body for acupuncture. There was heated debate as to whether all the associations should join the British Acupuncture Association, the longest standing body. In the end, because of a history of differences and squabbles, it was decided to form a completely new association, representing all the properly qualified lay acupuncturists, but not the medical acupuncturists.

Most of the lay homeopaths have similarly joined within the Society of Homeopaths as the accrediting body that keeps the register, with the UK Homeopathic Medical Association in parallel. The various herbalists have formed the combined Herbal Practitioners Association, still an infant, and the reflexologists are attempting to work together under the umbrella of the Therapy Group for Reflexologists, the aromatherapists and other therapies similarly. The outstanding unresolved issue is the rivalry between those therapeutic organizations whose members are medically qualified and lay therapist organizations. The medical osteopaths, acupuncturists, and hypnotists still hang on to the attitude that they should dominate the profession. The Faculty of Homeopathy has been more accommodating to lay homeopaths. However now that even the BMA has stated that medically qualified therapists need to be properly trained, and the medically qualified therapists cannot but agree that accreditation and standards are a good thing and there cannot be exceptions, it is possible that protagonists will also find themselves arguing over a boundary that has already vanished, and the historical conflict will peter out.

References

1. Burton, A. K. (1977). *A work study of the Osteopathic Association of Great Britain: Part I: the structure of practices; Part II: the characteristics of patients.* Osteopathic Association of Great Britain.
2. Sharma, U. (1991). Complementary practitioners in a Midlands locality. *Complementary Medical Research*, 5, 12–16.
3. Boven, R., Lupton, G., Najman, J., Payne, S., Sheehan, M., and Western, J. (1977). *A study of alternative health care practitioners.* Appendix 7 of the Committee of Inquiry, Parliamentary Paper No. 102. This is the second report by the University of Queensland team, based on interviews with 594 practitioners throughout Australia.
4. Fulder, S. J. and Monro, R. (1985). Complementary medicine in the United Kingdom; patients, practitioners and consultations. *Lancet*, 2, 542–5.
5. Szmelskyj, A. (1992). The qualifications and geographical distribution of practising osteopaths in England, Scotland and Wales. *Complementary Medical Research*, 6, 1–8.
6. Wharton, R. and Lewith, G. (1986). Complementary medicine and the general practitioner. *British Medical Journal*, 292, 1498–515.
7. Hadley, C. M. (1988). Complementary medicine and the general practitioner: a survey of general practitioners in the Wellington area. *New Zealand Medical Journal*, 101, 766–8.
8. Anderson, E. and Anderson, P. (1987). General practitioners and alternative medicine. *Journal of the Royal Society of General Practitioners*, 37, 52–5.
9. The Consumers Association (1992). Alternative medicine. *Which?* November 1992, 45–9.
10. Datamonitor (1993). *Opportunities in European herbal and homeopathic remedies.* Datamonitor, 106 Baker Street, London W1M 1LA.
11. Frost and Sullivan Ltd. (1987). *Alternative medical practices in Europe*, Report No. E874. Sullivan House, Grosvener Gardens, London SW1W 0DN.
12. Eisenberg, D. M., Kessler, R. C., Foster, C., Norlock, F. E., Calkins, D. R., and Delbanco, T. L. (1993). Unconventional medicine in the United States. *New England Journal of Medicine*, 328, 246–52.
13. Thomas, K. J., Carr, J., Westlake, L., and Williams, B. T. (1991). Use of non-orthodox and conventional health care in Great Britain. *British Medical Journal*, 302, 207–10.
14. Edwards, D. (1994). A personal perspective of the Osteopaths Act 1993. *Journal of Osteopathic Education*, 4, 120–3.
15. EU directive: CD/89/48/EC.
16. British Medical Association (1993). *New approaches to good practice.* Oxford University Press, Oxford.

17. Hooper, B. (1990). In: *Medicine: complementary and conventional treatments.* *Hansard*, **518**, 82 (5 May).
18. Cant, S. and Sharma, U. (1995). Creating boundaries and minimising dissent. The construction of homeopathic knowledge as a strategy for professionalisation. *Social Science and Medicine* (submitted).
19. Langford, M. (1995). Competence and clinical aspiration: the situation for complementary therapies outside the 'big five'. *Complementary Therapies in Medicine*, **3**, 16–20.
20. British Medical Association (1993). *Complementary medicine: new approaches to good practice.* Oxford University Press, Oxford.
21. General Medical Council (1993). *Tomorrow's doctors: recommendations on undergraduate medical education.* HMSO, London.
22. Reilly, D. and Taylor, M. A. (1993). Developing integrated medicine. Report of the RCCM research fellowship in complementary medicine, Glasgow University, 1987–1990. *Complementary Therapies in Medicine*, **1**, Supplement 1, 1–49.
23. Reilly, D. T. (1995). Clarifying competence by defining its limits. Lessons from the Glasgow Educational Model of Homeopathic Training. *Complementary Therapies in Medicine*, **3**, 21–4.
24. Shifrin, K. (1995). Squaring the circle: the core syllabus of the British Acupuncture Accreditation Board. *Complementary Therapies in Medicine*, **3**, 13–15.
25. Ernst, E. (1995). Competence in complementary medicine. *Complementary Therapies in Medicine*, **3**, 6–8.
26. Fielding, S. J. and Sharp, G. J. (1995). Competences: their development and value in contemporary health education. The experience of the osteopaths. *Complementary Therapies in Medicine*, **3**, 42–5.

4
Policy, law, and the National Health Service

PART 1 LEGAL AND POLICY ISSUES

The practice of medicine and the law

A complex ordinance introduced by Hammurabi, a king of ancient Mesopotamia, decreed that physicians mismanaging their patients could be punished by mutilation. In dynastic Egypt, a malpractising or incompetent physician whose patient died was arraigned for trial and might be executed. No doubt certain critics of the medical profession, such as George Bernard Shaw, would have delighted in these measures, but times have changed. Modern legislation controlling medical professionals has been instigated and influenced in part by the professions themselves. The result is that it protects the doctor as much as the patient. The doctor is given power over the patient, power over other auxiliary or paramedical professions such as nurses or pharmacists, part protection from the consequences of possible incompetence, and a virtual monopoly over health care decisions. The patient is given protection from quacks and charlatans, and from avaricious or unethical activities, and gross incompetence.

Until just over a century ago, the profession of medicine in the UK was largely self-regulating. Licences were issued by various established bodies, such as the Royal College of Physicians, to those who had completed the required course of instruction. Heavy pressure was brought to bear on doctors who practised unorthodox or unscientific methods, in particular homeopathy or hypnotism, but this was a struggle within the profession. It ran in parallel with a centuries-long jostling for power between physicians, apothecaries, and surgeons. Unlicensed folk practitioners of traditional medicine—bonesetters, herbalists, and healers—were not deemed a threat to the physicians. They treated the poor, who were anyway unable to afford the attentions of physicians. Indeed, many a country doctor would send cases to the local bonesetter.

Parliament has always been reluctant to map out the boundaries of professional activities, partly because such legislation cannot guarantee competence and public respect and partly because it is hard to enforce. However, Parliament was, and still is, drawn in to shore up the status of different professional groups or settle their squabbles, for example those between the drug prescribers (physicians) and drug dispensers (apothecaries). When legislation establishing a medical profession was eventually passed in 1858 it was intended to rationalize a chaotic system of multiple licensing, hierarchies, and rivalries, the end-result of centuries of self-regulation.

The 1858 First Medical Act laid down that all qualified doctors should be entered on a single register, and that only registered practitioners could practise conventional medicine or surgery. A General Medical Council (GMC) was established with powers to set standards, control entry to the register, and outline and enforce appropriate ethical requirements. In its first reading, the bill made it possible to strike off any doctor practising unconventional forms of therapy. This clause was rejected by Parliament, allowing doctors to practise as they wished. There are separate acts registering the profession of dentist (1956) and optician (1958) with their separate registration authorities. Nurses and midwives have their own legal mandate and licensing procedures, and eight other paramedical professions (radiographer, dietitian, occupational therapist, orthoptist, physiotherapist, remedial gymnast, chiropodist, and medical laboratory scientific officer) are grouped under the Professions Supplementary to Medicine Act (1960). This sets up a separate registration board to oversee standards in each profession, all of which report back to one council.

Registration confers on doctors the sole right to describe themselves as doctors, physicians, or registered medical practitioners. If they are struck off the register, they cannot use these titles, and though they can work outside the NHS, they would find it almost impossible to gain patients. Registration as a Profession Supplementary to Medicine does not provide closure of title, but is a condition for working within the National Health Service and receiving GP referrals. In some cases, such as those of dentists or midwives, an unregistered person may not practise at all.[1]

The lay complementary practitioner and the law

On his own ground, the lay practitioner has almost complete freedom: a customary right to practise any form of therapy apart from a few exceptions defined below. This right is part of common law; that is, a traditional freedom to carry out those kinds of activities which are not expressly restricted by Act of Parliament. The freedom under UK common law is an enviable freedom not shared by therapists in other European countries that largely follow the Napoleonic code, in which activities are generally restricted unless regulations expressly permit them. The restrictions that do exist are designed to protect the public from charlatanism and confusion and are of no great hindrance to the complementary practitioner. Certain functions are limited to those on the relevant registers, namely the practice of dentistry, midwifery, veterinary surgery, and the treatment of venereal disease.

Mental health legislation prevents any but registered medical practitioners and psychiatrists from carrying out certain procedures related to mental health such as electroconvulsive therapy. However, all kinds of verbal, hypnotic, or psychological techniques are not restricted.

It is illegal under the Cancer Act (1933) to advertise treatments or remedies for cancer, although it is not illegal to treat it. A clinic in the UK offering natural therapy and advice to cancer patients, calls itself a Cancer Help Centre and is therefore within the law. The law also prohibits the advertisement of treatments for certain specific diseases including Bright's disease, cataracts, diabetes, epilepsy, glaucoma, locomotor ataxy, paralysis, or tuberculosis. Legislation under the Companies Act (1982) now prevents any new centre, except those employing doctors and nurses, from describing itself as a 'health centre' to avoid confusion with the 1000 National Health Service health centres.

Naturally, complementary medical practitioners are subject to laws, both criminal and civil, which apply to all professions, for example, the laws concerning misrepresentation and trade description, health and safety at work, data protection, or professional negligence. Misrepresentation could arise if a practitioner attracted members of the public by announcing that he could cure a disease or achieve a result. If he is unsuccessful, he is laying himself open to civil action by those induced to take his services. This is normally avoided by practitioners observing voluntary codes of behaviour which prohibits advertising claims. Yet the author has seen many hypnotherapists advertising liberation from smoking or obesity, a claim which would seem to be most unwise. The Health and Safety at Work Act (1974) requires employers, professionals, and others to ensure that injury to employees or members of the public on their premises does not occur. On the other hand, the small inspectorate which enforces this law is unable to cover all possible premises to which the law applies. The Data Protection Act (1984) imposes certain limitations on the way private information on clients is handled by therapists.

Professional negligence, or malpractice, may arise if someone is injured as a result of inadequate care by a professional. When a client or patient visits a therapist he automatically enters into an agreement in which the practitioner, for his part, must observe a minimum reasonable standard of competence. This standard is difficult to define but is usually taken to be the quality of treatment 'professed', or normally expected, by the profession, and that expected from the qualifications of the therapist. Medical professionals have a duty of care not to harm their client, and can be liable to allegations of negligence if they breached that duty, resulting in proven harm to the patient. It may even be negligent to fail to disclose adequate information about the risks of a certain procedure.[2] Doctors and therapists are usually protected by professional indemnity insurance against actions for damages brought by their clients. Contrary to the USA, in the UK actions for professional negligence against therapists are rare, and this is reflected in the low level of insurance premiums which complementary therapists pay. For example, most therapists are insured through a special policy for complementary medicine which provides indemnity of £1 million, and divides therapies into groups, chiropractic being highest risk (£250 per year), osteopathy next (£150), then acupuncture, followed by herbalism and homeopathy, and the non-interventionist or psychotherapeutic therapies offering least risk. Such low policies are conditional on the therapist being a fully paid-up member of a known register. It is worth noting that although medical litigation is generally increasing, there have been no recent civil professional negligence cases against complementary therapies.

Approaches to registration of complementary practitioners

'I am free to practise as I wish, I have more patients than I can cope with, why should I bother to change my status?' 'Our therapy can make a unique contribution to health, and should properly take its place alongside other caring professions in national life.' These are frequent refrains from individual therapists showing a clear division in attitude among therapies. On the one hand, the more established and biomedical of the therapies, such as osteopathy and chiropractic, have always been eager to regularize their status by some form of statutory recognition. On the other hand, therapies such as naturopathy, which are further away from the medical model see neither prospects nor benefit in registration. Therapies such as acupuncture, which are split between medical and the traditional camps, are correspondingly split on the registration question. The advantages of registration are obvious. It gives status in the form of a 'Parliamentary-approved' persona to practitioners and therefore attracts the confidence of the public. It protects the profession from quackery (although not incompetence) and ensures standards. It secures for the profession a recognized niche or therapeutic territory, and it opens the door into the NHS. The disadvantages are not so obvious. Registration may result in:

- Official control over training standards and practices, and some supervision by the medical profession, who will sit on the Councils.

- Possible gradual medicalization of the therapy's basic tenets.

- The unification of the profession and standardization of education which will restrict the varieties of interpretation and practice, giving the consumer less choice and opportunity.

- more treatment and less health maintenance and instruction as therapists move closer to the sickness-orientation of modern medicine.

- more bureaucracy and many more costs in running the various supervisory councils and committees.

- additional problems when receiving medical referrals, in particular the loss of alternative diagnosis, the restriction of therapeutic role (such as chiropractic's acceptance of a new identity as the 'bad backs' therapy), and various other kinds of pressure to reduce holistic treatment.

No wonder, therefore, that practitioners are often loath to give up their current independence, an attitude which has some justification if one considers the way the medical profession first recognized, then swallowed up, osteopathy in the USA.

The osteopaths have always felt themselves closest to the medical establishment, to the point of emulation. They have also been the most persistent in approaches to the government, their abortive attempt in 1935 being only the first of several. This attempt proved most instructive as they were told that in order to attain registration, they must first put their house in order. This meant primarily upgrading the standard and rigour of their training, and introducing an acceptable corporate structure and professional body, with a register and voluntary self-regulation of standards and ethics. The osteopaths established the General Council and Register of Osteopaths in 1936. The lesson was not lost on the rest of complementary medicine. Therapists coalesced into professional bodies, however diminutive, with their own registers, codes of ethics, regulations, and infrastructure. In 1957, the osteopaths asked those involved in drafting the Professions Supplementary to Medicine Regulations whether they intended to include osteopathy. They were told that osteopathy was not envisaged as a Profession Supplementary to Medicine. Having come to terms with the notion of a somewhat humiliating professional destiny as auxiliary to physicians, and then being refused, osteopathy went back to exploring independent registration. In 1963 they were told informally by the Minister of Health that there were neither plans nor intentions of registering osteopaths, and that registration could only happen by 'natural processes', that is when a consensus existed between the profession, the public, and the Department of Health (DOH). In a House of Lords debate on registration in 1985 the government recorded its position that there was no reason to afford complementary medicine further powers nor to impose on it further regulations. In the 1980s, as long as alternative medicine was small and ineffectual, the government could cosily regard its position as 'benign neutrality'.[3] However when alternative voices became too strident, the Department of Health was forced to reveal its less friendly face, which was identical with that of the medical profession: before registration

. . . the practitioners themselves would have to demonstrate, by objective scientific evidence, firstly that their system of therapy was valuable, and secondly that registration was necessary for the protection of the public against persons not qualified to practise it.[4]

Herbalists, too, have sought independent registration several times by means of Private Members' Bills, presented in the nineteenth and early twentieth centuries.[5] Since they were all unsuccessful, the herbalists put their energy into defending their products rather than registering their practice.

However the momentum of consumer use of the therapies was eloquent and could no longer be ignored. In 1989 the King's Fund set up a working party to study osteopathy, chaired by the appeal judge Sir Thomas Bingham. The report came out in 1991, and strongly favoured the registration of osteopathy in the public interest, adding a Draft Bill in its appendix.[6] The report recommended that all osteopaths be eligible to join the register, but some would need a period of postgraduate training. The Bill, which turned out to be the largest Private Members Bill ever to succeed, became law in 1993. It was an historic event; the first full acceptance of a complementary therapy, implying the end of centuries of medical opposition. From now on, only registered osteopaths can use that name. The profession will be self-regulating, with four statutory committees: Education, Investigating, Professional Conduct, and Health. These are controlled by a new General Osteopathic Council, which is answerable to the Privy Council. Like the General Medical Council, it will oversee standards, maintain the register, and deal with problems created by sickness or unprofessional conduct of osteopaths.[7] Only students passing the validated accredited courses are eligible to join the register, and postgraduate education is mandatory. Chiropractic was hot on the heels of osteopathy, and went through much the same process, with a report from the King's Fund,[8] and subsequently a Bill (The Chiropractic Act, 1994) that gave chiropractic registration on much the same structural model as the osteopaths. There will be a statutory General Chiropractic Council to oversee education, standards, etc. So far, the registered therapies do not seem to have gained very much by registration, although it is early days yet. Doctors now have confidence to refer many musculoskeletal patients to a therapist that they know is properly trained and professionally accountable.[9] So medical referral is increasing, and there will be more likelihood (not yet visible) of work under the NHS and in hospitals.

The main conditions for registration in the above therapies seem to have been:

1. A unification of the profession.

2. Improved teaching standards and accreditation of courses.

3. Biomedical content of education.

4. Restriction of therapeutic area to one part of the body (as opticians).

5. Modern medicine's realization that it needed a helping hand (to deal with back pain).

The other major therapeutic systems are going through the process of fulfilling preconditions 1, 2, and 3, so that everything will be in place in case they wish to request state registration. But they are not at all sure that registration is advisable, and they are waiting to see what happens to the osteopaths and chiropractors after registration. It is also not so sure that government will so easily agree to state registration without conditions 4 and 5 to oil the wheels. Acupuncture will be first in the queue, followed by herbalism, and then, possibly, homeopathy and naturopathy.

In theory, registration as a Profession Supplementary to Medicine is open to complementary practitioners. The DoH has often recommended it in the past to one or other of the organizations representing therapists, and most have been tempted to apply, as it appeared to be an easier path to follow than full registration. However as the Professions Supplementary to Medicine are subsidiary to doctors, and receive their patients after diagnosis, complementary therapies would lose their independence to diagnose and treat their own patients, and would therefore become supplementary therapies. All the major therapies that applied in the past have been turned down for their pains, for which today they must be thankful. Currently, art and drama therapists have applied and succeeded in joining. Therapeutic modalities such as reflexology and aromatherapy have recently considered this route, but they came to the conclusion that the price is too great and the benefit too small. For the PSM registration does not after all, give protection of title, but only credibility and permission to work in the NHS, which these therapies are doing at present anyway (see below) without state registration, and with more autonomy. Their status can be ensured instead by independent self-regulation and accreditation of courses by the National Vocational Qualifications scheme.

The influence of the European Union on complementary professions

The Treaty of Rome specifically excluded health care. Therefore the basic medical legislation of the member countries stands independently of one another. However there are areas such as education, research, insurance, and the status of herbal and homeopathic products in which Brussels can and does have a significant influence within the UK. That relating to herbal and homeopathic products will be discussed later, on page 81. The general positions of the EU within the European complementary medicine stage is discussed in the next chapter.

Directive 89/48/EEC defines higher education diplomas and subsequent professional training and experience that qualify state-recognized professionals, including health professionals. It requires such training to be three years at university or similar establishment. The European Commission stated that the directive only related to professions which are regulated or statutory. Therefore the Directive only applies to osteopathy and chiropractic, which already has such education in place anyway, not to the other therapies which practise under common law. In other words, the European Commission encourages three-year tertiary courses for unregistered complementary therapists but does not require it. However if a complementary therapist wanted his/her Diploma to be recognized in another country, it would have to conform to the Directive.

There was also concern of the loss of common law rights after 1992. But the European Commission has confirmed, on more than one occasion, that it will not interfere with the status of complementary medicine in member states. In 1987:

'. . . the Commission has no plans to study or promote the widespread use of these methods in the absence of conclusive proof of their efficacy.'[10]

In 1988:

'. . . the practice of such professions is governed entirely by national law. The general system of recognition of higher education diplomas will apply to therapists moving between Member States in which the practice of their profession is permitted, provided that their qualification is based on at least three years' professional education and training at a higher level.'[11]

The detachment of the EU also works in the opposite direction too, and the European Court has upheld the right of Member States to restrict the practice of alternatives to doctors in accordance with their own legislation.[12]

Advertising standards

Almost all complementary therapists have imposed voluntary constraints upon themselves, preventing advertising of the benefits of their treatments. Like doctors, therapists usually limit their advertising to a name plate with a note of their specialty. The Advertising Standards Authority, in the British Code of Advertising Practice, today makes no mention of therapists. It only states that in respect of herbal, homeopathic, and other non-allopathic medicinal products, claims must be assessed in the light of expert opinion within the fields concerned.

Insurance

Private medical insurance in the UK is tightly within the medical mould, but is slowly and cautiously incorporating some complementary medicine into its insurance schemes. Western Provident Association and the Hospital Savings Association both admit the major therapies for reimbursement, provided patients are referred by their doctor, and up to a certain limit. The Private Patients Plan has announced that it will reimburse patients who are referred by their doctor to a complementary practitioner of approved status, provided that the patient has a recognized and admissible medical condition. Approved status implies state registration for an osteopath or chiropractor, and medical qualification plus several years of full-time experience in alternative practice for a homeopath or acupuncturist.

In relation to accidents, or insurance of life and limb, insurance companies expect a doctor's assessment of injury or incapacity. Therapists normally send patients to a medical practitioner for this purpose in order to avoid prejudicing the patient's claim. However, both chiropractors and naturopaths have on occasion supplied reports to insurance companies which have provided the basis for claims.

Sickness and death certificates

Sickness certificates are notes to the Social Security office that a named individual is sick, and therefore potentially eligible for sickness benefit. These certificates are traditionally signed by the individual's doctor. Can a lay complementary practitioner sign them too? Until recently, most complementary practitioners have assumed that they could not. Local Social Security offices and their medical advisers were happy to reinforce this assumption. The law, however, states otherwise. Sickness certificates can be supplied by any competent person who is in a position to state that an individual is sick. Complementary practitioners can supply sickness certificates. Under the Social Security and Housing Benefits Act of 1982 it is the responsibility of the employer not the Social Security office to decide whether or not to accept a certificate. In case the employer is in any doubt, the DHSS has issued specific instructions in its leaflet NI 227 that non-registered medical practitioners, including acupuncturists, osteopaths, and herbalists, are quite entitled to issue certificates.

Death certification differs, however. Although any person may furnish such a certificate, the coroner will not normally accept it unless it is provided by a medically qualified practitioner. Nevertheless, on occasions death certificates have been accepted from complementary practitioners.

The fees of chiropractors, osteopaths, and occasionally naturopaths are being reimbursed with ever greater frequency by the Criminal Injuries Compensation Board, the Industrial Injuries Board, and ex-servicemen's bodies. Certificates and reports from these practitioners are also being accepted as evidence in court cases.

Homeopathy—medicine's unwelcome bedfellow

With the rapid rise in public interest in complementary medicine, it is often forgotten that there has been a truly complementary medical dual system in place for generations, *within the National Health Service*. These are the homeopathic hospitals in which doctors who are also trained in homeopathy utilize both systems side by side. Medical procedures are performed where urgent need or seriousness of the health problem requires a more interventionist approach, and homeopathy is used alongside or as sole treatment where appropriate. Whether it is the provision of palliative care to cancer patients, or the use of homeopathy to control tissue damage and post-operative complication of surgery, or the experience of weaning patients off steroids for inflammatory conditions, the homeopathic hospitals have built an unparalleled experience in the side-by-side use of complementary and conventional medicine, with thousands of cases over many years, within the NHS.[13] Their experience could be invaluable today, and the homeopathic hospitals developed as a primary resource, as the NHS struggles to find ways of satisfying the public demand for complementary medicine.

In 1949, the Minister of Health gave an 'absolute guarantee' that homeopathy would be allowed to continue within the National Health Service as long as patients demanded it. Despite this assurance, there has been a catalogue of closures. In 1977, a homeopathic clinic was planned at the newly built Royal Liverpool Hospital, to replace an earlier facility which was closed down. At a meeting of the Area Health Authority medical consultants it was insisted 'unanimously' that

'. . . undergraduates should not be exposed to any unorthodox medicine before qualification, that the very existence of such a clinic in the hospital's prospectus would cause alarm and . . . under no circumstances would the Departments of Medicine of Clinical Pharmacology . . . accept a Homeopathist as a teaching hospital professional colleague.'[14]

There was an immediate response in the House of Commons where Tom Ellis MP stated that:

'for sheer blind prejudice and bigotry, crass ignorance and highly questionable ethical behaviour, it would be hard to find a better example, even from the minutes of the Wapping Bargees' Mutual Benefit Society, let alone a body of professional men!'[15]

Strong words.

The Liverpool clinic was opened, and has achieved an international renown. Yet even in 1986, the local District Health Authority requested it to close down two days a week. Eventually the hospital was sold, and the department moved to small premises in Mossley Hill Hospital. The Bristol Homeopathic Hospital has also been living on a knife-edge. In 1987, the Local Health Authority emptied the building, allowing only out-patients to continue their visits. These were moved to another site. The Glasgow Homeopathic Hospital has also been under threat, but was saved by public action. The Royal London Homeopathic Hospital itself has also been at risk. Only some frantic lobbying and marshalling of public support has managed to forestall drastic action by its Area Health Authority. The first occasion was in 1979, when the Area Health Authority decided to close down most of the hospital as part of a long-term plan. An Early Day Motion was signed by 230 MPs requesting that the hospital be saved, and later, a petition containing no less than 116 781 signatures was laid before Parliament. The result was successful. The hospital was kept open. Yet the Area Health Authority, followed by the District Health Authority Health persisted, and eventually succeeded in having its operating theatre and half its wards closed.

However the worst is over, and things are now looking up. After strong representations by the medical homeopaths that public demand requires the development of homeopathic NHS facilities, the health administration has turned. Glasgow has appointed a second consultant, Bristol has a secure future, with some in-patient beds. The Royal Homeopathic Hospital has become an official NHS Trust and is now financially secure. It receives GP patients on contract, has an academic research department, and can appoint good staff.

Unsuccessful steps to control hypnotherapy

It has been difficult to control the practice of professionals who treat the human body. It has been impossible to control the practice of those who treat the human mind. Apart from the Mental Health Acts (1959 and 1975), which have placed boundaries on the more forceful kinds of management of the mentally disturbed, Parliament has been unable to agree on the means by which psychotherapy can be controlled or even the desirability of doing so. There are fundamental issues at stake relating to personal freedoms of exploration and expression, and there are powerful ambiguities which, fortunately, make it absurd to draw lines between therapy and guidance, between psychology and religion, and between hypnosis and conviction.

Since the time of Mesmer, Charcot, Coue, and others, the medical profession has found hypnosis an uncomfortable subject. Hypnosis has a history of spectacular demonstrations, passionate converts, and emphatic denials from the medical world. Like homeopathy, it has largely been introduced by heterodox doctors, making it a subject for attempts at suppression from within the profession rather than for legislation from without. However, doctors no longer doubt that hypnosis works. Indeed the British Medical Association's Psychological Medicine Committee now regards it as a 'treatment of choice for psychosomatic conditions, psychoneuroses, and the removal of morbid patterns of behaviour'.[16] It recommends that hypnosis be taught to medical undergraduates although this has not yet happened.

In 1952, the Hypnotism Act, concerning stage hypnotism, gave responsibility to local authorities to supply licences for public performances of hypnotism. However, if Parliament could not decide whether hypnotism was harmful it is hardly likely that the local authority would be able to do so; some local authorities grant licences freely, others, particularly in the London area, never grant licences. In 1979, Lord Kinnoul introduced a bill which went further. It was intended to tighten up the control of stage hypnosis by including clubs, to control hypnotists' advertisements, and to ban the sale of hypnotic tapes or records. The Government stated that it could not see what all the fuss was about, and it had no evidence of harm, even from stage hypnotism.[17] Hypnotherapy emerged untouched and, without ammunition, there are no signs of inclination for further attacks. Recently the use of hypnotic regression to uncover memories, such as of childhood sexual abuse, and to use these memories in evidence, has created controversy. The British Psychological Society has proposed guidelines for the use of such material forensically. But Professor Weiskrantz, Emeritus Professor of Psychology at Oxford, has roundly criticised this practice because such hypnotically extracted memories are unreliable, and could easily have been placed there by suggestion.[18] Exactly the same criticism has, incidentally, been levelled at Freud in his psychoanalytically uncovered evidence of childhood sexual abuse.

Acupuncture needles

No therapy has taken the authorities by surprise in the way acupuncture has. In 1977, events in Birmingham forced acupuncturists into the limelight and the authorities to take them more seriously. An outbreak of hepatitis was traced back to a lay acupuncturist who had previously been denied entry to acupuncture associations. He had been using dirty needles. Questions were asked in the House of Commons about registering and controlling the practices of acupuncturists.[19] The Under-Secretary of State for Health answered that registration would not necessarily prevent dirty needles, and anyway might have the side-effect of giving statutory support to the acupuncture profession before it has established itself. It so happened that the West Midlands County Council had already put a bill before Parliament requesting powers to control standards of hygiene by licensing acupuncturists, tattooists, massage parlours, and similar activities. Parliament was glad to leave it to the local authorities to worry about, and supported the Bill. However, it met stiff resistance from acupuncturists, who forced the DHSS in committee to admit that they had no evidence that there was any health risk from a trained acupuncturist. The acupuncturists won the battle but lost the war when the House of Commons overturned its committee's recommendation for an exemption, and the Bill became law.[20] Fortunately, acupuncturists had another chance in the similar Greater London Council's General Powers Bill, and later the London Local Authorities (No. 2) Bill which would have given the local authorities power to grant or refuse licences to any acupuncturist or other complementary therapist who was not a medical or dental practitioner. The Council for Complementary and Alternative Medicine and also the Institute of Complementary Medicine fought successfully. An exemption was included in the Bill.[21] However the exemption applies only to those practitioners who belong to the main professional organizations with acceptable Codes of Practice. Other practitioners, including, for example, many massage therapists, must obtain a licence. These events have taught the acupuncturists to feel the political pulse with a little of the sensitivity that they normally reserve for wrist pulses.

Outside the London area acupuncturists practise without the need for licensing from local authorities, although they are inspected for cleanliness by Environmental Health Department officers, and their premises are registered under the Local Government (Miscellaneous Provisions) Act 1982. There is no requirement to use disposable needles, although most do so, and of course the standard of practice required by the professional bodies is very strict about needle sterility. The Blood Transfusion Service was concerned about the AIDS risk from acupuncture, and used to require a six month period after treatment, before blood can be donated. Today they have agreed to drop this requirement if acupuncturists follow their new Code of Practice.

Herbs and medicines

Government has trodden gingerly in the boggy territory of the licensing of the healing professions. But it has stepped more confidently to regulate the substances they use. An inscription on the Acropolis, dating from the fourth century BC, announces that one Evenor the physician had been appointed inspector of drugs. A similar function has existed in the West ever since. A pharmacopoeia, in which standards are defined for the preparation and purity of specific drugs and herbs, has existed in the UK from the early seventeenth century.

Medicines legislation is extremely complex, and will not be reviewed here other than where it relates to the complementary practitioner. A number of Acts, including the Pharmacy and Poisons Act 1933, the Therapeutic Substances Act

1956, and the Dangerous Drugs Act 1965, resulted in a system in which certain defined remedies were to be available from a pharmacist on prescription only, and some poisons were placed under special restrictions. The Acts also described the measures to be taken to ensure purity. In 1968, the Government sponsored the Medicines Bill which became law in 1971. This required manufacturers to prove to the Licensing Authority of the Medicines Division of the DHSS that a remedy was both safe and effective before a licence could be issued to supply it to the public. The claims made in the advertisement had to conform to those granted in the licence. These controls took effect immediately with new drugs. However, drugs that were already on sale before 1971 were given automatic Licences of Right, allowing sales using the previous claims. At the same time a Committee on the Review of Medicines was established to review the safety and efficacy of all pre-1971 remedies.

Prior to the Medicines Act, herbal medicines could be sold openly, with the exception of a few that were more or less accidentally found to be toxic. When the White Paper preceding the Medicines Bill was published, the herbalists mounted an unprecedented national campaign to ensure that herbalism was not drowned in a sea of medicines legislation, setting up the British Herbal Medicine Association for this purpose. They succeeded in obtaining substantial exemptions for herbal products, and undertakings to consult with herbalists before enacting the various subsequent orders embodied in the bill. A Herbal Remedies Subcommittee of the Prescriptions Only Committee examined the current use and dosages of herbs supplied by herbalists, and listed them in the Herbal Remedies Report. They were then incorporated into law in the Herbal Remedies Order of 1977.[22]

The Order listed three restricted categories of herbal remedies: Part I are full Prescriptions Only Medicines, and may only be prescribed by a doctor, for example ergot, scopalia, or digitalis. Those in Part II may not be retailed to the public; they include all the herbs for which any restriction exists. Those in Part III may be supplied by herbal practitioners (who are not defined, and would also include naturopaths) to their patients, within the dose levels indicated in the list. They include Atropa belladonna, Ephedra sinica, or Datura stramonum. They must be prescribed from the herbalist's private premises after personal consultation with the patient, and they must be labelled with names and addresses of the herbalist and patient, together with dosage details and directions. The herbalist must also keep records and notify his practice to the 'enforcement authority', the Secretary of State for Health and Social Security. Any herbs that are not entered on the above three lists can be freely supplied by herbal practitioners and sold in all retail outlets, provided that they are properly labelled. This was a good effort, but herbalists generally did not take any notice of the Order, and many herbs on the lists continued to be available. The Order was generally not enforced.

However it was used as a legal basis to ban occasional herbs that have come to the notice of the Medicines Control Agency or the National Poisons Unit because of possible toxicity. A total of 32 have been banned in various countries of the European Union because of fears of toxicity. The banning of such herbs that have been part of folk medicine for thousands of years has dismayed herbalists, particularly because the grounds for prohibition have often been irrational and unscientific. Mostly it has been because toxic constituents have been discovered which are present in small quantities. Yet these may be in plants which have been used widely without apparent adverse effects. The substances may not be toxic when used within the protective environment of the whole plant. The reports of adverse effects are rare and questionable. Comfrey root was withdrawn from use because of four cases reported in the medical literature in which individuals with existing health problems may have had an exacerbation from comfrey, and because it contains alkaloids which have been kown to be toxic in animals in large doses. But in normal does it is indisputably safer than paracetamol which is sold indiscriminately (see Chapter 13).

Substances are defined as medicines if they are supplied with a therapeutic intent, even if they contain nothing but salt. Many substances with a quasimedicinal value are sold in health food shops. Provided that the substances do not appear on the Herbal, Homeopathic, General Sale, or Prescriptions Only lists, and no medicinal claims are made for them, they are classed as vitamins and foods and are allowed on unrestricted sale. Eighty per cent of the herbs on sale are in this category. They are outside the Medicines Act altogether, and under the food regulations of Ministry of Agriculture Fisheries and Foods (MAFF). The food regulations are only concerned with purity and toxicity, and of course honest labelling. MAFF may intervene when it has evidence of toxicity, for example in its action against the amino acid tryptophan, sold as a sedative. There are no specific regulations concerning herbs sold under the foods laws, although a report by MAFF and the DoH highlighted a few areas of concern, such as the fact that certain substances had been removed from sale as medicines for safety reasons (such as mistletoe) but were still available as foods.[23]

A herbalist creates a medicine out of a herb or food supplement only when he opens the packet and supplies its contents to members of the public, with a therapeutic intent. The substances are then brought into the sphere of the Medicines Act. The herbalist is allowed to prescribe them because they would either be on the General Sale List or not mentioned on any list and therefore exempt, or on the list of prescribable herbs under the 1977 Act. However, the herbalist must obtain an Assembly Licence, normally granted automatically after his qualification.[22]

When a manufactured herbal product has a therapeutic claim on it, it automatically becomes a medicine. All manufacturers, wholesalers, and importers of medicines need to obtain licences, the most difficult being the Product Licence that the manufacturer or original supplier must obtain for each and every medicinal preparation, even those on the General Sale List. A huge amount of evidence on safety, purity, and especially effectiveness (including clinical trials) is needed for a new license, costing many millions of pounds. Obviously it is inappropriate to demand the same for each herbal and food supplement product, especially since herbs are basically unpatentable. But the Medicines Control Agency has so far been quite confused as to how much laboratory and clinical research to call for before granting a Product Licence. They have adopted delaying tactics and almost no new licences for herbal medicinal products have been issued since the Medicines Act became law.

In actual fact, most of the medicinal herbal products now on sale were given a Product Licence of Right in 1971, since they were sold before 1971. They were required to be fully assessed in due course. By 1990, 500 had been granted full product licences on review by the Committee on Review of Medicines. In relation to the problem of evidence, the Medicines Control Agency decided on a policy, outlined in their proposal MLX 133, which stated that the safety and quality of herbal and traditional products should be examined with the same rigour as conventional drugs. However, they recognized that they could not call for the same evidence of effectiveness for a herb as for a chemical drug. Therefore, effectiveness will be assessed on the basis of whatever information is available, including traditional experience. The amount of evidence will also be in proportion to the claim the manufacturer wished to make. For minor or 'self-limiting' conditions traditional evidence may suffice. For claims that relate to more serious conditions, much more scientific evidence will be required. In other words clinical trials would be required for a herbal blood pressure pill, but not for a herbal cough mixture.

A new label wording was introduced for 'mild' claims that were accepted on the basis of traditional use, for example: '. . . traditionally used for colds and catarrh . . .' for garlic capsules.   On the one hand this is a significant step forward. For the first time the DHSS has recognized that herbs are more subtle, long-term, and preventive; that the current pharmacological methodology may be inappropriate to assess them, and the herbal industry unable to do so. On the other hand none of the members of the various commissions are experts on herbs or herbal practitioners. Furthermore, the lenient attitude stops short of permitting all herbal preparations to pass easily through the net; only those for minor conditions. Worse was to come. The cost of a licence, even a shorter version for a herb that did not require a roomful of scientific documentation, was hiked tenfold in 1990 to £97 500. It is peanuts for a drug company launching a new drug, but would cripple a herb company. The herbal manufacturers formed a pressure group, the Natural Medicines Society, to lobby on these issues. They made the strong point that to make the licensing process so heavy, would only encourage unlicensed and unregistered 'cowboy' herbal products of poor quality and effectiveness. Indeed, the shelves of the health shops are full of herbal products of indeterminate species, origin, and purity, sometimes of quite inadequate amounts of active ingredients and of ineffective dosage.[24] An Early Day Motion requesting the Health Minister to include experts in the practice of natural, homeopathic, and herbal medicines on the expert committees that determine the fate of such remedies, was signed by more than 200 MPs. In 1989 the herbal groups went to the High Court to complain about inadequate consultation and the licence fees. The case was lost, but it achieved its result anyway, and from then on there was much closer consultation between the MCA and the herbal organizations, and the fee structure was changed.

The years of dialogue between herbal manufacturers and the MCA were paying off. The British Herbal Pharmacopoeia was recognized and used as a basis for quality, the PLR review process was proceeding, and the authorities acknowledged (for example in MLX 133) that herbal products reduce trivial consultations with doctors, and prevent people from using more toxic conventional remedies unnecessarily. But then a bombshell struck; from Europe. A circular from the MCA, MLX 206, was sent round in July 1994, which announced proposals to implement new EU product licensing procedures and 'to create a new legislative basis, separate from the Medicines Act 1968, for marketing authorisations and related controls on medicinal products.' It went with a new draft Statutory Instrument (SI) to bring UK law into line with the EU so as to create a single market in pharmaceuticals, to take effect by January 1995.[25] But it also removed the exemptions for herbs enshrined in the Medicines Act of 1968, indicating that all 'processed or industrially produced' herbs will need a licence, which would effectively wipe most herbal products off the shelves. The directive appeared in July, but the herbalists were unable to obtain clarification from the MCA until September, and what the herbalists heard confirmed their worst fears: not only were the exemptions to go, but even practitioners and health shop sales staff would need medicines licences to supply a herbal product to a member of the public. Since the SI was to be laid before Parliament in November, there were only days for the herbal industry to respond.

A lightning public campaign was mounted which resulted in a huge response. The media howled.[26] Tens of thousands of letters were received by MPs. One MP stated that he had received 2000, and Baroness Cumberledge, Secretary of State for Health, received 700.[27] More than 100 MPs also wrote to the DoH. Politicians found the response overwhelming. The MCA tried to negotiate a compromise but was turned down. An Early Day Motion was tabled. Finally, on November 11 the Parliamentary Under-Secretary for Health issued a statement announcing that the exemptions would continue. He had found a way to wriggle out from under the EC regulations. The term 'industrially produced' was not legally defined, so that the government could decide that herbal remedies made in traditional ways 'fall outside the interpretation of an industrial process'.[28] This was then confirmed in detail in Parliamentary discussions.[27]

Herbs had won a reprieve, but when the storm had passed the landscape looked completely different. Twenty-five years of a gradually constructed dialogue with the governemnt on the need to take herbs into account in legislation seemed to have vanished. Clearly the DoH did not take natural medicine's contribution to health care seriously. In addition the consultation process was absent when it was most needed. More fundamentally, it now appeared to herbal manufacturers and users that the sense of security that they had enjoyed since the Herbalists Charter of 1543 was gone. Herbs were now allowed by default. The whole herbal industry and herbalism itself as well as common law rights seemed to hang on an exception to regulations which were imposed from outside without due democratic consultation or debate.

The MCA safeguard does not, therefore, constitute the final status of herbs under the European and UK law. The situation is open again and there are many real concerns and uncertainties. The basic problem is that EU medicines legislation appears to be irrelevant to herbs, and serves against consumer interests. If herbs are classed as medicines they are severely discriminated against in the medicines legislation (for example in relation to licencing fees and issues of evidence). But if they are classed as foods, they will be under-regulated in terms of quality and safety. A great deal of work has already gone into improving standards of purity, safety, and manufacture, which will be lost if the herbs are downgraded to foods. The issue of safety has been very much in the public eye recently, and assessments on the safety of traditional medicines confirm that they are safe but that it is wise to keep a close eye on them which would be impossible if they were classed as foods.[29] There are no specific exemptions in place for herbalists. There is still insufficient representation of experts in herbs and natural remedies on the committees which assess them. There is a pressing need for a new defined category of traditional and herbal medicines with its own legislation. This will require a specific EU directive. Fortunately there is a precedence for this in the new homeopathic legislation which will be discussed below. The new European Herbal Practitioners Alliance, the European Scientific Cooperation on Phytotherapy (ESCOP), and the BHMA have all been pressing European legislators for a special status for herbs, placing them legally in between drug and food.

Homeopathic remedies

The position of homeopathic remedies is, by contrast, fairly simple. A precedent was set by the Medicines Commission who considered that any medicine which is diluted to one part per million (in homeopathic terms $6x$) or greater is harmless. Therefore they advised that, even where a medicine is on the Prescriptions Only List, at a $6x$ dilution or greater, it is exempt from restriction and can be supplied by lay practitioners and sold in shops. No proof of efficacy was required. This was incorporated into the Medicines Act of 1971, and was confirmed by the EEC in the EC Directive 75/319/EEC. The homeopathic products had a Product Licence of Right (PLR) which allowed them on sale: no less than 6000 PLRs were issued. However the status of homeopathic remedies came up for review in 1990, and has been the subject of new EEC Directives 92/73/EEC and 92/74/EEC which became UK law early in 1994. This takes the place of all the old regulations, and therefore the PLRs have mostly gone except for a few products which cannot be incorporated into the new laws. The new laws incorporate anthroposophical medicines into the homeopathic basket. They apply to products for sale, not to homeopathic prescriptions made up specially for patients, which are unrestricted.

The laws state that if a homeopathic product for oral or external use is sold without claims on the labels or literature that the product can treat a certain condition, then it is eligible for a very simplified registration procedure. It must have a licence, it must be made according to rules of Good Manufacturing Practice in relation to cleanliness and purity, and it must be sufficiently dilute (1: 10 000 or $4x$ of the mother tincture). However no evidence of effectiveness is required. On the other hand if a claim is made for a minor, non-serious, self-limiting complaint (such as upset stomach), then it must be substantiated by documented evidence according to certain criteria, still to be precisely defined. Ironically, the homeopathic organizations and the Medicines Control Agency are both aligned on the issue of the difficulty of making label claims for products, since it is fundamentally against the individualized nature of homeopathic prescribing. For major health problems, such as cancer, and for injectable homeopathics, such as Iscador, there are no simplified registration procedures, and they will be treated as drugs, with all that implies in terms of premarketing clinical and toxicological testing. Labels should define such things as dilution, scientific name of original stock (without brand name), etc., and should include a statement: 'Homeopathic medicinal product without approved therapeutic indications'. After much petitioning from homeopaths, the Medicines Control Agency also set up an advisory board which included homeopaths, to advise on uncertain cases.

The other part of the Directive sets in motion the preparation of a combined European Homeopathic Pharmacopoeia. This would create quality standards, and thus make licencing much easier for all parties. The creation of such a pharmacopoeia is complex. It is being carried out by the European Pharmacopoeia Commission which will produce an entirely new European Pharmacopoeia, of which only one section covers homeopathy. The French and Germans have produced their own candidate, combining earlier national homeopathic pharmacopoeias to reflect their own perspectives and approaches, and the British responded likewise with a new British Homeopathic Pharmacopoeia, the first since 1882. The MCA is using it at present for registration purposes until the European Homeopathic Pharmacopoeia is ready. The preparation of such a combined version is sensitive, as there are different interpretations and schools, and some classical homeopaths charge that there is insufficient consultation, and serious omissions in the draft versions. Hopefully these will be ironed out and an historic pharmacopoeia will emerge which will legitimize, encourage, serve, and draw together homeopaths all over Europe.

PART 2 COMPLEMENTARY MEDICINE WITHIN THE NATIONAL HEALTH SERVICE

Background

The National Health Service, though paid for by the public through their taxes, has not invited the public to contribute to the debate concerning what kind of medicine the Service should provide. Its policy in this regard is determined by doctors. The relationship of complementary medicine to the national medical system is thus a mirror of its relationship to the medical profession. In the past the medical profession has cemented an exclusive preserve for itself. The General Medical Council (GMC), set up by the Medical Act of 1858 to oversee the medical profession, set about ensuring its monopoly by instituting the harsh ruling that medical practitioners consorting with, or aiding, unregistered practitioners could be struck off. This spelled the beginning of a difficult period for complementary practitioners. Patients had to go to therapists more or less in secret for fear of jeopardizing their relationship with their medical practitioner. Therapists hardly dared advertise their existence for fear of exposure by the media or the threat of a malpractice case. Society as a whole, strongly influenced by the medical profession, created a negative stereotype of complementary practitioners, as semi-illegal, twilight, back-street, primitive, and suspect. Even though the Queen had a homeopath, this was regarded as a quaint foible of the Royalty; in fact homeopathy was in decline as the opportunities for education and practice, the corps of homeopathic professionals, and the homeopathic hospitals were restricted.

The founding of the National Health Service in 1949, under Aneurin Bevan, only augmented the physicians' monopoly. It did so by refusing entry to alternatives, besides medical homeopathy, and offering patients free treatment in orthodox medicine only, thus restricting freedom of choice. However, as we saw in Chapter 1, the attitudes of doctor, patient, and therapist to each other have been rapidly changing. The formal barrier was removed in 1974 when the GMC dropped its notorious clause preventing doctors from making contact with complementary therapists. The Council's position then became that a doctor may send a patient to someone who is not medically qualified, if it would benefit the patient, provided the doctor retains overall responsibility. The British Medical Association (BMA), could not, for many years, bring itself to adopt the GMC's more relaxed position, claiming ingenuously that since a doctor does not know what a complementary practitioner does, he cannot retain overall control of the patient.

Breaking the barriers

In 1983, the inaugural speech of its president, Prince Charles, forced the BMA to take another look at its position.[30] The BMA announced it was setting up a working party to consider ways in which the contribution of complementary medicine could be assessed.

'Our minds are open. Much success is being claimed for alternative therapy so we believe the time is right to gather information.[31]

The report of the working party, as seen in Chapter 1 (see p.18), did not reflect this open attitude to the slightest degree.[32] It was, as the Research Council for Complementary Medicine indicated, produced by a

'committee struggling to understand new concepts, failing to do so and falling back defensively upon what they were brought up with'.

Even the DHSS remarked, unofficially, that the report was premature, biased, and generally unhelpful.[33] But it did reveal clearly to the public and Government, that the conventional medical establishment did not respect freedom of choice or the new mood of patients as participants and consumers. Nor indeed did it respect the many GPs interested in complementary therapies. It appears that this report was a watershed. From then on the medical profession lost the driving wheel. Consumer pressure forced the Department of Health itself to take complementary medicine seriously. In 1991, Stephen Dorrell made a dramatic statement that opened the doors of the NHS to non-medically qualified therapists. After that, the BMA could only try and tidy up the mess. Its second report, discussed in Chapters 1 and 3, merely attempts to encourage an orderly relationship between the medical systems.

The Health Minister's statement[34] began:

'It is open to any family doctor to employ a complementary therapist to offer NHS treatment within his practice . . .'

It repeated the earlier ruling that the doctor must remain clinically accountable, and take overall responsibility for a patient's care.

'It is not a referral system, whereby one registered practitioner refers a patient for treatment to another. It is a 'delegation' system, where the GP asks another professional to provide care for which he remains clinically accountable. It is therefore for the individual GP to decide in the case of each individual patient whether the alternative therapist offers the most appropriate care to treat that patient's condition.'

This clarification does not introduce any new rules. However its importance is that it spells out for the first time that lay therapists can work in the NHS, and it invites complementary therapies into national medicine.

To some extent this came as a surprise. Although it is inevitable, given the current scale of use, that complementary medicine is and will be licenced in some way and legitimized, it could have done so with or without entry into the NHS. Patients could have gone to therapists as much as their pockets would allow, doctors would have referred where necessary, and the two systems would be autonomous and parallel. There are specific reasons why the NHS is interested. Something is happening to the health service, a deeper process, that is sweeping away the old habits and professional compartments. It is the rise of a new commercial culture, and it is this, more than any other consideration, that is creating a level field in which various competing medical systems can sell their wares. The current slogan is no longer 'scientific credibility' but the 'buying of services' which have to be cost-effective. It is indeed ironic that the centuries old struggle between Hygeia and Aesculapius has been resolved, for the moment, by shopping. On a purely commercial basis, complementary medicine has a lot going for it. Consumers want it. It may be able to reduce expensive drug and hospital bills, and it may help to treat chronic problems, such as back pain, which currently bleed health service resources.

There are other reasons. One is the current attempt to shift the emphasis of medicine from Secondary to Primary Care—out of the hospital into the local GP's office. The GP, at the forefront of health care, is on the lookout for new tools for use in Primary Health Care. As we saw on page 17, most doctors want to learn more about the therapies, the majority refer patients to them, and three out of four want them on the NHS. The main problem for doctors has been that it is hard to know to whom to refer, and why. What kind of therapist would help a certain patient, how can his level of education and competence be relied upon, how long should he be treated and what would be the expected outcome? The doctors are required to be clinically accountable but this is impossible without real familiarity with the therapies and therapists. Moreover, GPs do not feel comfortable referring a patient to a therapist who charges fees. A new book has been published which discusses these problems and can help to inform doctors as to how to incorporate complementary medicine into general practice.[35] From the doctor's point of view, all of these problems can be substantially reduced by bringing the therapies into the NHS fold.

First steps to integration

There are several ways in which this can be done.[36] A GP in a fund-holding practice, who has a good deal of flexibility in the way he can allocate resources, can decide to offer a wider range of services in his practice, including complementary medicine. In other practices, the GPs will request or bid for complementary therapy sessions or staff from the Family Health Service Authority, just like any ancillary staff, for example physiotherapists. The FHSA will allocate funds to the GP for this purpose according to its priorities, from its General Medical Services budget, or its Research and Development budget. Complementary therapists may be employed directly by the District Health Authority or FHSA, and then seconded to those practices that are able to make use of them, or employed in a complementary therapy referral centre as a service to local GPs.

In 1992, a national survey was carried out among district health authorities, FHSAs, and GP fundholding practices, that is all those administering primary health care in the UK, to examine their attitudes to complementary medicine and their current usage of it.[37] This found that approximately 70 per cent wanted complementary therapies on the NHS, mostly homeopathy, acupuncture, osteopathy, and chiropractic, which are perhaps perceived as most legitimate and useful. Aromatherapy and reflexology were mentioned, but of less interest, 'perhaps perceived as relative 'new age' therapies'. Those that did not want the therapies on the NHS were mostly concerned with what they perceived was a lack of proven effectiveness/cost-effectiveness. Most of the FHSAs and 83 per cent of the District Health Authorities were funding complementary therapies, usually on an experimental basis. The FHSAs generally were in the dark about how exactly the relationship should work. A few had agreed a policy that required a brief review of the therapies and the indications for use, recommendations about education and qualifications, where the money should come from, and the need for evaluation and audit. Many FHSAs regarded the health promotion clinics as an opportunity for complementary therapies to contribute to smoking cessation, stress management, and pain control, and most had approved such clinics, but others felt that complementary medicine was therapeutic not preventive. The main factors restricting the buying of complementary medical services were lack of information on the therapies, lack of evidence on their effectiveness, and lack of resources.

Evidently, as the report stated, the single most important factor holding back further integration of the therapies into the NHS was the lack of good quality information on effectiveness, cost-effectiveness, training, and so on. It is not that the information does not exist. The amount of research into the therapies is actually impressive and probably convincing. However it has not arrived at its destination. Does each FHSA in the country need to carry out the massive review of thousands of reports and papers, and at the same time, to fully grasp some challenging issues such as the limitations of the trusty old double-blind controlled trial, and then to understand what education and training standards are and what they mean, and so on? It is clearly up to the therapies to explain themselves to the NHS, to see the NHS in its new clothes as 'prospective purchaser' and provide it with the information it needs. In other words, as one NHS Development Officer put it, 'to market themselves pro-actively.'[38]

But it is not so easy. The reason for the hesitation is that at the present time it is hard for most therapists to know if integration is at all possible or desirable. The exceptions are modalities like chiropractic whose restricted mission would accommodate them to the role of an NHS service, and are keen to be employed in that way. The problem is that the NHS, as the employer, sets the agenda, and does not feel the need to change its entire way of operating to adapt to the few therapists it tentatively employs. There are some deep differences that leave guests dancing at two weddings, not one. These arise from the essential nature of the therapies, as defined in Chapter 1. For example, insofar as the therapies attempt a more radical and deeper cure, they will require far more time and contact than the NHS is accustomed to or will pay for. Moreover, as the therapies invoke self-healing, they attempt to empower the patient to heal himself, for example by lifestyle measures and attitude changes; whereas the NHS sees itself as providing a repair service which disempowers patients. Untreated cases are left hoping for the next miracle drug rather than girding their loins for the healing journey. So expectations are as far apart as methods, and they prevent doctor and therapist from working together, and often from talking together.

Examples of complementary medicine in primary care

The experiment at the Liverpool Centre for Health, a complementary health centre set up by Liverpool FHSA as a service to local GPs, is a good example. The therapists were at first very pleased to be part of an integrated system, receiving referrals from doctors and treating patients, some of whom had serious and complex conditions that they would not often see. But there were some big disappointments in store:[39]

- The doctors failed to discuss cases with the therapists or even send sufficient referral data. They had minimal contact or dialogue with the centre, which felt depressingly marginalized: 'as if the debate about complementary medicine could be dealt with by employing therapists, whereas the therapists saw it as the starting point of the debate.'[39]

- Doctors sent over (less politely: dumped) their chronic and failed cases, rather than acute and easily treatable cases. In consequence the entire service was taken up with lengthy treatment of few cases. The FHSA however did not appreciate the reasons for the log-jam, and continued to evaluate the service on the usual basis of patient throughput. There was a pressure for rapid results, which arose from a lack of understanding of the holistic nature of the therapies. In general the complementary therapists were attempting quality, the NHS was assessing quantity.

- There was a failure to respect the need for deeper contact between therapist and patient, for example, in providing the appropriate quiet facilities and ambience.

- The therapists always felt constrained by the system, for example they were unable to go beyond the contracted therapy into preventive education (such as stress reduction) which was, in their view, an essential part of therapy. In general the bureaucracy, especially the contracts, were imprisoning.

From the GPs perspective it was more positive. After only three months into the project, GPs found that the majority of the patients could have reduced drug regimes in the future, particularly analgesics, NSAIDs and antidepressants. In addition, more than half of the patients referred to the centre would otherwise have been referred to hospital out-patients.[38] In both cases, there were substantial financial savings.

Therapists are concerned that insofar as the NHS management model dominates complementary treatment, patients may come to see it as little different from their GP clinic. A revolving door—quick in and quick out. However from the patient's perspective, things were not so bad at Liverpool. He or she internalizes both systems, and is dancing at only one wedding. Patients were pleasantly surprised and very satisfied with the complementary treatment, the only problem being that there was never enough of it. The quality of life questionnaires (SF 36) that the patients filled out revealed extremely positive results, especially in the categories of pain, mental health, energy, change in health perceptions, and in general health. As an acupuncturist in another FHSA pilot study reported, patients learn to get the best from both worlds. Chronic 'failed' arthritis cases sent for treatment by the GP experienced a deeper sense of well-being that is, from the holistic perspective, the beginning of the journey back to health, but was of little interest or importance to the doctor. Therefore they began to talk in two languages.

'When questioned by the doctor they would describe improvements in the symptoms for which they had been "officially" referred to the acupuncture clinic. In the acupuncture clinic they would report qualitative changes, e.g. "I feel like my real self again".'

Since to the doctor, the qualitative, non-specific changes were unimportant,

'patients sometimes invented fictitious quantitative changes to ensure continued access to treatment.'[40]

This says it all. Doctors and therapists are eyeing each other warily from both sides of the divide, while patients are busily getting on with building bridges.

There is a small but growing collection of reports of how complementary therapists get on within an NHS general practice, and some major MRC-funded studies on the issue are in the pipeline. They generally reflect the problems and opportunities outlined above. Therapists often say how pleased they are to see different kinds of patients from those in private complementary practice—an older age range, more serious conditions, and generally of lower socio-economic status. It is clear that if free on the NHS, complementary medicine would be tried by many more people than can now afford it.[41] All therapists are faced with a potentially infinite demand and long waiting lists, and yet are referred patients with late-stage chronic diseases who need lengthy treatment, which delays treatment for others with more recent or acute problems who would respond more quickly.

Some of the problems described above can be gradually solved through daily contact between therapists and doctors who begin to understand the way the therapists work, and, for example, resist the temptation to refer only the difficult cases.[41] Workshops and intensive dialogues between doctors and therapists would be an excellent way of developing that rare faculty: the wisdom to be able to see what the world looks like from the other party's perspective.[42] A good model is that of the Lewisham Hospital NHS Trust Complementary Therapy Centre. This benefited from four years of preparatory training and workshops, in which complementary therapies became familiar to medical staff. The success of this project lies in the specific referral guidelines which were established through intensive dialogue between doctors and therapists, and continually revised taking into account outcomes. Practitioners utilized an established computer system to monitor practice, which records clinical information, summaries, outcomes, assessments, and audit, and this greatly aids evaluation.[43]

As discussed in the previous chapter, it would be very positive to include classes in complementary health education, such as diet, yoga, relaxation, and other self-care approaches, within NHS primary health care settings. This is an essential part of holistic health care, and one of the most effective and inexpensive ways of improving health. Yet there is little effort to formally encourage self-care even within complementary NHS practices, and little effort to set up evaluations. Even the conventional NHS health promotion campaigns, concerned with smoking, obesity, and exercise, have been cut back. One well-known example of the use of holistic self-care instruction within an NHS practice is the Marylebone Health Centre, part of the Department of General Practice of St Mary's Hospital Medical School. Here patients are referred by therapists or doctors for classes within the centre on relaxation, stress education, diet, and meditation. The results, which have been monitored, are improved health awareness and reduced medication for the patients, with half reporting that their symptoms were much or somewhat improved. There were spin-offs—the staff too felt better and it even helped the ambience in the centre.[44]

Complementary medicine in secondary care

Complementary therapies are trickling into hospitals too. Some from the top down, from specialists employing osteopaths in orthopaedic clinics, acupuncturists in pain clinics, and hypnotherapists working with anaesthesiologists. This has been going on for some time, but there is now a greater readiness to employ lay therapists. Again there is a strong commercial motive here, for lay therapists are more cost-effective. Take the example of irritable bowel syndrome (IBS). Studies have shown that even with chronic intractable IBS, most patients could be substantially cured by hypnotherapy. A lay hypnotherapist achieved as successful an outcome as the gastroenterologist but at much less cost.[45]

Most complementary medicine enters secondary care from the bottom up, brought in by nurses. Many nurses have shown great interest in complementary medicine, partly because they, rather than doctors, supervise patients' healing and recovery yet have frustratingly little influence upon it. Nurses have generally been keen to extend their professional boundaries and complementary medicine gives nurses an opportunity to do so in a peaceful, harmless, and holistic manner. Indeed there is a considerable overlap between the holistic, patient-centred approach of complementary medicine, and the central concepts of patient care in nursing.[46] And many nurses find in complementary medicine an antidote to the lack of caring and coldness of modern technological medicine. Over 2000 nurses have joined the Royal College of Nursing Special Interest Group on Complementary Therapies. There have been some very promising trials of complementary nursing, for example within holistic cancer care.[47] Nurses report that the quality of their care increases, and patients feel better and are less stressed.[48] Generally, nurses have found that the most suitable therapies are those which are adjunctive, palliative, or restorative, which include touch, and which are intended to restore the general well-being of the patient. These are massage, reflexology, aromatherapy, and healing (therapeutic touch).[49] Specific studies on the outcome of using these therapies as part of nursing care are discussed in the relevant therapy chapters (especially Chapter 16 p. 221). Many nurses feel that these therapies have given them a genuine healing craft for the first time, and their heartfelt enthusiasm may make nursing the main profession within the NHS to bring the therapies into the heart of modern medicine.[50] It has also given the nurses themselves a way to stop 'doing good while feeling bad'; the new Holistic Nurses Association in the UK concentrates particularly on the way that complementary medicine can help to recharge carers as well as patients, to

'help nurses to develop a greater sense of themselves and raise bruised and damaged selfesteem . . . an awakening into 'being' and not constantly striving to 'do'.'[51]

Nurses can be champions, and demonstrate to other health professionals how compassionate complementary medicine can be to patients and carers, and how complementary.

References

1. Stone, F. J. and Mathews, J. (1995). The effective regulation of complementary medicine. *Complementary Therapies in Medicine*, **3**, 175–8.
2. Dimond, B. (1995). Competence and indemnity in complementary medicine. *Complementary Therapies in Medicine*, **3**, 28–31.
3. Editorial (1985). Lords debate alternatives: no action until BMA report. *Journal of Alternative Medicine*, **3**(4), 2. Baer, H. A., (1984). The drive for professionalism in British osteopathy. *Social Science and Medicine*, **19**, 717–25.
4. Trumpington, The Baroness (1987). Alternative medicines and therapies and the DHSS. *Journal of the Royal Society of Medicine*, **80**, 336–8.
5. Fletcher-Hyde, F. (1978). The origin and practice of herbal medicine. *MIMS Magazine*, **2**, 127–36.
6. King's Fund Centre (1991). *Report on the Working Party on Osteopathy*. King's Fund Centre, London.
7. Standen, C. S. (1993). The implications of the Osteopaths Act. *Complementary Therapies in Medicine*, **1**, 208–10.
8. Maxwell, R. J. (1993). The Osteopaths Bill. *British Medical Journal*, **306**, 1556–7.
9. King's Fund Centre (1993). *Report of Working Party on chiropractic*. King's Fund Centre, London.
10. *Official Journal of the European Communities* (9/2/1987). No C 31/63.
11. *Official Journal of the European Communities* (12/6/1989). No C 145/15.
12. *Official Journal of the European Communities* (23/10/1990). No. C 267/9.
13. Clover, A., Last, P., Fisher, P., Wright, S., and Boyle, H. (1995). Complementary cancer therapy: a pilot study of patients, therapies and quality of life. *Complementary Therapies in Medicine*, **3**, 129–33.
14. Meeting of the Medicine Division of the Liverpool Area Health Authority Central District, March 1977.
15. House of Commons Adjournment Debate. 7 April 1977.
16. Asher, R. (1956). Respectable Hypnosis. *British Medical Journal*, **1**, 309–13.
17. *Hansard*. Hypnotism Bill. 20 November 1979, Column 54.
18. Morton, J. *et al.* (1995). *Recovered memories: report of the Working Party of the British Psychological Society*, London. Weiskrantz, L. (1995). Comments on the report of the Working Party of the British Psychological Society. *Therapist*, **2**, 5–8.
19. *Hansard*. 16 December 1977, Column 1174.
20. *Hansard*. 19 February 1980.
21. Anon. (1990). Threat still exists for Londoners. *Journal of Complementary and Alternative Medicine*, **8**, 12.
22. Ministry of Agriculture Fisheries and Foods/ Department of Health (1991). *Dietary Supplements and Health Foods*. HMSO, London.
23. The Medicines (Prescription Only) Order 1977, No. 2127; The Medicines Act 1968 Order 1977, No. 2128; The Medicines (Supply of Herbal Remedies) Order 1977, No. 2130; The Medicines (General Sale List) Order 1977, No. 2129.
24. Fulder, S.J. (1986). Ineffective herbal remedies in the UK market. *Journal of Alternative Medicine*, (February 1986). 4–5.

25. The Medicines for Human Use (Market Authorisations, Pharmacovigilance and Related Matters) Regulations 1994. Statutory Instrument SI 3144. The package of EU legislation consists of Regulation 2309/93, Directive 93/41/EEC and 93/93/EEC (which amends 65/65/EEC, 75/318/EEC, 75/319/EEC).
26. *Daily Telegraph*. 7 November 1994, p.12.
27. *Hansard*, **250**, 29 November 1994, 538–40.
28. *Hansard*, **249**, 11 November 1994. *Hansard*, **250**, 21 November 1994 p.26.
29. Perharic, I., et al. (1994). Toxicological problems resulting from exposure to traditional remedies and food supplements. *Drug Safety*, 11, 284–94. Atherton, D. J. (1994). Towards the safer use of traditional remedies. *British Medical Journal*, **308**, 673–4.
30. Physician heal thyself. *The Times*, 10 August 1983.
31. British Medical Association (BMA). 16 August 1983.
32. Board of Science and Education (1986). *Alternative therapies*. British Medical Association, London.
33. Editorial (1986). Pressure grows in parliament. *Journal of Alternative Medicine*, 4, (7), 1.
34. Press Release, Department of Health, 3 December 1991. *Hansard*, **200**, 3 December 1991.
35. Hill, R. and Gould, A. (1995). *Complementary medicine: its practice in the Health Service*, submitted.
36. Pietroni, P. (1992). Beyond the boundaries: relationship between general practice and complementary medicine. *British Medical Journal*, **305**, 564–6.
37. Cameron-Blackie, G. (1993). *Complementary therapies in the NHS*. National Association of Health Authorities, Birmingham.
38. Whelan, J. (1995). Complementary therapies and the changing NHS: a development officer's view. *Complementary Therapies in Medicine*, 3, 79–83.
39. Donnelly, D. (1995). Integrating complementary medicine within the NHS: a therapist's view of the Liverpool Centre for Health. *Complementary Therapies in Medicine*, 3, 84–7.
40. Moore, C. (1995). A clash of cultures. *Journal of Alternative and Complementary Medicine*, 13, 24–5.
41. Budd, C., Fisher, B., Parrinder, D., and Price, L. (1990). A model of co-operation between complementary and allopathic medicine in a primary care setting. *British Journal of General Practice*, 40, 376–8.
42. Swayne, J. (1995). Homeopathy in the NHS: a holistic and interprofessional challenge. *Journal of Interprofessional Care*, 9, 53–9.
43. Richardson, J. (1995). Complementary therapies on the NHS: the experience of a new service. *Complementary Therapies in Medicine*, 3, 153–7.
44. Pietroni, P., McLean, J., and Walton, N. G. (1987). A self-care programme in general practice: a feasibility study. *The Practitioner*, 231, 1226–30.
45. Taylor, E. E. and Whorwell, P. J. (1993). Cost effective provision of hypnotherapy in a hospital setting. *British Journal of Medical Economics*, 6, 75–9.
46. Rankin-Box, D. (1993). Innovation in practice: complementary therapies in nursing. *Complementary Therapies in Medicine*, 1, 30–3.
47. Burke, C. and Sikora, K. (1992). Cancer—the dual approach. *Nursing Times*, 88, 62–6.
48. Tattam, A. (1992). The gentle touch. *Nursing Times*, 88, 16–17.
49. Stevenson, C. (1992). Appropriate therapies for nurses to practice. *Nursing Standard*, 6, 51–2.
50. Pfeil, M. (1994). Role of nurses in promoting complementary therapies. *British Journal of Nursing*, 3, 217–19.
51. Benor, R. (1994). Holistic nursing 1. Reaching into the foundations of society. *Caduceus*, Issue 24, 10–13.

5

Complementary medicine internationally

In this chapter the social and legal positions of the therapies in several countries are reviewed. No attempt is made to give a classified and comparative survey. Instead countries have been picked out either because they are Western countries in which the status of complementary medicine is undergoing critical changes (Europe and Australia) or because their treatment of complementary medicine carries particular weight throughout the West, or because they have an ambivalent attitude to complementary medicine which it is instructive to consider (Russia), or because they have been notably successful in welding traditional and modern medicine together and so exemplify solutions to the perennial problem of incompatibility between the systems (China and India).

The United States

The legal, social, and political situation of complementary medicine in the USA is exceedingly complex and volatile, with each state deciding its own independent policy, and with sets of definitions which may be unfamiliar to Europeans.[1] In most cases these describe complementary medical techniques as the practice of medicine, which is proscribed to non-physicians under various Medical Practice Acts. However, in each therapy there are some states that have introduced some kind of regulatory or licensing arrangements. Chiropractic has won universal recognition only after a hard and bitter fight which culminated in hair-raising court actions leading to the Supreme Court finding the American Medical Association guilty of criminal conspiracy. Today doctors are obliged to refer to and receive referrals from chiropractors. Many states only allow acupuncture practice by physicians. In some cases physicians are required to demonstrate some acupuncture training or even a licence. Other states (for example, Massachusetts) only permit lay practitioners to practise under medical supervision and of these a few states (for example, Washington) require them to have a licence as well. Many states do allow the independent practice of acupuncture by lay therapists, but in every case only after a recognized course of training and an examination. The new New York State Alternative Medical Practice Act recognizes all the therapies and supports freedom of choice in health care. Naturopathic medicine is now recognized and licenced in 10 states.

Since the publication in 1993 of data showing that one third of the US population use some kind of alternative health care annually, at an out-of-pocket cost of nearly $14 billion,[2] there has been rapid development of research on alternative medicine. The National Institutes of Health opened an Office of Alternative Medicine, with a $7 million budget to explore areas such as the effectiveness of acupuncture in asthma, and naturopathic treatment of AIDS. The legitimization implied by such a commitment has resulted in a cascade of other projects by the NIH (currently spending $13 million on 90 small studies on alternative therapies) and other agencies. Nearly half of the US's Health Maintenance Organisations (HMOs) cover chiropractic, and many private health insurers cover acupuncture and other alternatives because it is so much cheaper than high-tech medicine.[3] Medical students at Harvard and 30 other US medical schools now take courses in alternative medicine, and there are 6–8 major centres being set up for research and evaluation of the therapies such as the University of Maryland School of Medicine's major *Centre for the Integration of Orthodox and Complementary Medicine*.[4]

Western Europe

Anyone looking for consistency in the relationship between European governments and their complementary practitioners will find only a frustrating chaos. Each country has moved into the final years of the twentieth century carrying its own special brand of historic friction between medical and non-medical healing traditions. Membership of the EEC has not led to a common policy. On the other hand the use of complementary medicine in Europe has grown rapidly, and again far outstripped the capacity of policy makers, scientists, and the medical infrastructure to accommodate to it. Europe-wide, from one quarter to one half of the population now use complementary medicine at some time, and this proportion has doubled in the last 10 years.[5] The majority of the medical profession in European countries is also interested in, if not already using, complementary techniques. And the vast majority of the public, 60–80 per cent in various countries, believe it should belong to the national medical system.[5] For summaries of the European situation, see references 5 and 6.

The legal position of individual therapies in each country is summarized in Table 5.1. Countries which adhere to the Napoleonic Code (where an action is generally forbidden unless specifically permitted) have allowed complementary medicine to remain illegal except where it is practised by registered medical professionals, such as doctors or physiotherapists. However, circumstance, culture, and political

Table 5.1 The legal position of therapies in some West European countries and Scandinavia (1986)

Therapy	Denmark Scandinavia	Belgium Italy, Spain	The Netherlands	Germany, Luxembourg	France	Switzerland
Chiropractic	Legal but restrictions	Illegal	Legal: registration in process	Illegal unless also a Heilpraktiker	'Recognized' but formally illegal except in Alsace-Lorraine	Legal
Naturopathy	Legal but restrictions	Illegal	Legal: registration in process	Legal as Heilpraktiker	Illegal	Illegal except in the Canton of Appenzell
Acupuncture	Legal but restrictions	Illegal	Legal: registration in process	Illegal unless also a Heilpraktiker	Illegal but substantially taken up by doctors	Illegal except in the Canton of Appenzell
Homeopathy	Legal but restrictions	Illegal	Legal: registration in process	Illegal unless also a Heilpraktiker	Illegal but substantially taken up by doctors	Illegal except in the Canton of Appenzell
Herbalism (phytotherapy)	Legal but restrictions	Illegal	Legal: registration in process	Illegal unless also a Heilpraktiker; substantially taken up by doctors	Illegal but substantially taken up by doctors	Illegal except in the Canton of Appenzell

history have resulted in exceptions such as nature-cure in Germany or chiropractic and anthroposophy in Switzerland.

Germany

In relation to medicine, Germany is one of the most liberal countries in Western Europe. There has been a cultural trend away from the dehumanizing extremes of science ever since the German Romantic philosophy movement of the last century. Legislation has incorporated natural medicine into the state system, and it is partly covered by state medical insurance schemes. There is a strong cultural trend of therapeutic freedom, and nature-orientation in medicine. Naturopaths have been licensed as a special class of health care professionals (Heilpraktiker) since the Second World War. New Heilpraktikers were forbidden to practise by the Nazi government but the edict was repealed in 1956. Today the Heilpraktikers, who are basically nature cure/hydrotherapy practitioners, are trained in accredited colleges and granted a state licence after examination. Acupuncture, homeopathy, herbalism (phytotherapy), chiropractic, etc., thrive under the banner of Heilpraktik. Any practitioner may use these therapies without restriction provided he first trains as a Heilpraktiker.

There is no easy way in for doctors. If they wish to be Heilpraktikers they must also obtain the qualification. But alternative medicine is now taught at universities, for example acupuncture is taught at the Universities of München, Giessen, and Düsseldorf. Six to eight thousand doctors have taken these courses and now practise acupuncture. In addition many more doctors explore complementary therapies within their conventional medical practice without being Heilpraktikers. Indeed herbal and homeopathic remedies are so much part of the average German doctor's armamentorum that a recent survey found that 95 per cent of German doctors used them. Nearly all doctors also believed that complementary medicine should be integrated within national medicine. The study confirmed the demand by showing that patients were more interested in receiving complementary treatments than their doctors were to provide them.[7] All medical undergraduates in Germany are now obliged to learn something about complementary medicine. There is one large homeopathic hospital and several homeopathic sanatoria. Medical homeopathy in the land of homeopathy's foundation flourishes and is certainly much stronger than in the UK.

A powerful nature-cure organization, the Kneipp system, organized by medically qualified practitioners, flourishes in Germany. These doctors have set up a national health and therapy movement, based on the teaching of Father Sebastian Kneipp over a century ago. This movement is basically a spa-orientated mixture of water, exercise, and diet cures. It is large indeed. Its main spa is a virtual hydrotherapy town. Bad Worishoesen has about 50 Kneipp doctors, 80 masseurs, and 120 trained bath attendants.

Herbalism, or phytotherapy, is also much stronger in Germany than in the UK. Most pharmacists have displays of natural product remedies which rival those of conventional drugs. Germany is the centre of the international herb trade, and the main traditional source of herbal teas and tisanes. The German market for natural remedies is over \$2 billion, 10 per cent of the total pharmaceutical market and far more than any other country in Europe.[8] The Federal Health Office has relaxed its strict pharmaceutical registration laws. Committees on anthroposophical, herbal, and homeopathic remedies include practitioners as members, and have been working to establish monographs for all remedies which form the basis for market authorizations. The herbal monographs of Kommission E have become world-famous as authoritative guidelines on quality, safety, and efficacy of over 300 herbs.[6] Research into complementary medicine has developed by request of the German parliament. The Federal Ministry of Research and Technology is making a serious commitment to upgrade the level of research in alternative medicine, and a unit at the University of Witten/Herdecke has acted as a resource and information centre, a kind of RCCM with state support, to prepare the ground and suggest strategies.[9]

France

France does not have authorized exceptions to the rules against non-medical practitioners, and alternative medicine remains firmly in the hands of the medical profession, which is strongly organized to resist any lay practitioners daring to invade their patch. Nevertheless the law is widely flouted, giving support to the view that the Napoleonic Law provides an ideal to be attained or a contest to be won, rather than a commonsense boundary. Chiropractic, especially, is in a very strange position of Gallic indeterminacy. Thirteen per cent of the French population go to chiropractors, and they are reimbursed by the state social security and private insurance schemes. Despite this de facto recognition, chiropractic remains illegal.

The law has deterred laymen from careers in complementary medicine, and there are no accredited courses for lay students in French tertiary education institutions, thus leaving it open for French doctors to add a good deal of complementary medicine to their exclusive domain. Almost half of all doctors practise some form of complementary medicine. The medical profession in France are determined. On the one hand this has helped the practice of complementary therapies because, unlike the USA, they have retained the purity and independence of the therapies and taken their principles seriously. On the other hand those that are against these therapies are not above taking their colleagues to the disciplinary committees, for example for prescribing natural remedies to seriously ill patients.[10]

Acupuncture was brought to the West by the French, 10 000 doctors are trained in it, and it has been practised widely in France in hospitals and clinics for almost 50 years.[11] A brand new hospital devoted exclusively to Chinese medicine has just opened.[12] The international acupuncture body (SIA) was started in France by Dr J. Schatz, who is a major figure in the development of acupuncture in the

West on rational yet traditional lines. Acupuncture too is reimbursed by the state social security system if it is performed by doctors. Doctors also practise extensively in phytotherapy and homeopathy. Five thousand doctors prescribe homeopathic remedies, many times more than in the UK.[10] Four schools train 1000 doctors a year in established three-year courses. There is a section on homeopathic remedies in the French pharmacopoeia. Almost every pharmacy is stocked with homeopathic remedies which are manufactured on a large scale by three pharmaceutical companies. Homeopathic prescriptions qualify alongside conventional ones for a state subsidy of 70 per cent of their price, and they are used by one in six of the population. Only the esoteric therapies, healing, and radionics, are rare compared with the UK.

The French spend extravagantly on health. Their health services cost some eight per cent of the Gross National Product, which is two per cent more than in the UK. Alternative medicine in France is part of living well, going with the ubiquitous herbal teas, and the serious attention to fitness programmes. But it remains ransomed to a monolithic medical profession.

The Netherlands

During the 1960s, a runaway public campaign for freedom of choice in medicine, made clear to the Government the anomaly of the promotion of natural health in a society that bans natural medicine. The Ministry of Health took their views seriously, and a 1970 State Commission on Medical Practice took the unprecedented step of recommending that only where public health was at risk should the unqualified be prevented from practising. This led to the drafting of a new Individual Health Care Occupations Bill, in 1977, which embodies this so-called 'Scandinavian' option. Wisely, the Secretary of State for Health wished to understand fully the social, legal, practical, and political dimensions of complementary medicine before actually putting the bill before Parliament. In 1977, the State Secretary for Health set up a Commission for Alternative Systems of Medicine. Its task was to investigate the significance of alternative medicine in The Netherlands and make recommendations to the Government on the basis of its findings.

Dutch law, as in all the European countries, stated that only qualified doctors were permitted to practise medicine, giving them effective monopoly. Professor Muntendam, the head of the Commission, pointed out in his introduction to the report that:

The consensus of public opinion is no longer behind the monopoly, and the law is broken a thousand times a day as sick and disabled people seek the help of people who are not legally authorized to provide it.[13]

Naturally, the medical profession was opposed to the Commission. It attempted to keep the monopoly by the argument that the therapies were not scientifically proven. The Health Minister boldly stated that the argument was not good enough;

that the public demand for freedom of choice in medicine was more important in generating new laws than scientific verification.

The Commission's report was comprehensive and powerful, reviewing subculture and mainstream literature, and incorporating legal, international, scientific, sociological, and statistical research.[13] No government has ever made such a comprehensive attempt to understand the practice of complementary medicine. Its basic conclusion was that: 'alternative medicine is such an important factor in health care in The Netherlands, that government policy cannot disregard it'. Accordingly, the Commission advised the Health Ministry specifically to include trained practitioners of complementary medicine as one of the qualified classes of health professionals defined in the 1977 bill. The report suggested state-sponsored courses in basic medicine for these practitioners to reduce any potential public risks. It saw expansion of training as the key to the successful integration of complementary medicine. As in the UK it proposes self-regulation by each profession, and strongly exhorted the squabbling complementary organizations to unify for this purpose.

It is taking a very long time to implement the recommendations of the Commission, and there are many problems still to be solved. The Health Council, which advised the Government on scientific aspects of alternative medicine, took 10 years to report! However finally the new Individual Health Care Professions Act (B.I.G.) is in place and allows freedom for lay practitioners and statutorily recognized registers, much like in the UK. The Government has instituted courses for complementary practitioners in tertiary educational institutions.[14]

The rest of Europe and Scandinavia

Of the other European countries, Belgium, Italy, and Spain tend to follow the French pattern, with Belgium the most conservative. In 1973, the complementary therapy world was shocked by dawn police raids on the premises of 28 Brussels chiropractors (it is said that the policemen who posted the closure notices arrived later for their usual treatment). Most of the Belgian practitioners in complementary medicine are doctors, who even now sometimes come into conflict with their colleagues on that account. Osteopathy is in the hands of physiotherapists and lay practitioners. Some 50 per cent of the population report going to homeopaths, the highest rate in Europe.[5] The Belgian Consumers Association found alternative medicine as popular in Belgium as elsewhere in Europe, with patients more satisfied with it than with doctors' treatment, but there is an enormous gulf between popular wish and state policy, which is controlled by the medical profession. Thus despite 80 per cent of the population wanting alternative medicine to be freely available within state medicine, at present no alternative medical expenses are reimbursable by the state social security system, even if a doctor carries them out. In practice doctors usually can obtain reimbursement by not specifying the actual treatment.[15]

Some Scandinavian countries, particularly Denmark and Sweden, have licensed lay practitioners and offer training at tertiary institutions, although there are certain forbidden areas, for example surgery, obstetrics, and anaesthesia. Denmark has, like Germany, the liberal principle that citizens are entitled to seek help freely.[16] Denmark has invested heavily in research, for example, the University of Odense, where much of this research has centred, has set up the International Network for Research on Alternative Therapies (INRAT) which specializes in the fascinating cultural and anthropological dimensions of the shift to alternative paradigms. Since 1975, Finland has included acupuncture as a standard part of its medical curriculum following the Soviet model, but it is mostly practised by doctors. In most of Scandinavia, chiropractic fees are partially reimbursed, in many cases without prior medical referral.

The EEC and complementary medicine

Britain's entry into the Common Market caused widespread alarm in the complementary medicine movement. The main fear, of course, was that the UK common law right would disappear under EEC harmonization plans. However this is not a threat to UK practitioners because health care is outside the Treaty of Rome, and thus the EU cannot harmonize medical practice legislation of member countries. It has merely restricted itself to requiring minimum education for diplomas of recognized professionals (see p.76). At the same time, herbalists of the UK and France, and the Heilpraktikers of Germany were worried that the special consideration won by herbalists and homeopaths would be lost under EU harmonization of medicines licencing, and this very nearly happened (see p. 85). Here we will present the EU position on general issues.

In the 1970s, the European Commission had said that they were not in any position to recognize any alternative profession, but that if it were to occur, it would be based on the Heilpraktikers in Germany, being the only profession whose training was formally accepted at that time by an EEC government. The matter surfaced briefly again in 1979 in the European Parliament. A question was put forward by French chiropractors who said that since their profession was still illegal in France, but not in certain other member states, they were discriminated against within the EEC.[17] The EEC's answer, predictably, was that as no harmonization of laws had occurred, member states were free to pursue their own policies; in those countries where chiropractic is legal, there should be no discrimination against chiropractors from any other member states. In those states where it was illegal, the law would apply to all nationals anyway.

In 1984, the Council of Europe issued a Directive on alternative medicine.[18] Its basic position is favourable to non-conventional medicine (which it found impossible to define):

'In view of the frequency with which sick people nowadays seek help from non-conventional practitioners, this phenomenon can no longer be regarded as a medical side-issue, it must reflect a genuine public need.'

The Directive requests member states to reimburse complementary medicine within each country's social security system:

'The emancipation of patients is resulting in the patient's right to choose the therapy and the therapist he considers best, and also the right to receive this health care on the same financial conditions as any other medical care.'

This appears to go beyond the issue of freedom of choice in medicine. However it is a statement of principles not law, and it has not been translated into legislation. Further it does not express any support for lay therapists, falling back on the conventional line that 'only those in general medical practice' (which is not defined) should be allowed to provide medical services under each state's social security system. Therapists at the time were justifiably nervous about moves that encourage more patients to consult them, but limit their freedom to treat these patients when they arrive.

In the intervening years, all European institutions, including the European Commission and the European Parliament held the non-interference policy in the way member states related to complementary medicine.[19] For example, the European Court of Justice in 1990 did not support the case of a French lay osteopath who was taken to court for illegal practice of medicine:

'In the absence of harmonisation at the Community level in relation to activities relating solely to the practice of medicine, Article 52 of the EEC Treaty does not preclude a member state from reserving a paramedical activity, such as, in particular, osteopathy, exclusively to those holding the qualification of Doctor of Medicine.'[20]

However there are interesting European initiatives in research that might bear fruit in the future, in particular the Committee for Science and Technology (COST) B4 project on unconventional/complementary medicine. It is a project to collect, assess, and encourage research in member nations, on

'the therapeutic significance of unconventional medicine, its cost-benefit ratio and its sociocultural importance as a basis for the evaluation of its possible usefulness or risks in public health'.

There appears to be a strong interest among administrators to check whether the therapies can indeed help to cut healthcare costs.

In April 1994, the Committee on the Environment, Public Health and Consumer Protection of the European parliament adopted a proposal put forward by the Belgian MEP Paul Lannoye. This repeated the call for complementary medicine to be freely available under all national social security systems, requested herbal remedies to be put back in the European Pharmacopoeia, and a research fund of $12 million per year for five years. It also called for European registration of all lay therapists using the registration of osteopaths in the UK as a model. The report was to have been debated in the whole European Parliament, but was blocked by 52 MEPs mostly French. It may well come up again, and if there is support and lobbying from the therapy world, succeed, in which case it would lead to watershed legislative changes throughout Europe.

Russia and Eastern Europe

Russia encompasses a diverse conglomerate of peoples: the Mongolians, the Siberian tribes, the Europeanized Slavs, and the Turko-Tartar Moslems of the south. Its medicine reflects this: it is a bizarre jumble of the unfulfilled intentions of central government and the unfulfilled desires of its constituent peoples. Like China, there are a large number of physicians and a system of rural paramedical health workers (Feldshers) to deal with primary care and preventive medicine. However, despite sophisticated centres of excellence in the major cities, conventional medicine is starved of resources. Drug supplies cover only about 20 per cent of patient needs and equipment is old and overloaded. Lifespan is going down and is now 10–14 years lower and infant mortality is double that of the West.[21]

All this leaves considerable scope for alternatives, and doctors are becoming increasingly interested in natural, low-cost, non-drug therapies, not so much because of the holistic vision but more from the practical concerns of delivery of primary health care in difficult circumstances.[22] Legally, only doctors are allowed to practise alternative medicine, such as acupuncture, to treat disease. There are departments for 'reflexotherapy' (Soviet style reflexology), acupuncture, and manual therapies, including massage, at medical colleges, where doctors and paramedics can learn. Lay therapists are allowed to practise under a general rubric of 'promotion of health', and there are schools to train lay therapists in the collectives and the cities. The organization of the therapies into professions is minimal.[22]

Traditional medicine is present in rural areas of Russia to an extent unparalleled in any Western country. Cupping, plasters, herbalism, and so on are regularly available, supplied by part-time, rural practitioners. Visits to spas are a national pastime. While the average British worker is enjoying an indulgent holiday in Blackpool or Palma Majorca, the Russian worker takes his break at a health spa on the Black Sea. One can still find strongly regional practices. The Mongols, who introduced yoghurt to the West, are still practising their version of Indo-Tibetan medicine and supplying 'Kumiss' (mare's-milk) cures to the chronically sick. Siberian semi-shamanistic folk medicine and the Arabic-Hippocratic Moslem medicine of Turkestan are thriving. Healers practise widely, treating even top officials. There is research into subtle energy phenomenon at some of the top research centres in the land, which has bemused many visiting scientists.[23]

In Eastern Europe there is also a rich herbal and natural medicine tradition. Bulgaria is the foremost exporter of herbs, and family medical chests are invariably herbal. UNESCO has its phytochemistry centre in Sofia. As in Russia, healing and parapsychology are demystified and secularized. The Sofia Institute of

Parapsychology and Suggestion Research is part of the university and teaches degree courses. There and at other places research is continuing on altered states of consciousness, healing, hypnosis, and yoga. Hypnosis has been shown to heal wounds more quickly, and as a result it is practised in sanatoria and neurological clinics all over the country.[24] Astonished journalists have even witnessed Bulgarian customs officers meditating over baggage to detect drugs by extra-sensory perception!

Legally, complementary medicine was not encouraged or prohibited. Although under the communist regimes homeopathy was illegal, that has now been lifted and homeopaths as well as other therapists are allowed to practise freely whether medically qualified or not. On the other hand in today's free-market climate, Eastern Europe, like Russia, has seen a tidal wave of quackery and charlatanism, without cultural or legal consumer protection. Most East European countries have a state medicine which lies some way between the hard official line of Russia and the open traditionalist attitude of Bulgaria. The future may see complementary medicine gaining strength in all Soviet bloc countries, both because of entry into the laboratories and because it takes the pressure off their overburdened medical systems.

Australia, New Zealand, and South Africa

'Back to it' ran the heading of a medical journal editorial on chiropractic and the medical profession.[25] The 'it' was the 'chiropractic problems' that the New Zealand Medical Association was having, arising from a thorough and now classical report of a Government commission of inquiry into chiropractic that recommended registration of chiropractors.[26] The chiropractors were registered, and so were the osteopaths; Australia, New Zealand, and South Africa became the first countries to formally register alternative therapists and establish formal education schemes, and acted as a precedent for other countries, in particular Britain, to follow.

Complementary therapies in Australia are enjoying a boom as great as in the UK and there are more consultations in relation to population than in the UK. For example the number of acupuncture clinics in one Australian city, Brisbane, rose from around 30 to around 200 in the years 1974–1988. This is partly because acupuncture was available free under the official Medibank insurance scheme.[27] There are now some 8000 practitioners on the register of the Federation of Natural Therapeutics. There are now some eight colleges training naturopaths (the general term used in Australia to cover alternative practitioners) and four of them have over 1000 students studying at any one time. Colleges train so many natural therapists that certain areas, such as Sydney, are already saturated.

Until various state Medical Acts were passed, complementary practitioners were free to practise in Australia under a common law right similar to that of the UK. However the medical profession were highly aggressive, and went as far as inducing patients to bring malpractice actions against complementary practitioners. In 1974, a committee was established by the Ministry of Health in response to the wide public usage of chiropractic. The Committee was adamant that chiropractic was a paramedical or auxiliary skill, filling a hole in modern health care, but not a system of therapy in its own right. It therefore recommended that chiropractic and osteopathy should be registered in each state by means of a Manipulative Therapists (Chiropractors and Osteopaths) Act, but not as alternative health systems. A registration board should be set up to supervise standards, ethics, and education. Existing practitioners should be registered providing they had sufficient past experience, and took a test of competence and an up-dating course. As far as education was concerned the Committee recommended that there should be a system of accreditation of colleges, and that a new four-year bachelor course in chiropractic and osteopathy at a tertiary institution in Australia would provide a standard qualification against which other attainments could be measured.[28] All of this has now happened. Australia became the first country to teach chiropractic at university level.[29]

The report regarded other complementary therapies very differently. The Committee described naturopathy as a 'minor cult system' and rejected herbalism in extraordinarily uncompromising terms, pronouncing that the pharmaceutical industry already knew all the plant chemicals of interest. The other therapists, grouped by the Government into Oriental medicine (acupuncture, Oriental herbalism), and naturopathy (the category for all the other therapies including homeopathy and herbalism) remain outside the law, though tolerated, apart from regulations relating to sterilization of needles and certain medical conditions such as cancer which may not be treated. However, the situation is very fluid. A major enquiry conducted by the Social Development Committee of the Victorian Parliament was sympathetic to the other therapies. It stopped short of recommending registration, as it feared the creation of 'self-centred and self-selected pressure groups', but encouraged accreditation.[30] Courses in acupuncture are now available at universities such as the University of New England. Various colleges have official accreditation of their diploma courses in everything from aromatherapy to Traditional Chinese Medicine. Medical insurance organizations are paying rebates for manipulative, naturopathic, and acupuncture therapies from selected colleges, but Medicare only reimburses chiropractic and osteopathic fees, as they are state registered. The Attorney General recently announced that natural therapists would be able to provide sick leave certificates, at which the Australian Medical Association reacted with charming forthrightness:

You might as well go to the hairdressers to get a sick leave certificate . . . This is a short-sighted knee-jerk response to the pandering of star-gazing public servants.[31]

Another interesting piece of legislation was born out of the State of Victoria's suggestions: the Therapeutic Goods Act. This Act sets up a licencing system for traditional remedies based on the advice of a Traditional Medicines Evaluation Committee which has among its members two herbal practitioners and two representatives of herbal manufacturers. The Evaluation Committee draws up monographs based both on traditional usage and research studies, and the licences are based on these monographs. Practitioner-only remedies are allowed to be handled by certified practitioners. The natural therapists have established a minimal standard of education, accepted by the Therapeutic Goods Administration, which allows them to prescribe practitioner-only remedies. The Thereapeutic Goods Act is a form of recognition of the value and uniqueness of natural remedies that European herbalists would love to bring to Europe.

Complementary medicine in New Zealand has developed in a similar fashion to complementary medicine in Australia. With the exception of chiropractors and osteopaths who are registered as medical auxiliaries in the manner of physiotherapists, complementary practitioners operate under common law but outside the statute book. Accreditation of courses is in place, and some complementary medicine is even taught in medical schools.

South Africa has also regularized complementary medicine in a set of laws that therapists regard as a mixed blessing. Act 63 of 1982 incorporates all complementary practitioners into a register supervised by the South Africa Associated Health Service Professions Board. This register has the same status as, and is independent of, the General Medical Council supervising the conventional medical profession. The register requires practitioners to be trained in a six-year university level course in alternative medicine, which runs parallel to the medical school course except that it replaces drug and surgical treatment in the later stages of the course, with naturopathy/manipulative methods or herbs/homeopathy. Some complementary practitioners were pleased with the new legalization. To others it was a disaster, and the profession was reduced from 3000 practitioners to 600 more or less overnight. One of the main problems is that they are not allowed to perform acts outside their defined profession. This encourages an unhealthy specialization which runs contrary to the natural eclecticism of complementary medicine; for example, it prevents a naturopath also prescribing homeopathic remedies where appropriate.[32]

Traditional and indigenous medicine—its worldwide fate

Third World countries

Many developing countries have only recently become aware of the fact that it is quite beyond their means to establish a sophisticated modern medical health structure, especially in rural areas. For example, the cost of maintaining 1 physician per 1000 population works out at roughly 1 per cent of the Gross National Product in the USA. In less developed countries such as Tanzania or Uganda, the cost would be around eight per cent of the Gross National Product and there is therefore very little chance of sufficient medical personnel being available to provide modern medicine for all. About 80 per cent of the world's population use traditional healing methods.

Traditional medicine is a designation that partly overlaps complementary medicine; it is usually applied to indigenous, non-conventional healing practices, including folk and village medicine. It may be primitive, like shamanism, or sophisticated like Chinese medicine. A World Health Organization (WHO) study group defined traditional medicine as:

the sum total of all the knowledge and practices, whether explicable or not, used in diagnosis, prevention and elimination of physical, mental or social imbalance, and relying exclusively on practical experience and observation handed down from generation to generation, whether verbally or in writing.

It continued:

The essential differences among various systems of medicine arise not from the difference in goal or effects, but rather from the cultures of the peoples who practise the different systems.[33]

Immersed in traditional culture, traditional medicine shares its changing fortunes.

Traditional medicine is not a panacea; among its collection of remedies and practices some are ineffective and even harmful, as in all medical systems. However there is now evidence that traditional healers have been unfairly blamed by doctors for supposed herbal toxicity, and that the dangers of inappropriate use of modern drugs are far greater.[34] It is also the case that traditional medicine is often overwhelmed by epidemics of infectious and contagious diseases, such as AIDS, often the result of poverty and the breakdown of the stable social milieu. Nevertheless, the effectiveness of much traditional medicine is not in doubt,[35] although there has been little research on the efficacy of traditional medicine outside of Chinese Medicine and Ayurveda. (Refer to the traditional medicine section of the Bibliography (p.275) for texts on its role and effectiveness). The value of traditional practitioners is that they are a part of a people's own health system, with the social standing necessary to reach everybody. They can readily deal with culturally based health problems arising, for example, from diet. They are acceptable and affordable. They have authority and respect. Above all, they are already there, present in the villages where they are needed, and where modern medicine is noticeably absent.

Obviously traditional practitioners can be a crucial aid to the delivery of primary health care for the majority of the world's population. For this purpose they need to be seen as a healthcare resource. This perspective is very hard for developing countries. In Africa, missionaries have for centuries branded the indigenous healers as 'witch doctors', representing a backward and even Satanic quasi-religious competition to modern Christian culture. Western development planners, the modern medical fraternity, and local officials see indigenous medicine as useless and an obstacle to progress. And there is the usual incompatibility between the languages and concepts of traditional healers and that of modern scientific medicine, which has allowed traditional medicine to be labelled by the urban western-oriented professional and middle classes as 'mumbo jumbo'. Nevertheless, it is becoming quite clear that it is impossible to do without traditional healers. Health care goals cannot be achieved by modern medicine alone. There simply is not the personnel, the facilities, or the money.

The WHO has long recognized this fact. A series of conferences led to a resolution at the 29th World Health Assembly to take into account 'the manpower reserve constituted by those practising traditional medicine'. A Working Group on Traditional Medicine was established at Geneva in 1976, and has been highly active in support of programmes to research and develop traditional medical resources. The International Conference on Primary Health Care at Alma-Ata in 1977 laid down the guidelines for the WHO policy of primary health care. It envisaged a worldwide movement of barefoot doctor or feldsher-type community health workers bringing low cost public health and first-line treatment to the villages, a reverse of the expensive, sophisticated, and inadequate medicine dispensed by specialists to the privileged few.[36]

A WHO meeting in 1977 proposed a programme to recruit traditional practitioners into primary healthcare:[33]

1. Give recognition to traditional practitioners and incorporate them into community development programmes.
2. Retrain traditional practitioners for appropriate use in primary health care.
3. Acquaint professional health personnel and students of modern systems with the principles of traditional medicine in order to promote dialogue, communication, mutual understanding, and eventual integration.
4. Educate the community to believe that the provision of traditional remedies is not second-rate medicine.
5. Catalogue all medicinal plants in a country or region and disseminate this information.
6. Retain the traditional forms for prescriptions used in primary health care and carry out relevant research into the traditional systems of medicine.

Actually, this is a top-down approach which simply has not worked. The problems are both political and cultural.[37] In many developing countries traditional medicine is excluded or illegal. Only three out of 19 African countries possess legislation for traditional medicine, while 15 do not even recognize traditional birth attendants, who are, perhaps, the spearhead of acceptable traditional medical personnel. This lack of interest in traditional medicine is usually the result of physicians' fears of loss of status and of competition for resources, or governments' fears of turning the clock back on modernization programmes.[38] Pilot collaborative programmes set up on the lines suggested by WHO in countries like Nigeria, Ghana, and Swaziland have failed or petered out for the reasons cited above, and especially because of the cultural gap between the indigenous practitioners and their magico-religious world view, and that of the modern trained professionals.[39] Then there are the patients themselves. Most prefer modern medicine if they can get it and afford it, not so much because they perceive it to be better but because it works faster and it bears the myths of comfort of the modern world. Patients may still use traditional practitioners in preference for certain health problems such as rheumatology and neurology.[40]

Traditional practitioners also have doubts about the WHO programme, arguing that it would turn them into paramedical health workers and destroy traditional medicine in the process. It is quite clear that contact with modern medicine often leads traditional practitioners hastily to abandon ancient practices in favour of fast-acting Western drugs. These bring speedy relief of symptoms and easily ensnare folk practitioners and their patients into dependence. Sulphonamides and aspirin are now used by most Third World healers. Sometimes, indeed the arrival of modern medicine creates such a cultural shock wave that in a few short years it leads to alienation and destruction of an entire sophisticated and ancient medical teaching. When this happens, as it has with Bedouin, Persian, and Eskimo medicine, reconstruction is virtually impossible.

Biomedicine is such strong medicine that integration can mean destruction. As with complementary medicine, traditional medicine thrives best and contributes most to primary health care when it is allowed to develop in parallel with biomedicine not enmeshed within it. Healers know this and have formed national associations to protect their practice in most countries. Countries which have had most success in drawing on traditional medical resources have been those in which traditional practitioners have been given a secure and independent status. For example in South Africa there are 200 000 healers, 8 times the number of doctors. They serve 80 per cent of the black population. There are basically three types: skilled herbalists, shamans, and Christian-oriented faith healers. Although there is a law against them; it is defunct, and the healers have several national associations to protect their interests. Doctors recognize their importance and effectiveness, especially in psychiatric and psychosomatic diseases. Doctors may send such patients back to their village, knowing that the traditional healers may do a better job, especially since they recruit the family and the community in a combined effort to restore the patient's health. Doctors would like to have more contact with healers, especially when they have common patients. However they are not yet ready to give healers greatly increased status, and they are worried by charlatanism. The medical view is summed up by an editorial in the *South African Medical Journal*:

'We need to know what training is required, how they actually certify themselves. Then we just have to recognise them because the are indeed part of the health care delivery system.[41]

In neighbouring Mozambique there are 80 000 healers compared with only about 350 doctors. They are already the backbone of rural health care. They should receive the respect that they deserve.

China

China can claim to have the most ancient and sophisticated medical system in the world. It stretches back at least as far as Egyptian medicine, and has been developing in an unbroken line since then. In contrast, Western medicine is the result of cycles of growth, destruction, and renaissance. The unique Chinese techniques of acupuncture, herbalism, and moxibustion have folk and shamanistic origins overlaid with Taoist and imperial theory to produce a unique, elaborate, and sensitive system of physiology, pathology, and medical skills. Chinese medicine is discussed in Chapter 6.

Western medicine entered China with the missionaries at the end of the seventeenth century. Jesuit doctors confounded and entranced the imperial court with the novelties of Western anatomy and drug treatment, a mirror image of the captivation of French doctors by the mysteries of acupuncture some 200 years later. One early Chinese emperor used to pit the wits of European, Chinese, and Tibetan doctors against each other. Another locked up Western anatomy charts as the potential dynamite that indeed they were, for by the end of the nineteenth century hospitals and Western doctors were so pervasive in the main cities of China that traditional medicine, or *Chung-i*, was on the brink of disappearing altogether. Lack of resources and communication saved it, for it persisted in the rural hinterland as the sole medical resource.

The Communist Party was originally committed to the final eradication of traditional medicine. It was seen as a superstitious feudalism, standing in the way of progress into the modern world. During the Civil War both sides relied heavily on traditional medicine, the Nationalists willingly, the Communists grudgingly. Subsequently, the Communists had to admit that traditional medicine had proved itself in the ultimate test: the epidemics, injuries, and chaos of the war. As early as 1944, Mao stated,

'to surrender to the old style is wrong; to abolish or discard is wrong. Our responsibility is to unite those of the old style that can be used, and to help, stimulate and reform them.'[42]

This was the embryonic stage of a movement 'to unite the old and the new' that Mao pursued throughout the development of the People's Republic. The cardinal principles of the Chinese health care system were defined at the First National Health Conference in Peking in 1950 as follows:

1. Medicine should serve the masses.
2. Prevention should come first.
3. Health work should utilize mass campaigns.
4. Chinese traditional and Western medicine should be integrated.

Traditional doctors were brought back into society, and the barriers of secrecy lifted. Dual clinics were set up in the countryside. Traditional doctors were included in Western hospitals and clinics, and new hospitals, colleges, and research facilities were established exclusively for traditional practitioners; finally, in the midst of the Great Leap Forward, traditional doctors were included in the Chinese Medical Association. Medical doctors were encouraged to study traditional medicine, although this was later discouraged when it was realized that this would undermine the strength of the traditional practitioner.

In fact integration was much more difficult to achieve than any of the party ideologues imagined. Western-trained doctors shirked their duties to research and upgrade traditional practices, and dumped their impossible cases on traditional practitioners. The conceptual basis of Chinese medicine proved to be completely untranslatable in scientific terms. Years after the call to integration, Chinese experts still cannot agree on whether the traditional term for 'kidney' (one of the five main viscera) corresponded to the Western anatomical kidney, the testes, or some physiological function that included both. A further step in integration happened, in a drastic way, during the Cultural Revolution. While sowing doctors in the fields along with other urban elites, the Cultural Revolution did establish the barefoot doctor programme, the most successful community health system in the world. Barefoot doctors (who are neither barefoot nor doctors) are trained paramedical health visitors who carry on medical work for one-third of their time and agriculture for the rest. They offer primary treatment, first aid, public health, preventive medicine, and family planning, and they refer more serious cases to clinics and hospitals. They carry a medicine chest of basic drugs as well as traditional herbs and acupuncture needles. In many cases they are traditional practitioners who have been retrained. They have been given most of the credit for the remarkable increase in health and life expectancy during the last 25 years in China, which now rivals any Western country. Barefoot doctors are the main inspiration for the World Health Organization's vision of community health workers bringing primary health care to the world's poor. But it may need the dictatorship of the proletariat to achieve it.

While traditional medicine remains popular today, especially in the countryside, it has taken second place to the echelons of new health workers. There is now a feeling that true integration can damage both systems, and they are essentially separate. The Chinese Medical Association does not now accept traditional practitioners, who have their own All China Association of Traditional Chinese Medicine. Thirty per cent of medical education includes traditional medicine but this proportion is not reflected in the number of doctors skilled in it. There are not many highly experienced doctors of traditional medicine in China and Taiwan. The current view is that integration is possible in the future, but it will be a much slower process than was first thought. It can occur by a gradual retraining of both physicians and practitioners at the grass roots level.[43]

All hospitals have a traditional medicine out-patient clinic, but few have proper in-patient facilities for traditional practitioners. In the Western hospitals medical doctors mostly assign serious cases to medical departments, often despite patient preference for traditional medicine. In traditional hospitals, traditional medicine is often found alongside departments which carry out surgery, radiology, ENT, obstetrics, and other modern specialties. The traditional doctors in charge of traditional in- or out-patient facilities are Western-trained doctors with a subsequent traditional training. They use traditional techniques for the less serious conditions and cases such as liver diseases, the treatment of bone disorders, kidney and gall bladder stones, acute abdominal syndromes, or cardiovascular diseases, where Chinese research or experience has shown that traditional medicine is highly effective.[44] The tandem usage of western medicine and a somewhat modernized version of traditional Oriental medicine in hospitals and health centres is also happening in countries like Vietnam.[45]

More surprising is the fact that modern scientific terminology and the classification of diseases has taken over in traditional treatment centres. Because it has been largely left to doctors and paramedical health workers to bring traditional medicine into the twentieth century the doctors have of necessity imposed their language. For example, the original Chinese pathological designations, such as hot, cold, moist, full, empty, have been universally mapped onto Western nosology, so that doctors now diagnose a condition as a hot or cold, yin or yang, version of, say, high blood pressure.

Traditional methods of increasing the health and lifespan of the individual through delicate adjustments to organ systems by means of diet and herbs, is an ancient art that is unique to Chinese medicine. Yet it has no place in the modern Chinese doctor's use of traditional techniques, in the functional therapeutic 'TCM' approach of the medical schools of Beijing. Though there is the beginning of a revival of Qigong and ancient self-care in China today, traditional acupuncturists in the West are often of the opinion that true Chinese traditional medicine is now more authentically practised in places like Hong Kong and Taiwan than in mainland China. The political upheavals and pressing immediate public health problems may have forced traditional medicine into a subsidiary mode. As Marilyn Rosenthal asks:

'Is this integration or is it Western medicine assimilating selected treatment modalities and traditional medicine grasping for a future by enmeshing itself in the structure of Western medical explanation?'[44]

China can be justifiably proud of its medical achievements. It has achieved its health goals, and set a precedent of co-operation rather than destruction of the old by the new. China wishes to export its medical knowledge. It is supported by the World Health Organization in its belief that acupuncture is a powerful health weapon for the Third World. Traditional medicine is still very strong in China. The attempt to bridge the gap between systems is continuing, and given time, more of the old knowledge will be found useful and applicable. Chinese investigations into their medical heritage are 'redolent with the balmy air of spring, budding with life and energy', according to the head of the Shanghai Chinese Traditional Medical Institute, who also reminds us that there are more than double the number of Chinese traditional doctors in Shanghai today than at the time of liberation. The evidence shows, however, that when the ancient cultural base is destroyed and traditional medicine is squeezed into a modern health care role, it may be weakened in the process.[46]

India

Traditional medicine in the Indian subcontinent consists largely of Ayurveda, an ancient healing system derived from the Vedas. Like Chinese medicine, it represents a complete guide for health, well-being, and spiritual energy which dates back several thousand years. Siddha medicine is an offshoot of Ayurveda and practised almost exclusively in Tamil Nadu and Sri Lanka. Unani-tibbi is a mixture of Ayurvedic medicine and Arabic or Persian medicine, largely in use in north-west India and Pakistan. Ayurveda is discussed more fully in Chapter 9.

Statistics relating to the practice of traditional medicine in India are amazing. In a country of 800 million population there are no less than 400 000 Ayurvedic practitioners, 242 Ayurvedic hospitals, some 11 000 dispensaries, and more than 100 officially accredited colleges, many of which are attached to universities, to train practitioners. Unani medicine in India is also strong, with 19 hospitals and 903 dispensaries, while Siddha medicine, although local, boasts 65 hospitals and 392 dispensaries.[47]

Ayurvedic medicine used to be the centre of considerable and often violent controversy. Traditionalists saw Ayurveda as part of the rootstock of Indian culture and had been lobbying strongly to preserve and expand it. The rural poor and Indian intellectuals had supported this approach, as had local politicians whose promises of universal health care could only be realistically fulfilled by expanding the traditional Ayurvedic corps. Ranged against them were the Health Ministry and the medical profession, who were adamant that modern medicine would eventually provide exclusive health coverage in India. However, it was transparently clear that modern medicine was, if anything, getting worse rather than better. By 1973, the Primary Health Centres, government rural clinics, provided two doctors per 100 000 population, 90 per cent of whom did not find reason to use the centres. While 80 per cent of the population live in the countryside, 80 per cent of the doctors work in the towns.[48] Ayurveda was itself in a poor state, for without controls on standards or education, incompetent practitioners had free reign. Students who were rejected by medical school became partly qualified Ayurvedic practitioners as a soft option. The traditional apprenticeship system gave plenty of opportunity for quackery.

Necessity forced the Indian Parliament to pass legislation recognizing and controlling Ayurveda for it continued to be the only medicine serving a large proportion of India's population. The 1970 Indian Medicine Central Council Act set up a Central Council for Ayurveda which was charged to establish a register of current established and qualified practitioners, and to ensure proper training. Under this Act, new colleges were established and old ones accredited. The qualification was called Bachelor of Ayurvedic Medicine and Surgery; it was a three-year course, and included a basic study of Western medicine. A further three years postgraduate study was required for full qualification. Separate bodies were set up to govern research and development of Ayurveda, and new legislation was introduced to control the manufacture of Ayurvedic and Unani medicines. Each state had a Directorate of Indian Systems of Medicine, in parallel with the Directorate of Medicine and Health Services, which operated the accreditation.

The Act has not solved the problem of incompetent practitioners, as there are no real measures in the law to prevent the unregistered from practising, and there is therefore a free for all. A survey of Ayurvedic practitioners has found that only 12 per cent of practitioners had obtained the degree diploma of a recognized teaching institution, 54 per cent had obtained diplomas at unrecognized institutions, and the remaining 33 per cent had no formal qualifications.[49] Although there is much room for improvement, considerable progress has been made in upgrading standards since the setting up of the register, and 75 per cent of Ayurvedic practitioners are now registered.

Following the example of the Chinese, the Government introduced an alternative rural health scheme which attempted to use traditional practitioners to distribute medical services. However, only about one-sixth of these practitioners were willing to join the scheme, as it involved some additional training in modern medicine, family planning, and public health. Those that wished to join the scheme were mostly the unregistered practitioners. Although the rural health scheme was not a great success, it turns out that a large number of traditional practitioners were using modern medicines anyway, largely at the insistence of their patients. Those Ayurvedic practitioners who were using modern medicine said that if they did not do so they would face extinction.[50] Ninety per cent of practitioners prescribed modern scientific medicines, and over half used these medicines most of the time. Less than a third, however, had training in their use.[50] A recent survey in Sri Lanka sent 'pseudo-patients' to 764 ayurvedic and allopathic physicians and found that most prescribe only modern medicines, with Ayurvedic physicians preferring milder, less specific drugs.[51] This data has shown that rural communities like modern medicine but not the doctors that administer them.

'Traditional practitioners have shown a considerable degree of adaptability to fill this vacuum though at no cost to the Government but considerable cost to the consumer.'[49]

India has the largest homeopathic establishment in the world. A separate Central Council for Homeopathy was established alongside that for Ayurveda. It has now registered some 200 000 homeopathic practitioners. There are 104 colleges running undergraduate courses for school leavers, with four years to a diploma and five and a half years to a degree. Postgraduate degrees are awarded by a new National Institute of Homeopathy in Calcutta, which is developing and evaluating homeopathic teaching. It carries out an extensive research programme in which clinical research as well as drug provings in the Hahnemannian fashion are carried out. There are 130–150 homeopathic hospitals and some 1500 homeopathic dispensaries, all supported by the Government. Each state has its homeopathic board. There is also a Central Council for Research in Homeopathy which undertakes standardization, prepares a homeopathic pharmacopoeia, and co-ordinates drug 'provings' (that is, homeopathic checking of remedies) and clinical trials.

Homeopathy in India is respected and taken seriously, although it must be said that it is also considered a soft option for those that cannot be medical students. It is interesting that even doctors must start more or less from scratch and study for several years if they wish to become homeopaths. The practitioners practise pure Hahnemannian homeopathy with some admixture of naturopathic instruction. The extent of homeopathy in India ensures that it is taken more seriously world-wide, although Indian homeopaths are chagrined that they are not recognized by the Faculty of Homeopathy in the UK.

Like China, India is a country with a powerful and sophisticated ancient pre-existing medical tradition. This is now under serious threat because of the ready availability of modern medicine and its overwhelming cultural attraction. The Government does nothing to encourage traditional medicine, and what still exists survives more by default than by intention. When I taught at an Indian boarding school for 6 months in 1993, I was surprised to find that in none of the official educational books on health was the word Ayurveda even mentioned. When I taught students and teachers about their own indigenous Ayurvedic tradition, it was clear that they, like much of the great Indian middle class, thought it was backwards and irrelevant—a bit of a joke. Their role model was an American doctor or engineer. Many feel that the lack of encouragement by central government could result in Ayurveda becoming extinct before long.[52] However in my experience of rural primary health care in India, the rural poor do flock to obtain Western medicines which are readily available, but their heart is still within the indigenous system and their views of health and healing derive from it. Other observers have commented how patients weave modern drugs into traditional Ayurvedic explanations about health.[53] Modern medicine is an enchantment, against which their herbal tradition is boring, but in the end, more trustworthy. And Ayurveda is aligned with the deeply ingrained Indian cosmic and religious view, giving it a hidden strength and durability.[54]

Indian medicine represents an accommodation between traditional and bio-medicine, compared with their official marriage in China. Perhaps the ideal solution would be a combination of Indian and Chinese strategies. Indigenous practitioners could be encouraged to train in the lengthy and rigorous traditional manner, supported if necessary by Government funding comparable to that offered to medical students. At the same time, community health workers in each village could provide public health, family planning, and simple healthcare, activities that would waste the talents of highly skilled traditional and modern practitioners. The community health workers would be drawn from the villages and could provide mixed, integrated primary care using traditional and modern techniques pragmatically, in the style of the barefoot doctor. Conventional doctors would have their role to play. However, if the sophisticated but fragile traditional medical wisdom is to be preserved it is essential that medical schools teach the limitations of conventional medicine as well as its potentials, and ensure the respect for time-tested therapeutic systems that is their due.

References

1. Wardwell, W. I. (1994). Alternative medicine in the United States. *Social Science and Medicine*, **38**, 1061–8.
2. Eisenberg, D., Kessler, R., Foster, C., Norlock, F., Calkins, D., and Delbanco, T. (1993). Unconventional medicine in the United States. *New England Journal of Medicine*, **328**, 246–52.
3. Carton, B. (1995). Health insurers embrace alternative therapies. *Alternative Medicine Journal*, **2**, 16–18.
4. Berman, B. and Anderson, R. W. (1994). Improving health care through the evaluation

and integration of complementary medicine. *Complementary Therapies in Medicine*, 2, 217–20.

5. Fisher, P. and Ward, A. (1994). Complementary medicine in Europe. *British Medical Journal*, 309, 107–11.

6. Lewith, G. and Aldridge, D. (1991). *Complementary medicine in the European Community*. C.W. Daniels, Saffron Walden. Aldridge, D.(ed.) (1990). Complementary Medicine in the European Community. *Complementary Medical Research*, 4, 1–35.

7. Himmel, W., Schulte, M., and Kochen, M. M. (1993). Complementary medicine: are patients' expectations being met by their general practitioners? *British Journal of General Practice*, 43, 232–5.

8. Steinhoff, B. (1994). The legal situation of phytomedicines in Germany. *British Journal of Phytotherapy*, 3, 76–9.

9. Rosslenboich, B., Schmidt, S., and Matthiessen, P. F. (1994). Unconventional medicine in Germany: a report on the situation of research as a basis for state research support. *Complementary Therapies in Medicine*, 2, 61–9.

10. Bouchayer, F. (1991). The role of alternative medicine: the French experience. In: *Complementary medicine in the European Community*, (ed. G. Lewith and D. Aldridge), pp. 45–60. C. W. Daniel, Saffron Walden. Bouchayer, F. (1990). Alternative medicines: a general approach to the French situation. *Complementary Medical Research*, 4, 4–7.

11. Bossey, J. (1985). Practice, training, and legal status of acupuncture in Western Europe. *Alternative Medicine*, 1, 45–54.

12. Dorozynski, A. (1995). French to get hospital for Chinese medicine. *British Medical Journal*, 310, 1285.

13. Alternative medicine in The Netherlands (1981). *Report of the Commission for Alternative Systems of Medicine*. Ministerie Van Volks Gezondheid en Milieuhygiene. Available from Staatsuirgeverij, C. Plantijnstraat 2, Is Gravenhage, The Netherlands.

14. Menges, L. J. (1994). Beyond the anglophone world. Regular and alternative medicine: the state of affairs in the Netherlands. *Social Science and Medicine*, 6, 871–3.

15. Sermeus, G. (1990). Alternative health care in Belgium: an explanation of various social aspects. *Complementary Medical Research*, 4, 9–13.

16. Rassmussen, N. and Morgall, J. (1991). The use of alternative treatments in the Danish adult population. In: *Complementary medicine and the European community*, (ed. G. Lewith and D. Aldridge). C.W. Daniel, Saffron Walden.

17. Commission of European Communities (1979). Written question No. 100/79.

18. Council of Europe (1984). *Legislation and administrative regulations on the use by licensed health service personnel of non-conventional methods of diagnosis and treatment*. Strasbourg.

19. *Official Journal of the European Communities C*, April 22 1992, 102/23–24, (92/C 102–55).

20. *Official Journal of the European Communities C*, October 23 1990, 267/9.

21. Holden, C. (1981). Health care in the Soviet Union. *Science*, 213, 1090. Razumov, A. (1994). Systemic problems of health in the workplace. *Journal of Comtemporary Health*, 1, 9.

22. Agnew, T. (1991). Moscow backs the alternative. *General Practitioner*, 11, 53. Andrews. L. (1991). USSR friendly. *Journal of Complementary and Alternative Medicine*, 9, 11–12.

23. Moody, L. (1992). The Soviet health care system. *Journal of Holistic Nursing*, 10, 47–61. Fulder, S. (1980). The hammer and the pestle. *New Scientist*, 87, 120–3.

24. Brelet, C. (1979). *Traditional medicine in Eastern Europe*. Report submitted to Traditional Medicine Section, World Health Organization, Geneva.

25. Editorial (1980). *New Zealand Medical Journal*, 91, 345.

26. Commission of Inquiry (1970). *Chiropractic in New Zealand*. Government Printer, Wellington.
27. Stephenson, D. (1990). Acupuncture in Australia: past, present, future. *Complementary Medical Research*, 4, 18–20.
28. Committee of Inquiry (1977). *Chiropractic, osteopathy, homeopathy and naturopathy*. Parliamentary Paper No. 102, Government Printer, Canberra.
29. Walker, W. G. (1990). A world first: chiropractic as a university discipline. *Journal of Australian Chiropractic Association*, 20, 152–4.
30. Parliament of Victoria, Social Development Committee (1986). *Inquiry into alternative medicine and the health food industry*. The Government Printer, Melbourne.
31. Anon. (1994). Doctors defend their power to be sole arbiters of 'sickies'. *The Natural Therapist*, 9, 37.
32. Kayne, S. (1995). Training for homeopaths in the New South Africa. *Homeopathy*, 45, 12–13.
33. World Health Organization (1978). *The promotion of traditional medicine*. Technical Report Series No. 622, Geneva.
34. Savage, A. and Hutchings, A. (1987). Poisoned by herbs. *British Medical Journal*, 295, 1650–1.
35. Scarpa, A. (1981). Pre-scientific medicines: Their extent and value. *Social Science and Medicine*, 15A, 317–26. Harrison, Ira E. and Cosminsky, Sheila (1976). *Traditional medicine: Implications for ethno-medicine, ethnopharmacology, maternal and child health, mental health, and public health; an annotated bibliography of Africa, Latin America, and the Caribbean*. Garland, New York.
36. World Health Organization (1978). *Primary health care*. A Joint Report by WHO and UNICEF, International Conference on Primary Health Care, Alma Ata, USSR.
37. World Health Organization Document, SEA/OMC/Traditional Medicine Meeting. *Interregional consultation on traditional medicine programme*, New Delhi (October 1976). World Health Organization Document EB/57/21. *Training and utilisation of traditional healers and their collaboration with health care delivery systems*. (November 1975).
38. Velimirovic, B. and Velimirovic, H. (1977). *The utilisation of traditional medicine and its practitioners in health services: a global overview*. Modern Medicine and Medical Anthropology. Pan-American Health Organization, Washington. Imperato, P. J. (1995). Western and traditional medicine in Africa: a century of encounter. *Pharos*, 58, 43.
39. Green, E.C. (1988). Can collaborative programs between biomedical and African indigenous health practitioners succeed? *Social Science and Medicine*, 27, 1125–30.
40. Carpentier, L., Prazuck, T. Vincent-Ballereau, F., Ouedraogo, L.T., and Lafaix, C. (1995). Choice of traditional or modern treatment in West Burkina Faso. *World Health Forum*, 16, 198–202.
41. Kale, R. (1995). Traditional healers in South Africa: a parallel health care system. *British Medical Journal*, 310, 1182–5.
42. Crozier, R. (1968). *Traditional medicine in modern China*. Harvard University Press, Cambridge, Mass. Hillier, S. and Jewell, T. (1987). Traditional medicine in China, pragmatism and holism. *Holistic Medicine*, 2, 15–26. Fulder, S. (1993). *The book of ginseng, and other Chinese herbs for vitality*. Healing Arts Press, Rochester, Vermont.
43. Chi, C. (1994). Integrating traditional medicine into modern health care systems: examining the role of Chinese medicine in Taiwan. *Social Science and Medicine*, 39, 307–21.
44. Rosenthal, M.M. (1981). Political process and the integration of traditional and western medicine in the People's Republic of China. *Social Science and Medicine*, 15A, 599–613.

45. Ladinsky, J.L., Volk, N. D., and Robinson, M. (1987). The influence of traditional medicine in shaping medical care practices in Vietnam today. *Social Science and Medicine*, 25, 1105–10.

46. Bibeau, G. (1985). From China to Africa: The same impossible synthesis between traditional and western medicine. *Social Science and Medicine*, 21, 937–43. Connett, G. J. and Lee, B. W. (1994). Treating childhood asthma in Singapore: when West meets East. *British Medical Journal*, 308, 1282–4.

47. Bannerman, R. H., Burton, J., and Wen-Chieh, C. (1983). *Traditional medicine and health care coverage*. World Health Organization, Geneva.

48. Ministry of Health and Family Planning (1973). *Pocket book of health statistics*. Government of India, DGHS, CBHI.

49. Bhatia J. C., Vir, D., Timmappaya, A., and Chuttani, C.S. (1975). Traditional healers and modern medicine. *Social Science and Medicine*, 9, 15–21.

50. Doyal, L. (1987). Health, underdevelopment and traditional medicine. *Holistic medicine*, 2, 27–40.

51. Waxler-Morrison, N.E. (1988). Plural medicine in Sri Lanka: do Ayurvedic and Western medical practices differ? *Social Science and Medicine*, 27, 531–44.

52. Srinavasan, P. (1995). National health policy for traditional medicine in India. *World Health Forum*, 16, 190–3.

53. Sachs, L. (1989). Misunderstanding as therapy: doctors, patients and medicines in a rural clinic in Sri Lanka. *Culture, Medicine and Psychiatry*, 13, 335–49.

54. Thomas, L. E. (1992). Identity, ideology and medicine: health attitudes and behaviour among Hindu religious renunciates. *Social Science and Medicine*, 34, 499–505.

Part 2
The Therapies

6

Acupuncture and Oriental medicine

Background

Traditional Chinese medicine is a system of medicine which uses not only acupuncture but herbs, diet, and exercise for the prevention and treatment of disease. The theory of acupuncture is drawn from an ancient Chinese text—*The Yellow Emperor's classic of internal medicine (The Nei Ching)*—probably compiled during the warring states period (770–476 BC), although the mythical Yellow Emperor referred to in the text belongs to a much earlier period (2000 BC). The theories of medicine expounded in the *Nei Ching* remain to this day the most authoritative guide to traditional Chinese medicine.[1]

There is also archaeological evidence which shows that acupuncture dates back to the Stone Age: instruments called *bian* found in China were thought to have been used as very primitive needles. By the Bronze Age acupuncture was already quite well developed, and needles were made of bronze. Today the needles are made of high quality stainless steel.

Throughout its history acupuncture has experienced periods of popularity and neglect. However, in China today many hospitals offer treatment by Western and traditional methods, according to the doctor's judgement of which is more suitable for the individual patient (see Chapter 5, p.114). Sometimes the systems complement each other, for example the use of acupuncture for anaesthesia or for the relief of pain. However, traditional Chinese medicine stands on its own as a complete system of healing, and its complex theories of diagnosis and treatment are currently beyond explanation by modern scientific analysis.

Fundamental concepts

The Chinese medical system embraces a philosophy very different from that of the West.[2] This philosophy springs from a sensitive awareness of the laws of nature and more particularly of the order of the universe. Life is activated by what the Chinese call *Qi*, roughly translated as life force. *Qi* pervades all things: in man this energy is derived partly from heredity and partly from the air we breathe and the food we eat. As long as *Qi* flows freely through the body, health is maintained.

The emphasis of traditional Chinese medicine is on the prevention of disease. Every morning in China today, ordinary people practise T'ai-chi: exercises to encourage the free flow of *Qi*. The practitioner of traditional Chinese medicine aims in the first instance to detect subtle changes in the flow of energy before these changes become gross and give rise to disease.

The principal premise of the *Nei Ching* is that health is achieved through a balance between opposing forces, represented by *yin* and *yang*. *Yin*, originally signifying the shady side of the mountain, implies coldness, darkness, passivity, interiority, and the negative. *Yang* the sunny side, implies warmth, light, activity, expressivity, and the positive. When either *yin* or *yang* quality predominates, disorders of health result. Thus an organ that is too *yin* is too sluggish, and static, and accumulates waste.

Chinese medicine employs other polarities by which all diseases and disharmonies can be described. Together with yin-yang, these are known as the eight principles: yin-yang, empty-full, hot-cold, excess-deficient. They are used to group symptoms. For example, red face, dark urine, fever, and pain increased by warmth, are hot symptoms; while slower movements, slow pulse, pale tongue, thin clear urine, and pain lessened by warmth are symptoms of a cold condition. Such a classification of diseases in itself suggests suitable methods of treatment: for example, if a patient is diagnosed as too hot, treatment will aim to disperse this heat; if too weak, it will aim to build up strength.

Alongside this system of opposing principles stands another tradition known as the theory of the five elements (or five transformations), which like the Greek system distinguishes qualities such as solidity, heat, fluidity, etc., metaphorically described as earth, fire, water, wood, and metal. These provide a qualitative understanding and classification of thousands of body signs, attributes, and symptoms. The relationship between these five elements is subject to certain laws that govern the flow between them; these cyclical laws can be applied to the working of the body, enabling the practitioner to treat disorders.[3]

Another important tenet of traditional Chinese medicine is that it regards man as a 'whole being', i.e. as an indivisible combination of mind/body/spirit, where it is impossible to treat one aspect without affecting the others. The patient is also seen as an inextricable part of the environment. Disease is interpreted either as originating within man himself (internal) or as being derived from environmental factors (external).

The internal causes of disease may be constitutional ('the hereditary energy') or the somatic consequence of unwise actions such as overindulgence, or of an emotional nature. Normally a person's natural emotions dictate an appropriate response to a given situation. However, when such responses become too intense or prolonged, disease may develop; this would be discernible at first as a distortion of the energy balance and eventually as a distortion of the organs themselves. Conversely, if an organ becomes diseased, there will be a corresponding imbalance in the emotion associated with that organ. It is entirely consonant with the holistic view of the patient that emotional problems can be traced to a physical origin and physical symptoms explained as emotionally induced. For example, excessive anger allows the energy to rise up and may cause stiff shoulders, headache, tinnitus, sinusitis, etc., and diseases of the lung may cause periods of deep melancholy, crying, rigid ideas, etc. According to the ancient classics: 'Joy and shock injure the heart, anger injures the liver, worry and overconcentration injure the spleen, grief injures the lungs, fears injure the kidneys'.

The external causes of disease are largely associated with climatic conditions. A healthy constitution should be able to withstand changes in the weather, but in extreme cases or where the person does not take adequate precautions (e.g. by wrapping up in cold winds), certain conditions can enter the body and cause disease, an obvious example being epidemics of colds and flu in winter.

Climatic conditions are not the only external causes of disease; poisoning and traumatic experiences are other examples. These categories are not simple or discrete, and in reality disease may be caused by any combination of factors. This considerably complicates the process of diagnosis. In understanding disease the emphasis is not on a germ invading the body but rather on the individual's ability to cope with changing internal and external factors.[4] Thus, the quality of the patient's *Qi* is vital for the prognosis.

The role of traditional Chinese medicine is two-fold: to prevent disease and recognize pre-disease conditions, and to treat disease according to a patient's needs as well as his symptoms. This may involve advising on diet or lifestyle and promoting general health education. Eventually the emphasis shifts from treating a disorder to supporting good health.

Diagnostic and therapeutic practices

The main application of these elaborate theories lies in the techniques of acupuncture. To treat a disorder the practitioner can manipulate the patient's *Qi* at certain points along the body in order to balance the subtle energies. Close to the surface of the body runs a network of pathways known as meridians; these connect with the inner organs and constitute channels through which energy can pass. For example, the meridian of the colon runs from a nail point on the index finger along the arm and over the shoulder and neck to the nose; from there it follows a deep pathway down to the colon itself (Fig. 6.1). Because the meridian system connects the exterior of the body by pathways to the viscera, external factors can penetrate and produce symptoms such as abdominal pain, migraine, etc. Conversely, diseases of the internal organs will produce superficial symptoms which may appear along the lines of the meridians. Thus, kidney disease can induce back pain, while disease of the gall bladder can bring pain to the shoulder, these being areas through which the respective meridians run.

There are 12 basic meridians which are named after the organs or functions to which they are attached.[5] Six are predominantly *yin*: heart, heart protector, spleen, lungs, kidney, and liver; and six are predominantly *yang*: small intestine,

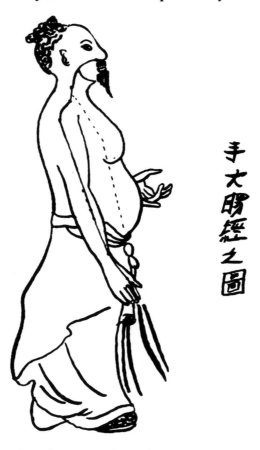

Fig. 6.1 Illustration from the ancient classic showing the meridian pathway of the great intestine (colon).

triple heater, stomach, colon, bladder, and gall bladder. The *yin* organs are those of storage, while the *yang* organs are regarded as 'hollow' and are organs of activity. Two extra meridians are the Conception Vessel which runs up the centre-front of the body, and the Governor Vessel which runs up the spine and over the head. Emphasis is placed on the relationships between organs and functions; for example, the spleen is included in the digestive function, and the kidneys are regarded as involved in the production of marrow. Traditional Chinese physiology also recognizes two functions which are more general; the heart protector protects the heart from external pathogenic factors, and the triple heater has connections with all the organs and regulates the body's temperature.

In order to ascertain the nature of a patient's disorder, the acupuncturist will employ traditional methods of diagnosis. These include the observation of significant features of the patient: the appearance and colour of the face, the sound quality of the voice, the distinctive odour of the body, the quality and texture of the skin, and the emotional disposition. The practitioner will also take a full history from the patient, measure his blood pressure, palpate the abdomen, and take a reading of the pulses. Finally, there is a whole system of diagnosis based on observation of the colour, shape, coating, moisture, etc., of the tongue. These techniques of diagnosis all require an acute perception on the part of the practitioner which is acquired through years of careful training and practical experience.

The technique of reading the pulses has a special importance and calls for further explanation. Chinese medicine recognizes 12 different pulses (as opposed to the single pulse in Western medicine). The 12 pulses correspond to the inner organs and are palpable on the wrists of the left and right hands, 6 being deep and 6 superficial. From reading the pulses the experienced practitioner is able to diagnose illnesses the patient has previously suffered, illness now present, and future illnesses. Refinement of the technique takes many years, and by mastering it the acupuncturist obtains insight into the degree of seriousness of a disorder. For example, a tight pulse can indicate heat, a hasty pulse extreme heat, while a weak pulse reflects an empty flaccid or atrophied condition. In all there are 28 qualities which can be recognized from the pulses. The *Nei Ching* defines different types of pulses qualitatively and figuratively. For example:

The pulse is the store house of the blood. When the pulse beats are long and the strokes markedly prolonged, then the constitution of the pulse is well regulated. When the pulse is small and fine, slow and short, like scraping bamboo with a knife, then it indicates that the heart is irritated and painful.

It should be remembered that there is no easy formula in traditional Chinese diagnosis: no patient will fall exactly into a textbook category, and no single diagnostic tool will be absolutely conclusive. An understanding of the subtle permutations of normal physiology and pathology is thus essential for correct treatment. While using the traditional methods of diagnosis (listening, smelling, looking, asking, and touching) the acupuncturist is attempting to analyse the disorder according to the laws of the five elements and eight principles (i.e. interior-exterior, hot-cold, deficiency-excess, *yin-yang*). Thus he is looking for certain signs that indicate that an organ is out of balance.

For example, in terms of the five-element model a disorder in the liver may manifest itself by wood-type characteristics: greenish colour in the face, shouting voice, angry disposition, rancid smell with perhaps symptoms of migraine, anorexia, and insomnia. The pulse may be full, indicating that the energy needs dispersion. In terms of the less diffuse eight principles model, the acupuncturist has to ask if the disorder is *yin*-type or *yang*-type, cold or hot, etc. The patient might then be classified as a liver-*yang*-full, of the wood-type. A symptom such as a headache can arise from any kind of imbalance. It should disappear as a matter of course when treatment is applied according to the patient's general needs and his system is restored to balance.

Once a patient's problems have been diagnosed, treatment normally proceeds by one of two methods; these are respectively the dispersion and the 'tonification' (meaning both stimulation and gathering) of energy in the meridians. Certain conditions require the use of moxa (see below) as well as needle techniques. There are numerous points along each meridian where needles or moxa can be applied. The points are chosen according to their action and relevance to the patient's condition. For example, 'wind gate' on the gall-bladder meridian can be used to dispel the external factor in disease, wind points may also be used for their cooling action, for their action on the Qi, on the blood, or on the element in need of help.

The *Nei Ching* explains in detail the techniques of inserting, withdrawing, and manipulating the needles. To tonify the energy the needle must be inserted at a 45° angle to the required depth, aligned with the flow of the meridian, and rotated in a clockwise direction; when the needle is removed the 'hole' is closed by rubbing the skin firmly. Different techniques of tonification are described poetically in the classics, but usually tonification is a quick manipulation to stimulate the energy and takes less than 30 seconds. To disperse the energy the needle is inserted rapidly against the flow of the meridian at 45° and rotated in an anti-clockwise direction; it is left in place until the energy is dispersed. This can take between 10 and 60 minutes and is gauged by reading the pulses and by the flesh 'letting go' of the needle. The needle is withdrawn slowly and the 'hole' left open. The needles enter pathways of energy and naturally no blood is lost during the procedure.

Acupuncture needles are made of stainless steel of varying length, the most commonly used being approximately 12 cm, 25 cm, or 37 cm. The handles are of twisted stainless steel. Each point has its specific depth measurement, which varies with the size of the patient; however, the needle will usually only penetrate a few millimetres beneath the skin. For treating children a special '7 star' needle may be used which pricks the skin superficially by tapping and thus manipulates the energy. The needles are always sterilized to avoid risk of viral infection, particularly after one or two reported cases of the transmission of hepatitis from unsterilized acupuncture needles. Today most acupuncturists use sterile disposable needles.

The technique of moxibustion involves burning a herb, 'moxa'. The traditional moxa is made from the pressed and dried leaves of mugwort, *Artemisia vulgaris*. Moxa may be used in various ways. A small cone of it may be placed on the blunt end of an acupuncture needle while it is in place. It is lit, transmitting the heat down the needle into the acupuncture point. Or a cone may be placed directly, or over a slice of ginger, on the acupuncture point. It is lit at its apex, and burnt down until the patient is able to feel the heat; it is then removed before it burns the skin. Moxibustion tones, stimulates, and supplements energy in the meridians, and is useful in the treatment of chronic ailments and cold conditions such as rheumatic or arthritic problems.

Acupressure is another supplementary technique that uses fingers instead of needles. It involves a steady penetrating manual pressure for some time at acupuncture points, and is useful for self-treatment, or at times when needling might be too strong or inappropriate. Examples include self-treatment of nausea or pain, or first aid. Acupressure has been found highly effective at rapidly halting epileptic convulsions. Shiatzu combines acupressure with general massage, and massage of trigger points in the Japanese tradition, and is described in Chapter 16.

Oriental herbal medicine is a crucial part of the basket of therapies within Oriental medicine, and is gradually becoming more available in the West.[6] It is included here because the principles are essentially those of Oriental medicine; Western herbal medicine has its own chapter (Chapter 13). It involves literally thousands of remedies which have been used since ancient times. The herbs are often more powerful than acupuncture, and can be taken daily, so they tend to be used for deep-seated, chronic, or serious conditions, as well as preventive health maintenance. The herbs are used in mixtures that are often boiled for some time. The art of the herbalist is to design the mixtures to fit the physiological and energetic condition of the patient and his symptoms. Each component of the mixture has one or more functions in an exceedingly complex concert of interrelated and overlapping actions which is so difficult to orchestrate, that it used to be said that it took 50 years to become a master herbalist. The plants may for example, drain or supplement the 'fire' or 'cold', or other energetic conditions just like acupuncture, and may, by means of carrier plants, direct their power at specific organs. The plants themselves are classified in different ways. One way is by the five tastes: bitter, sour, salty, sharp, or sweet, which correspond to the five elements. Sweet tasting plants, for example, have a mild 'earthy' character and affect the function of the spleen—pancreas system. Plants are also graded according to their safety, those which are mild, adjustive, and preventive, such as ginseng are the 'kingly' plants, and those which are stronger and more toxic, such as aconite, more like modern drugs, are merely the 'servants'.

Taking the 'six remedies' (*lu-wei*) as an example. This is a formula containing *Rehmannia glutinose* root, *Cornus officinalis* fruit, *Dioscorea batatas* root, *Paeonia suffruticosa* root, *Alisma plantago aquatica* tuber, and *Pachyma cocos* tuber. One of these is determined to be the 'master' and its dosage is set, and the other accessory plants fall into place around it. Rehmannia might be the master if the blood is poor and Yin weak, Cornus if there are mental symptoms such as giddiness, Alisma if there is too little urination, Paeonia if the heart needs strengthening and Dioscorea if the digestion is weak and there are skin problems. The plants also balance each other in the mixture, Rehmannia stimulating the kidney and Alisma, the water plantain, bringing water to clear the 'fire' or waste products of such powerful action so that no damage is done. Dioscorea stimulates the spleen and Pachyma disperses the consequent humidity, and so on. In all cases the vital energy of the patient is respected and enhanced, for example a stomach infection may be treated by stronger antibiotic and anti-inflamatory plants, which clear the 'fire', together with plants that remove poisons from the infection. But if the infection has already weakened the patient's constitution, resulting in lassitude, poor appetite, and weak circulation, herbs will be given to recharge his batteries first, herbs which work on the immune system and vital reserves.

Tibetan herbalism is a variation of Oriental herbal medicine which employs the same basic principles. However the herbs used and the way they are prepared are slightly different. There has been some influence from Ayurveda, and the Tibetan herbalist will often use little pills or dried powdered herbs with honey and spices, and Himalayan mountain herbs which would also be familiar to an Ayurvedic doctor. Japanese herbalism (Kanpo) is another variation of Oriental herbal medicine. It has, in recent years, become relatively scientifically developed and industrialized. There are a large variety of pre-prepared formulae made by Japanese pharmaceutical companies for specific health problems, something like the Chinese patent herb mixtures.

Besides herbalism, other therapeutic modalities within Chinese medicine have been steadily introduced into the West in recent years. T'ai-chi has been available for a long time. As a system of psychophysical exercises used for personal growth and development, for balance and well-being, it is essentially outside the scope of this book. However it is worth mentioning that Qigong is an ancient system of meditational movements, newly introduced into the West, and is becoming very popular. It is, in a way, the basis of T'ai-chi and all the Oriental therapeutic exercises. It involves simple movements which cultivate and harmonize Qi in the body. It increases awareness and control of Qi, encouraging its free flow throughout the body and its organs. It helps to maintain health, vigour, energy, and peace, and is also used therapeutically.

Applications and contra-indications

Acupuncture aims to re-balance vital energy and restore normal functioning to the body-mind. Since energy is partly derived from food, simple dietary changes may be enough to restore balance and eliminate disorders. Acupuncturists will always encourage good diet as this improves the quality and quantity of energy, and thereby aids in the treatment of the disease.

Because traditional Chinese medicine treats the individual as a whole person, including both susceptibilities and symptoms, acupuncture can help most ailments. However, there is no such thing as an instant cure: disease has to work its way out of the body, and a longstanding illness may take considerably longer to do so than one recently contracted. It is unrealistic to expect immediate alleviation of symptoms, whereas it is realistic to expect to feel changes within oneself such as a feeling of general well-being and ability to cope with or shake off the symptoms. The patient's attitude is itself important: even the confirmed sceptic will experience changes, but clearly a positive attitude to health will allow treatment to work more effectively. Acupuncture is generally harmless. In the rare cases where a complication has occurred,[7] this can usually be traced back to a badly trained practitioner.

There are certain situations in which treatment should only be administered by the experienced practitioner, for example in pregnancy, where points which may affect the fetus must not be needled. Cranial points are similarly forbidden in the treatment of infants, although they may be massaged safely and to good effect. Needles should also never be inserted into tumours or glands. If a practitioner suspects certain gross underlying diseases such as cancer, the patient is always referred to his GP for a thorough investigation. Even if there is a serious condition or injury which the patient elects to have treated with modern medicine, acupuncture can be of immense value in the relief of pain, in preventing the spread of disease, in supporting the immune system and reducing symptoms during the medical treatment.

An acupuncturist should always take into consideration any other forms of treatment the patient may be undergoing, whether conventional or otherwise. For example, drugs may mask symptoms and complicate diagnosis, but awareness of their use may guide the practitioner towards the proper course of treatment. Standard practice dictates that treatment should not be given to patients who are intoxicated or in an extreme state of emotional excitement. Although it is not expressly forbidden, it is wise to avoid treatment immediately after a meal. Finally, it is generally considered that a practitioner who is not in good health should not treat patients, a key Oriental principle which accords with common sense.

Theoretically, it should be possible to treat any disease with a reversible physiological process, to treat many psychiatric problems, and to alleviate symptoms in certain other cases such as chronic arthritis. In 1979 the World Health Organization listed 40 major diseases that could find relief by acupuncture treatment. These ranged from diseases of the respiratory tract (common cold, asthma) and of the gastro-intestinal tract (duodenal ulcer, colitis) to addiction,[8] nervous disorders (neuralgia, Bell's palsy, enuresis, sciatica, osteoarthritis, tinnitus),[9] migraine, and period pains. Because traditional Chinese medicine considers the body-mind to be a complete unit, it is able to link physical and mental disorders and to achieve a degree of success with problems such as depression, hypertension, and angina,[10] anorexia, and asthma, which elude Western medicine. All psycho-physiological problems are particularly suitable for acupuncture treatment.[2,11] Today, acupuncturists also treat many cases of immunological and energetic dysfunction including HIV positives and AIDS, chronic fatigue syndrome (ME), and allergies.

Research

Acupuncture and related forms of treatment are subtle and cannot easily be assessed in Western terms. Therapeutic acupuncture uses processes which have so far defied measurement by scientific instruments: meridians and the flow of energy along them are examples of this. However, acupuncture has caught the imagination of many Western scientists[5,12] and there are now both theories and experimental evidence to explain some limited aspects of acupuncture, particularly its effect in pain relief.

The first model that was put forward to account for acupuncture's success in treating pain was the 'gate theory of pain', put forward by Melzack and Wall in 1965. It suggests that stimulation of larger nerve fibres (A fibres) can block off pain impulses from the smaller C fibres when the impulses are integrated in the spinal cord and brain.[13] This theory does seem to fit experiments in which electrical impulses can block pain, however it does not explain chronic pain relief nor, of course, therapeutic effects. It is superseded by the finding that after acupuncture treatment, a variety of natural opiates, endorphins, are released in the brain providing natural pain relief: antagonists to opioids partially block the analgesic effects.[14] Other brain messengers are also known to be involved. For example research at the Beijing Medical College in China has demonstrated that susceptibility to acupuncture anaesthesia is related to serotonin levels in the brain, and that tiny amounts of the neurohormone cholecystokinin can block acupuncture anaesthesia completely.[15]

These are short-term effects, as the brain hormones come and go in a matter of hours. There is also evidence of long-term local reduction in pain that builds up over weeks or months. This may be related to the responses of the autonomic nervous system near the acupuncture site as well as, perhaps, gradual changes in the content of neurohormones in the brain.[16] For acupuncture analgesia can also be induced by needling at skin trigger points that are in nervous connection with muscles and deeper tissues but which are nothing to do with classical acupuncture points.[17] Indeed some practitioners use only trigger points and tender points for pain relief, although it may no longer be correct to describe this as acupuncture.

Both the autonomic nervous system and the brain neurohormones have a profound effect on health and well-being. For example the autonomic nervous sytem controls the blood supply to organs and how hard they work (one might even say their 'heat' in the Chinese sense) while neurohormones strongly influence immunity. In other words, some of the therapeutic or energetic effects of Chinese medicine could be the result of adjustments to the hormone and nervous messengers of the mind and body, which then in turn manipulate or balance organ function. However this is as yet unresearched territory. Indeed there is no published research on how acupuncture might achieve therapeutic results as opposed to pain control.

There is an interesting research debate in progress at present that concerns whether acupuncture at the classical sites is necessary for it to work. In the area of pain control it seems clear that although acupuncture has a stronger analgesic effect at classical points, as laid down in the traditional theory, non-classical points can work nearly as well.[18] In fact some clinical studies that find that acupuncture helps back pain have found no difference between acupuncture at the true and at false sites.[19] In the control of addictions too, it has been found that acupuncture can be somewhat effective, at least as effective as other methods, in helping people to give up smoking or alchoholism.[20] But again, both true and false points seem to work, and in this case as the false points are used as placebo, it has given apparently negative results in many trials and thrown this field into doubt.[11,21] On the other hand in more therapeutic situations, particularly that of nausea, acupuncture only works at the true, traditional points.[22] George Lewith and Charles Vincent have put forward the idea that the closer one gets to a purely endorphin process, in particular short-term analgesia, the less point location is relevant; the more the autonomic nervous sytem is involved, the more precise the points need to be.[23] However it could also be said here that the reductionist paradigm of such research is leading us away from the truth not towards it. That is, the relative effectiveness of pricking with a needle anywhere in the body, tells us something about pain, but nothing about acupuncture. The subtle energetic changes produced by acupuncture may be manifest in various biological systems in ways typical of those systems.

There has been a little progress in investigating the nature of the meridians and acupuncture points, although we do not know how messages actually get from the needle point to the neuromodulator-producing tissues of the brain, or what, in fact, meridians are. Assiduous dissection and anatomy has failed to find any correspondences between the body's physical structures and the meridians. The meridians do run along nerves at times, particularly in the limbs, but they soon branch off them and wander their way across and along every other kind of tissue.[24] It does appear that there are concentrations of skin receptors at acupuncture points, including tendon organs, free nerve endings, and muscle spindles. However there is nothing consistent, and different points are rich with different kinds of receptors.[25] Perhaps the most interesting area of research on the meridians at present focuses on their electromagnetic properties. Acupuncture points are known to be of low electrical skin resistance and there are a number of devices available which locate them exactly on that basis.[26] They can be located in animals and even in recently dead bodies. They have been clearly photographed by Kirlian electrophotography[27] and shown to change after acupuncture treatment and during disease. For example, an investigation at the Californian College of Acupuncture has shown that if heart rate is increased or decreased there is a precisely matching change in electrical conductivity at heart acupuncture points, but not at other acupuncture points, nor at random points on the skin.[28] Patients with tuberculosis have low electrical resistance on the lung meridian on the upper arm compared with healthy people.[29] It has been suggested that acupuncture points are trigger points,[30] areas on the skin which become sensitive when there are problems in underlying tissues. Chinese medicine uses them in diagnosis. Occasionally they do correspond to acupuncture points; but they are not acupuncture points.[24] Some tantalizing research exists on propagated channel sensations (PCS), or *Dequi*, which are the sensations patients feel running along the meridians. They can be followed closely on an electromyogram,[31] and they have been found to move at around 10 centimetres/second, a tenth of the speed of nerve conduction.[24] These sensations can be blocked by anaesthetics or cooling the area. This hints that acupuncture may be inducing local small electrical currents, and changes in the local electromagnetic fields in the surrounding tissues.[32]

Clinical evaluations of acupuncture are beset with difficulties, as has been indicated in Chapter 1. Clinical studies without a placebo are unacceptable and cannot demonstrate anything conclusive about the treatment in scientific terms: acupuncture could all be an elaborate placebo. If a weak or inadequate placebo is used, such as a vague pretence at acupuncture, a study might only show that real acupuncture may be a stronger placebo. If a more powerful placebo is used, such as sham acupuncture at non-classical points, it will have a therapeutic effect. So the study may prove nothing about acupuncture, proving only something about point location. If acupuncture is judged against such a placebo it will give a false negative result, and many potential areas of acupuncture use may have been abandoned for this reason.[18] An excellent critical analysis of acupuncture in pulmonary disease (mostly asthma) has shown how research presents acupuncture with an unequal playing field against conventional medicine.[33] It shows that of 16 properly conducted clinical trials of acupuncture only 10 were positive if sham acupuncture was used as a placebo. But if all acupuncture (true + sham acupuncture) was compared to baseline in these studies, then 14 out of 16 gave significant results. Even worse, the treatment tested was often not proper traditional Chinese medicine which must include an individual diagnosis and treatment by an experienced traditional therapist. In some trials it was simply needle insertion in specific formula points by a briefly trained practitioner; equivalent, the author suggests, to testing someone's treatment of asthma who had only spent a week learning chest medicine. It is also virtually impossible to carry out a true double-blind study as the acupuncturist must know all the time what he is doing.

Despite these problems, there are certain specific clinical areas where acupuncture has undergone proper clinical trials, allowing some conclusions. Its use in pain relief has been most thoroughly tested of all, and this research has been well reviewed,[18] and also surveyed in two recent critical meta-analyses.[34] Though there are, inevitably, many methodological criticisms, these reviews show that acupuncture has a 50–80 per cent success rate in acute and chronic painful conditions, especially low back pain and head and neck pain. Interestingly, patients who had classical acupuncture at individualized sites did better than patients who had formula acupuncture based on a specific point that was similar for all the patients. The results on migraine are also encouraging and show a much larger improvement in symptoms with true acupuncture than sham acupuncture. The benefits remained for a year. Results were equivalent to those with conventional drugs, though without the side-effects.[35] A survey of 12 clinical trials on pain relief that used an appropriate placebo (electroacupuncture with the machine switched off, or minimal acupuncture at irrelevant locations) found that almost all showed positive results compared with placebo, though they sometimes used too few patients to achieve statistical significance.[18] However, it has not been possible, so far, to determine how traditional acupuncture compares with various kinds of electrical or electro-acupuncture treatments for pain, nor ascertain for how long the relief lasts.[36] In China, the success of acupuncture anaesthesia and analgesia has been clearly demonstrated in exhaustive studies.[37]

There is an extensive clinical research literature of thousands of reports, on therapeutic acupuncture. Most of these studies are simply clinical observations carried out in the Far East intended not so much to test if acupuncture works which is obvious to Oriental therapists, but to guide its application. Evaluative research using controlled studies have been carried out in several therapeutic areas. There has been a focus on asthma, which is an enormous and sometimes disabling health problem affecting around two million people in the UK alone. A review in 1987 found eight controlled trials. These studies all showed very positive results compared with placebo in the majority of patients, who felt relief and in many cases complete remission.[38] Objective measures, including the freedom of passage of air during breathing, were not however noticeably changed. Since that time several more clinical studies have appeared which confirm that subjective improvements, and improvements in actual human function such as capacity to exercise, can be dramatically improved, as can breathing capacity but again, without obvious 'objective' physical changes.[33] This could be as much a result of the research methodology (such as the short time period of the trials) as the actual outcome.

Nausea has been intensively studied, especially by Professor Dundee and his group. These studies involve the symptomatic use of acupuncture, acupressure, or a 'Sea Band' device which stimulates a single point, the pericardium 6 point. Both acupuncture and acupressure have shown reductions in nausea at least equivalent to conventional drugs, in some careful placebo-controlled clinical studies in UK hospitals.[39] Nausea derived from morning sickness,[40] surgery,[41] or cancer chemotherapy[22] were all equivalently reduced. There was less effect on vomiting. Interestingly, these studies, along with others involving pain control, demonstrate that acupressure can match the power of acupuncture, perhaps because of continuous stimulation of a single point.

Chinese herbal medicine is a truly vast field, and there has been an equally huge amount of research on its use in Chinese hospitals and clinics. The clinical reports from China have been largely ignored in the West, although they suggest some fascinating potential new uses of herbs. For example there have been surveys of the safe use of herbal mixtures to eliminate kidney stones and gallstones, which could otherwise only be removed by surgery. It is impossible to review this research here, and readers are referred to reference 42. There are two aspects which have concerned Western researchers. One is the use of specific Chinese herbs in conventional research, as a source of novel active principles for the treatment of disease such as cancer.[43] The other is the occasional flurry of interest when a particular treatment happens to catch the public imagination. This happened recently when some patients with 'incurable' atopic dermatitis were cured by a Chinese herbalist in London. It came to the notice of researchers at various London hospitals who carried out research on one of the herbal mixtures used and found it extremely effective,[44] although they saw it as a happy accident, and could not allow that it derived from a different system of medicine. Such research may eventually lead to an appreciation that it is the treatment that is effective, and not just the formula. There has also been some concern about possible toxic effects of Chinese herbs. In ethnic Chinese communities where such herbal mixtures are taken regularly there are few cases of side-effects (1 in 500 in one report), nevertheless the possibility should be borne in mind.[45]

There is little research on Qigong and other Chinese psychophysical self-care methods. Yet a recent report to an international conference sets one thinking. A team from Shanghai medical centre studied more than a thousand people with blood pressure over no less than 20 years. Mortality in the Qigong group was 17 per cent in this period, 11.5 per cent from strokes. Mortality in those not doing Qigong was 32 per cent, with 23 per cent from strokes.[46]

New types of therapy

The influence of the West on Chinese medicine over recent years has led to the adaptation of certain techniques and to the introduction of new ideas. One of these is a complete system of treatment by needling the ear only. Organs and parts of the body are said to be represented on the ear and by puncturing specific areas on the external ear, disease can be treated in the body. Other forms of ear acupuncture are used in the treatment of pain, obesity, and addictions. In these cases a small staple is inserted into the ear and stimulated by the patient when he/she desires to eat or smoke. Ear acupuncture is not particularly Oriental. It was developed in France by Dr Nogier with new points added pragmatically to the traditional ones. It is symptomatic and relatively easy to learn, thus finding favour with medical doctors in pain and addiction centres in the West.

Electro-acupuncture is a developing field, used by technologically minded doctors though not by traditional acupuncturists. The surface of the body is seen as an electromagnetic map of the interior, with the meridians as the major, though by no means the only, features. The best known system is electro-acupuncture (EAV) developed by Dr Voll. The acupuncture needle is replaced with a stylus carrying a controlled electrical charge at the microvolt level at its tip. The machine is used both to diagnose and treat disease at acupuncture points.[13] Another kind of apparatus is a laser needle, a machine delivering a thin infrared laser beam to the acupuncture points. Though it seems elegant and sophisticated, its real therapeutic effect is questionable. Another new system (MORA) measures the frequencies of the patient's own bio-electricity, then it purifies and amplifies the electromagnetic wave before returning it to the patient via acupuncture points.

Some of the equipment used to deliver electric pulses to the body surface was developed with acupuncture in mind but does not involve acupuncture points at all, and one does not need to be an acupuncturist to use it. Transcutaneous nerve stimulation (TENS) stimulates nerve fibres which block pain messages. It is used in various kinds of chronic pain, including post-operative, low back, arthritic, or phantom limb pain. It has the advantage that the patient can take it home and use it frequently there, although it is acknowledged to be less effective than acupuncture. The pads deliver a pulse to acupuncture points, points that are tender, or simply areas close to the pain site. Like the other electronic systems, TENS has not been adequately evaluated as yet, and its application involves a certain amount of trial and error.

Other adopted forms of therapy developed over recent years include scalp acupuncture, for treatment in brain damage diseases, and the injection of drugs into acupuncture points for the alleviation of pain in such diseases as arthritis. These new techniques have developed under the influence of Western ideas and technology and contain an allopathic approach to medicine. The acupuncture points are regarded as buttons which help certain symptoms when manipulated. There is often little connection to the basic principles of traditional complementary medicine, which attempt to find and treat the causes of disease.

Obtaining treatment

Acupuncture is now widely available in the UK, but the quality of treatment is variable. When seeking treatment a person should be sure that the practitioner is properly qualified. Besides acupuncturists treating patients according to traditional therapeutic principles, it is possible to receive symptomatic acupuncture, particularly for the relief of pain. Acupuncture is now available on the National Health Service in Britain in special clinics for chronic pain, detoxification, and HIV and AIDS. GPs are now becoming more used to referring patients for acupuncture in certain areas, particularly asthma and chronic digestive problems such as irritable bowel syndrome.

During the first visit to a traditional acupuncturist the patient will be given a traditional diagnosis; this may take between an hour and an hour and a half. The course of treatment will vary from person to person and it is generally said that a month of treatment is needed for every year of illness. As a rule the acupuncturist can assess if the patient can be helped by acupuncture after the diagnosis and first few treatments. Once the energy begins to be balanced the patient will experience changes in himself and his symptoms.

To stimulate the energy successfully, the acupuncturist must obtain *Dequi* (or needle sensation) which is experienced both by the patient and the practitioner. *Dequi* can be different for each person and the sensation varies from a temporary painful feeling, burning, or prickling sensation to numbness. This sensation can be felt in different parts of the body as the energy travels along the meridian. The effects of a single treatment may be observed immediately or several days later.

Any age group can receive acupuncture, although young children, in whom energy levels fluctuate rapidly, should be treated only by an experienced practitioner. Acupuncture is also a preventive medicine. The subtle system of diagnosis allows for the correction of minor disturbances in patients who have no obvious illness but feel a little below average; if treated at this stage, the later development of obvious disease can be prevented. Because of seasonal variations in the activity of different organs different imbalances are more evident and more readily treated in particular seasons. Thus, a change of season is usually the best time at which to make an evaluation of an individual's condition with a view to deciding whether treatment is required.

In ancient China the physician gave his patient seasonal examinations to maintain his health, and was only paid while his patients were well. The wise physician would only accept as patients those who paid heed to the Laws of Nature. Such laws are still applicable today; they include sensible eating habits, exercise, and rest, the avoidance of toxins and self-abuse, and learning to live in harmony with the environment.[47] Such natural laws are basic to traditional Chinese medicine.

References

1. Needham, J. and Gwei-Djen, I. (1980). *Celestial lancets: a history and rationale of acupuncture and moxa.* Cambridge University Press, Cambridge.
2. Shanghai College of Traditional Chinese Medicine (1991). *Acupuncture: a comprehensive text.* Eastland Press, Chicago. Kaptchuk, T. (1991). *The web that has no weaver: understanding Chinese medicine.* Rider, London.
3. Pokert, Manfred (1974). *The theoretical foundation of Chinese medicine: systems of correspondence.* MIT Press, Cambridge, Mass. Maciocia, G. (1989). *The foundations of Chinese medicine.* Churchill Livingstone, Edinburgh.
4. Plummer, J. P. (1981). Acupuncture and homeostasis: physiological, physical (postural) and psychological. *American Journal of Chinese Medicine,* 9, 1–14.
5. Bensoussan, A. (1991). *The vital meridian: a modern exploration of acupuncture.* Churchill Livingstone, Edinburgh.
6. Songhyi, C. and Fei, L. (1993). *A clinical guide to Chinese herbs and formulae.* Churchill Livingstone, Edinburgh.
7. Carron, H., Epstein, B. S., and Grand, B. (1978). Complications of acupuncture. *Journal of the American Medical Association,* 228, 1552–4.
8. Bullock, M. L., Culliton, P. D., and Olander, R. T. (1989). Controlled trial of acupuncture for severe recidivist alchoholism. *Lancet,* i, 1435–9. Clement-Jones, V., McLoughlin, L., Lowry, P., Besser, G. M., Rees, L., and Wen, H. L. (1979). Acupuncture in heroin addicts: changes in met-enkephalin and β—endorphin in blood and cerebrospinal fluid. *Lancet,* ii, 380–2.
9. Marks, N. J., Emery, P. and Onisiphorou, C. A. (1984). A controlled trial of acupuncture in tinnitus. *Journal of Laryngology and Otology,* 98, 1103–9. Ellis, N. (1984). A pilot study to evaluate the effect of acupuncture on nocturia in the elderly. *Complementary Therapies in Medicine,* 1, 164–7. Liu, X. (1981). Psychiatry in traditional Chinese medicine. *British Journal of Psychiatry,* 138, 429–33.
10. Tam, C. and Yiu, H. H. (1975). The effect of acupuncture on essential hypertension. *American Journal of Chinese Medicine,* 3, 369–75. Chen, G.S. (1977). Treatment of angina pectoris with acupuncture. *American Journal of Acupuncture,* 5, 341–6.
11. Vincent, C. and Richardson, P. H. (1987). Acupuncture for some common disorders: a review of evaluative research. *Journal of the Royal College of General Practitioners,* 37, 77–81.
12. Blackwell, R. (1992). Acupuncture research in the 1990s. *European Journal of Oriental Medicine,* 1, 47–52.
13. Melzack, R. and Wall, P. (1965). Pain mechanisms: a new theory. *Science,* 150, 69–83.
14. Malizia E., Andreucci, G., Paolucci, D., Crescenzi, F., Fabbri, A., and Fraioli, F. (1979). Electroacupuncture and peripheral β-endorphin and ACTH levels. *Lancet,* ii 535–6. Editorial (1981). How does acupuncture work? *British Medical Journal,* 283, 746–8. Pomeranz, B. (1991). The scientific basis of acupuncture. In: *The basics of acupuncture,* Stux, G. and Pomeranz, B. (eds.) Springer Verlag, New York.
15. Han, J.-S. (1990). Personal communication.
16. Price, D. D., Rafii, A., Watkins, L. R., and Buckingham, B. (1984). A psychophysical analysis of acupuncture analgesia. *Pain,* 19, 27–42.

17. Macdonald, A. J. R. (1989). Acupuncture analgesia and therapy. In: *Textbook of pain*, Wall, P. D. and Melzack, R. (eds) Churchill Livingstone, Edinburgh.
18. Vincent, C. A. (1993). Acupuncture as a treatment for chronic pain. In: *Clinical research methodology in complementary medicine* Lewith, G.T. and Aldridge, D.A. (eds). Hodder & Stoughton, London. Lewith, G.T. and Machin, D. (1983) On the evaluation of the clinical effects of acupuncture. *Pain*, 16, 111–27.
19. Mendelsohn, G., Selwood, T. S., Kranz, H., Kidson, M.A., and Scott, D.S. (1983). Acupuncture treatment of chronic back pain: a double blind placebo controlled trial. *American Journal of Medicine*, 74, 49–55.
20. Lao, H. H. (1995). A retrospective study on the use of acupuncture for the prevention of alchoholic recidivism. *American Journal of Acupuncture*, 23, 29–33.
21. Schwartz, J. L. (1988). Evaluation of acupuncture as a treatment for smoking. *American Journal of Acupuncture*, 16, 135–42. Ter Riet, G., Kleijnen, J., and Knipschild, P. (1990). A meta-analysis of studies into the effect of acupuncture on addiction. *British Journal of General Practice*, 40, 378–82.
22. Price, H., Lewith, G., and Williams, C. (1991). Acupressure as an antiemetic in cancer chemotherapy. *Complementary Medical Research*, 5, 93–94.
23. Lewith, G. and Vincent, C. (1995). On the evaluation of the clinical effects of acupuncture: a problem reassessed and a framework for future research. Unpublished paper available from Research Council for Complementary Medicine, London.
24. Bensoussan, A. (1994). Acupuncture meridians—myth or reality? *Complementary Therapies in Medicine*, 2, 21–6.
25. Bossy, J. (1984). Morphological data concerning the acupuncture points and channel network. *Acupuncture and Electrotherapeutic Research*, 9, 79–106.
26. Bergsman, O. and Woolley-Hart, A. (1973). Differences in electrical skin conductivity between acupuncture points and adjacent skin areas. *American Journal of Acupuncture*, 1, 27–32. Voll, R. (1975). Twenty years of acupuncture diagnosis. *American Journal of Acupuncture*, 3, 7–17.
27. Moss, L. and Wei, L. Y. (1975). Brain response and Kirlian photography of the cat under acupuncture. *American Journal of Acupuncture*, 3, 215–23.
28. Rosenblatt, S. (1980). The electrodermal characteristics of acupuncture points. *American Journal of Acupuncture*, 10, 131–7.
29. Seisawa, K. (1978). An approach on meridians and acupuncture points in modern medicine. *Journal of Comprehensive Rehabilitation*, 11, 789.
30. Melzack, R., Stillwell, D. M., and Fox, E. J. (1977). Trigger points and acupuncture points for pain: correlations and implications. *Pain*, 3, 3–23.
31. Research Group of Acupuncture Anaesthesia, Fujian. (1986). Studies of phenomenon of blocking activities of channels and collaterals. In: *Research on acupuncture, moxibustion and acupuncture anesthesia*, (ed. Zhang, X. T.). Science Press, Beijing.
32. Bensoussan, A. (1994). Acupuncture meridians—myth or reality? Part 2. *Complementary Therapies in Medicine*, 2, 80–5. Milburn, M.P. (1995). Bioelectromagnetics: implications for Oriental medicine and acupuncture. *American Journal of Acupuncture*, 23, 53–62.
33. Jobst, K. (1995). A critical analysis of acupuncture in pulmonary disease: efficacy and safety of the acupuncture needle. *Journal of Alternative and Complementary Medicine*, 1, 57–85.
34. Ter Riet, G., Kleijnen, J., and Knipschild, P. (1990). Acupuncture and chronic pain: a criteria based meta-analysis. *Journal of Clinical Epidemiology*, 11, 1191–9. Patel, M., Gutzwiller, F., Paccaud, F., and Marazzi, A. (1989). A meta-analysis for acupuncture for chronic pain. *International Journal of Epidemiology*, 18, 900–6.
35. Hesse, J., Mogelvang, B., and Simonsen, H. (1994). Acupuncture versus metoprolol

in migraine prophylaxis. A randomised trial of triggerpoint inactivation. *Journal of International Medicine*, 235, 451–6. Vincent C.A. (1989). A controlled trial of the treatment of migraine by acupuncture. *Clinical Journal of Pain*, 5, 305–12.

36. Richardson, P. H. and Vincent, C. A. (1986). Acupuncture for the treatment of pain: a review of evaluative research. *Pain*, 24, 15–40.

37. Peking Children's Hospital (1975). A clinical analysis of 1474 operations under acupuncture anaesthesia among children. *Chinese Medical Journal*, 1, 369–74.

38. Aldridge, D. and Pietroni, P. C. (1987). Clinical assessment of acupuncture in asthma therapy: a discussion paper. *Journal of the Royal Society of Medicine*, 80, 222–4. Jobst, K. A., Chen, J. H., McPherson, K., Arrowsmith, J., Brown, V., Efthimiou, J., Fletcher, H., Maciocia, G., Mole, P., Shifrin, K., and Lane, D. J. (1986). Controlled trial of acupuncture for disabling breathlessness. *Lancet*, ii, 1416–19. Fung, K. P., Chow, O. K. W., and So, S. Y. (1986). Attenuation of exercise-induced asthma by acupuncture. *Lancet*, ii, 1419–22.

39. Dundee, J. W. and Yang, J. (1991) Non-invasive stimulation of P6 antiemetic acupuncture point in cancer chemotherapy. *Journal of the Royal Society of medicine*, 84, 210–12. Dundee, J. W. (1990). Prolongation of the antiemetic action of P6 acupuncture by acupressure in patients having cancer chemotherapy. *Journal of the Royal Society of Medicine*, 83, 360–2.

40. Belluomini, J., Litt, R. C., Lee, K. A., and Katz, M. (1994). Acupressure for nausea and vomiting of pregnancy: a randomised, blinded study. *Obstetrics and Gynaecology*, 84, 245–8. Bayreuther, J., Lewith, G. T., and Pickering, R. (1994). A double blind cross-over study to evaluate the effectiveness of acupressure at pericardium (P6) in the treatment of early morning sickness (EMS). *Complementary Therapies in Medicine*, 2, 70–6.

41. Barsoum, G., Perry, E. P., and Fraser, I. A. (1990). Postoperative nausea is relieved by acupressure. *Journal of the Royal Society of Medicine*, 83, 86–9. Phillips, K. and Gill, L. (1994). The use of simple acupressure bands reduces post-operative nausea. *Complementary Therapies in Medicine*, 2, 158–60.

42. Tang, W. and Eisenbrand, G. (1992). *Chinese drugs of plant origin*. Springer Verlag, New York. Chang, H. M. and But, P. P. H. (1987). *Pharmacology and applications of Chinese materia medica*. World Scientific Publishing, Singapore.

43. Han, R. (1994). Highlight on the studies of anticancer drugs derived from plants in China. *Stem Cells*, 12, 53–63.

44. Sheehan, M. P., Rustin, M. H. A., Atherton, D. J., Buckley, C., Harris, D. J., Brostoff, J. *et al.* (1992). Efficacy of traditional Chinese herbal therapy in adult atopic dermatitis. *Lancet*, 340, 13–7.

45. Wang, Y. M. and Hu, Y. J. (1985). Toxicity and side effects of some Chinese medicinal herbs, In: *Advances in Chinese medicinal materials research*, World Scientific Publishing Co., Singapore. Chan, T. Y. K., Chan, A. Y. W., and Critchley, J. A. J. H. (1992). Hospital admissions due to adverse reactions to Chinese herbal medicines. *Journal of Tropical Medicine and Hygiene*, 95, 296–8.

46. Chongxing, W., Dinghai, X., Yusheng, Q., and Ankun, K. (1994). *Research on 'anti-ageing' effects of Qigong*. Presented at the First International Conference of Qigong, Beijing.

47. Ionescu-Tirgoviste, C. (1980). Proper nutrition in the concept of traditional Chinese medicine. *American Journal of Acupuncture*, 8, 205–13.

7

Alexander and Feldenkrais Techniques

Alexander Technique

Background

Born in Australia in 1869, F. M. Alexander found his promising career as a young Shakespearean actor beset by vocal troubles. Finding no assistance from medical practitioners he concluded that the problem lay within. So began years of painstaking self-observation and experimentation. During this time he noticed that while reciting he tended to stiffen his neck and pull his head back and down, thereby depressing his vocal cords and shortening his spine. The correct posture, he found, could only be achieved by consciously allowing the head to assume its correct orientation in relation to the neck and torso. Of course the new posture was easily lost as force of habit made him revert to his usual stance. However he realized that if he did not compel himself to reach the end result directly, but attended only to the means for achieving it, he could break his habitual pattern.

His own success encouraged him to teach his discoveries to other actors. When he saw improvements in voice, in other functions, and in health, he concluded he had come across a fundamental approach to improving the use of the human organism as a whole. Encouraged by doctors, he came to London at the turn of the century and taught his technique both in England and America until 1955.[1]

Concepts and research

It is often held that man is still not perfectly adapted to the upright posture. However, it can be readily demonstrated in Alexander work that there can be perfect balance and poise with the minimum degree of tension. The way we use our body is faulty, not the mechanism itself: 'Mis-use' is one of the major factors in 'dis-ease'. This concept is largely unacknowledged in medicine and the effects of misuse can be more insidious even than nutritional factors.

Dr Wilfred Barlow,[2] a student of Alexander Technique, has investigated postural defects as an indication of misuse. Surveys of college students showed substantial defects in most of them. He then compared the efficiency of standard methods of postural re-education (admonishments to correct particular faults) with Alexander re-education, and found that the conventional approach produced deterioration, whereas the Alexander pupils improved markedly during their course. Nikko Tinbergen,[3] on being awarded the Nobel Prize for Physiology and Medicine in 1973, devoted half of his oration to the Alexander Technique, which he described as one of the true epics of medical research and practice. He recommended it for autism and stress diseases. Professor Tinbergen, an ethologist, assumed that a precise assessment of improvement in posture would be a sufficient demonstration of the value of the Technique. However in practice it has proved difficult to assess posture objectively.

Frank Pierce-Jones,[4] recognizing these limitations, proposed that the movement pattern itself should be the criterion of effectiveness of Alexander Technique. By means of multiple-image photography he was able to record the trajectory followed by the head during movement. He recorded a greater area underneath the trajectory in an Alexander-guided movement, compared with 'normal', showing greater efficiency of use.

The instruction

Alexander lessons powerfully confirm the need and possibility of changing one's habitual pattern of movement and bearing. They are a technique of re-education. In individual lessons, the pupil is made aware of what he is doing, and how this interferes with the head-neck-torso relationship in rest and activity. The teacher conveys through his hands the fact and sense of a new manner of use, and the pupil is encouraged to think with the teacher so that he learns increasingly to create this improved co-ordination for himself. There is an experience of lengthening, expansion, and ease in movement, although it almost certainly feels strange at first. A slight touch may be all that is necessary to allow an effortless change from sitting to standing, such is the extraordinary freedom and lightness when the head is allowed to lead the body.

The teacher is careful about correcting specific defects and postural faults. These usually arise out of poor general conditions which must be put in order first. Alexander deprecated breathing exercises, relaxation (collapse!), and other specific 'cures'. He was very concerned about the integrity of the psychophysical organism and therefore did not give 'treatment' or promise instant relief.

The range and application of the Alexander Technique is as wide as human activity itself; indeed John Dewey, the American educational philosopher, thought it bore the same relation to education as education does to living. It has great potential in all manner of psychosomatic and mechanical disorders, particularly back and neck problems, and in rehabilitation following accidents or injury.

Experience has shown that it is almost impossible for the individual by himself to break through the circle of habitual doing, and unreliable postural awareness. In a few lessons from a competent teacher the pupil can cover the same ground that Alexander took years to establish. Many come to lessons after years of chronic pain to find its cause. Ideally one should learn how to *prevent* the distorting effects of modern life on the way we use our body from an early age.

Feldenkrais Technique

Like F. Mathias Alexander, Moshe Feldenkrais is a founder of a technique for restoring full efficiency and function of the body. He synthesized this technique from Eastern and Western body concepts, combining some aspects of the Alexander Technique with knowledge of Oriental body training in the martial arts—he was a Judo teacher for 30 years. The result is a sophisticated and well thought out series of exercises which facilitate awareness of the body in movement.[5] Habitual movements are reduced to their component parts, games are played with gravity, new types and ranges of movement are explored, and the body is retaught its basic language of natural, pleasurable, and instinctive action. Its focus on gradually training awareness and sensitivity puts the Feldenkrais Technique in the same class as Alexander Technique, although it differs in its concentration on the body in motion rather than the body in space. In that sense one might liken it to a Western T'ai-chi. The teaching includes, for example, new perceptions of walking, crawling, the natural movements of babies, the consciousness of breathing while moving, self-image, the way the head, eye, pelvis, spine, and limbs move in relation to each other and so on. It has a directly therapeutic side in which the therapists re-train patients with musculoskeletal or neurological problems, particularly the ubiquitous bad back.[6]

Research

Jones pioneered research into Alexander Technique. He used photographic, mechanical, and even electromyographical methods to demonstrate that when a person is guided by Alexander Technique, his muscles work more effectively and efficiently and there is less tiredness.[4] Classical placebo controlled medical research is inappropriate to evaluate Alexander Technique, since the whole process is instructional and the tools are subjective awareness and intention. However there is a basic knowledge in science of the relationship between awareness of posture and position in space (proprioception) and patterns of muscular function.[7] Unblinded outcome measures are of course possible, although rarely carried out. A recent study has examined respiratory function using spirometry in healthy subjects after only 20 lessons in Alexander Technique compared with matched controls without lessons. There was a significant increase of 6–9 per cent in peak expiratory and inspiratory flow of air, and in several measures of breathing capacity, compared with the control subjects.[8] Since Alexander Technique involves awareness, not exercises, this may be due more to co-ordination and release of muscular tensions in the chest and abdomen rather than increased muscular strength. Long-term studies of the effect of Alexander Technique on various body functions including breathing would be of great interest and value.

There has also been some interest, especially among nurses, concerning the use of the Alexander Technique to help them cope with the considerable stresses of working with their bodies, for example lifting and supporting patients, while under emotional tension. It is highly recommended as a technique to help nurses with the great demands that their professional life places on them.[9]

References

1. Alexander, F. M. (1985). *The use of the self*. Gollancz, London.
2. Barlow, W. (1982). *The Alexander principle*. Gollancz, London.
3. Tinbergen, N. (1974). Ethology and stress diseases. *Science*, **185**, 20–7.
4. Jones F. P. (1976). *Body awareness in action: a study of the Alexander Technique*. Wildwood Press, London.
5. Feldenkrais, F. (1972). *Awareness through movement: health exercises for personal growth*. Harper & Row, New York.
6. Elsasser, M. B. (1991). The Feldenkrais method in ambulatory geriatric nursing and the nursing of the sick. *Deutsche Krankenpflegezeitung*, **44**, 538–41.
7. Garlick, D. (ed.) (1982). *Proprioception, posture and emotion*. University of New South Wales Press, Kensington, New South Wales, Australia.
8. Austin, J. H. M. and Ausubel, B. A. (1992). Enhanced respiratory muscular function in normal adults after lessons in proprioceptive musculoskeletal education without exercise. *Chest*, **102**, 486–90.
9. Anon. (1993). The Alexander technique. *Nursing Times*, **89**, 49–52. Maitland, J. and Goodliffe, H. (1989). Fit for nursing—the Alexander Technique. *Nursing Times*, **85**, 55–7.

8

Anthroposophical medicine

Background

Anthroposophical medicine constitutes an extension of medical thought and practice based on and inspired by the work of Rudolf Steiner (1861–1925). Steiner first created a philosophical basis for what he later termed anthroposophy in *The philosophy of freedom* (1894),[1] his fundamental work on the theory of knowledge. He went on to elaborate a description of the nature of man as a being of soul and spirit, as well as body,[2] and to outline the method and discipline which this research involves. At the same time he worked towards a renewal of the arts, including a new art of movement, eurythmy, which he later also developed for therapy.

After the First World War, the implications of anthroposophy for practical life and work began to be more widely recognized. Steiner was approached by people in various vocations seeking a new basis for their work. These included physicians, teachers of normal and handicapped children, farmers, scientists, and architects. In 1923, 15 months before his death, Rudolf Steiner founded the School of Spiritual Science, which had the task of providing the training and social framework for continued research and its application in cultural, economic, and social life. The School is divided into sections, each responsible for one field of practical work, e.g. a Natural Science Section, a Medical Section, etc. It is based at the Goetheanum in Dornach near Basle, Switzerland, which is also the centre of the worldwide Anthroposophical Society, founded at the same time for the furtherance of this work.

It was only in the latter years of Rudolf Steiner's life that his work took him into the field of medicine. He was not himself a medical practitioner, but worked with doctors who saw that anthroposophy could have a real contribution to make in the sphere of medicine. Amongst the doctors who worked with Rudolf Steiner was the Dutch physician Dr Ita Wegman. Their close collaboration led to the founding of a clinic in Arlesheim, Switzerland.

Anthroposophical work in Germany was suppressed by the Nazis, but after the Second World War further specialized clinics and general hospitals were founded.

At present, anthroposophical medical work is most widely developed in Germany, The Netherlands, and Switzerland, where there are two general hospitals in which anthroposophical work is integrated with modern medicine. and eight specialized hospitals using these methods. In addition there are many hundreds of general practitioners and specialists. These hospitals are fully recognized and funded by state and private medical insurance schemes, as are most of the individual practitioners. By comparison, in the English-speaking world the number of practitioners and the range of services and institutions is still very limited. In the UK, individual practitioners work both within the National Health Service and privately. A number of anthroposophical doctors offer their services as medical consultants to Rudolf Steiner Schools for normal, maladjusted, and mentally handicapped children. There is a residential therapeutic centre in Worcestershire where more intensive anthroposophical medical treatment is offered.[3]

Anthroposophical medicine is one aspect of a wider movement responsible for innovative work in education, agriculture, the arts, social development, and finance. Best known are the Waldorf Schools (some 200 world-wide, including 12 in the UK) and the homes and schools for children and adults in need of special care, including the Camphill Villages and communities.

Fundamental concepts

In order to understand anthroposophical medicine, its relationship with conventional medicine must be considered. The latter is based on physical experiment and observation guided by hypotheses. Only hypotheses about tangible and measurable phenomena are admitted as legitimate. The consequence is that all living, emotional, and mental phenomena must ultimately be reduced to physical events.

Steiner's challenge was not to the *spirit* of science, which he vigorously upheld, but to the self-imposed limitations of its practice. He contended:

1. The phenomena of life, of feeling, of consciousness, are not explained by reductionism which simply diverts attention from our actual experiences of them.
2. While physical perception is by definition confined to physical realities, awareness is not so confined.
3. Other forms of perception can be developed which reveal other levels of reality. These may also be permeated by disciplined thought. It is then apparent that we do not, in fact, yet have an adequate science of life, sentience, or consciousness.
4. The outline of a science of life can be grasped conceptually irrespective of whether the appropriate modes of 'supersensible' perception are available to a particular individual.

Such insights can then show us many apparently familiar experiences in nature and in human life in a new light, thus allowing the systematic development of new approaches in therapy, education, agriculture, etc. They are the foundations for an approach to therapy, which aims to be not an alternative to, but an *extension* of, scientific medicine.

Health and disease

To define the human being as a 'naked ape', E. F. Schumacher once remarked, is like defining a dog as 'a barking plant or a running cabbage'. A proper understanding of man must include his relationship to the mineral, plant, and animal kingdoms of nature, but must also acknowledge his uniqueness—notably a capacity to understand nature and change it.

Anthroposophical medicine is founded on a recognition of four distinct aspects of the human being, as outlined by Steiner: the physical body (shared with all other kingdoms of nature); the life or 'etheric' body (shared with plants and animals), which is the force that establishes and sustains life similar to the Chinese 'Qi' and Indian 'prana'; the sentient or 'astral' body (shared with animals) which is the soul aspect; and the 'I', the human intelligent self. The last three principles are each to be understood as a net of forces or energies different from each other and from those constituting the physical body. While inter-related, none is reducible to the laws of another. It is in terms of these four sets of activities, and their particular modes of inter-relation in a sick person, that the doctor seeks to understand an illness.

Life depends on maintaining a dynamic balance within the contrasting metabolic processes of catabolism (breaking down and using energy) and anabolism (building up and storing energy). Anatomically, this polarity is manifest in the contrast of nerves indicating nervous activity, and blood indicating nutritive processes; psychologically, in the contrast of waking and sleeping. For example the 'I' and 'sentient body' are to be conceived as working from 'outside' the physical and life bodies in sleep, and from 'inside' when we are awake. Degenerative and sclerotic illnesses may be pictured as a consequence of excessive activity of the 'I' and the sentient organizations shutting down the physical body. Inflammatory conditions and mental illnesses manifesting as manic and schizophrenic symptoms may be pictured as an excessive activity of the life forces and physical bodies.

The physical bearers of the day-time consciousness which come to dominate the life of the organism are the nerves, the senses, and the skin. While extending throughout the body their activity is particularly centred in the head. The physical bearers of the restorative and nutritive functions, in contrast, are the metabolic organs (e.g. the liver, digestive organs generally, and the muscles), centred particularly in the abdominal region and the limbs. Between the activities of these two polar systems lies the rhythmic organization, centred in the region of the chest and expressing its functions through the heart, the lungs, and the circulatory and respiratory systems as a whole. Within this rhythmic system the contrasting nerves and senses on the one hand, and the metabolic functions on the other, interpenetrate, producing all bodily rhythms. This system is of particular importance to the physician in that pathological processes within any region of the body may first show themselves as disturbances of rhythms, for example, in the pulse and respiration.

Such a picture of human physiology represents a radical departure from the generally accepted view that all functions of the mind and soul are centred in the brain. Although the conscious functions of thought and perception are centred in the nervous system, these represent only a part of our inner life. Steiner recognized explicitly what we often apprehend intuitively, that the life of feelings and emotions is centred physiologically in the rhythmic system, and the will in the system of metabolism and limbs. (To say that someone has 'no stomach for a fight' then ceases to be a mere figure of speech.)

In human beings, the realm of 'instinct' includes the unconscious working of the 'I', which guides individual destiny. Steiner was concerned that modern medicine should begin to include some awareness of this realm in its work. The outward expressions of this deeply hidden activity are found in individual biographies or in important illnesses or 'accidents', which may be recognizable not simply as unfortunate events requiring suppression or elimination, but as landmarks in personal development.

This picture of illness gives the anthroposophical physician and his patient the task of uncovering any potential meaning and purpose of an illness while using treatments to promote healing.

Diagnostic and therapeutic practices

Diagnostic procedures include conventional history taking, physical examination, and appropriate laboratory and radiographic investigations. In addition, special attention may be given to forming a picture of the patient's biography and social context, including a search for underlying patterns which may be seen in the light of an anthroposophical understanding of the phases of development.[4] It may also be important to observe some or all of the following signs: characteristic body shape and formation, tissue fluid distribution in skin and soft tissue, muscle tension, distribution of body warmth (the special field of observation for the masseur), posture, movements and gestures (the special province of the eurythmist), modes of artistic expression (e.g. too much or too little form), awareness of colour (the field of the artistic therapist), social behaviour (e.g. outgoing, inward-looking). A central motif underlying these phenomena is then sought. This represents a 'qualitative diagnosis', which includes but transcends the conventional medical diagnosis. It may be described in terms of the four-fold picture of the human being as outlined above. Such a procedure represents the 'ideal case' which may be realized in a residential clinical setting. An ordinary medical consultation will normally only include some of these aspects.

Anthroposophically developed medicines may be prescribed in addition to some of the following: special diets, massage, hydrotherapy, therapeutic movements (eurythmy), and artistic therapies such as painting, drawing, modelling, music, and speech formation. These therapies can be composed into an integrated therapeutic programme.

Medicines

Most medicines used in the practice of anthroposophical medicine are derived from natural sources—mineral, plant, and animal.[5] They may be used at homeopathic potencies or in material dosages. The anthroposophical approach sees the essential nature of a potential medicinal substance in terms of the forces and processes which have produced it. In order to derive a medicine from a plant source, for example, the plant itself must first be studied in connection to its unique form, its particular life-cycle and the way it relates to its environment. Its one-sidedness or peculiarities are noted. A qualitative picture of the plant may then be built up which includes its life in time as well as its form in space.

The influence of a medicine on the human organism is not seen as being limited to chemical processes and reactions, but may directly stimulate more subtle processes and bring about changes in life energy. It may have a facilitating or 'catalytic' effect. For example, through an appreciation of the relationship between silica and nerve—sense processes on the one hand, and between iron and sulphur and metabolic processes on the other, a preparation containing these substances has been formulated for the prophylaxis and treatment of migraine. Pharmaceutical laboratories which had started in order to meet the requirements of the first doctors working with this approach developed into an international pharmaceutical manufacturing company, Weleda. Later the Wala company was founded, and pioneered new methods to prepare biologically stable products without the use of preservatives such as alcohol.

Following up Rudolf Steiner's suggestion that mistletoe (*Viscum album*) should be developed as a treatment for cancer, several cancer research institutes were founded which have developed medicinal preparations for this illness.[6] The best known is Iscador. Other medicines have been developed from similar considerations, including medicines used in the treatment of psychiatric illnesses, based on Steiner's indication that many such illnesses stem from disturbances in the functioning of internal organs.

Physical treatments

Out of an understanding of the life body and its activity in the tissue fluids and the fluid organization as a whole, a special method of rhythmical massage was developed by Dr Margarethe Hauschke[7] and Dr Ita Wegman. A method of hydrotherapy using plant oils finely dispersed in water—oil dispersion baths—has also been developed. These baths allow the warming, stimulating, or relaxing effects of various oils on the skin to be enhanced.

The arts and therapy

Steiner's work has encouraged the development of a number of artistic therapies which may restore deformations within man's four-fold organization as described above and therefore have a central role to play in the practice of anthroposophical medicine.

Therapeutic eurythmy

Eurythmy, an art of movement created by Steiner, has been called 'visible speech' and 'visible music'. The performing eurythmist seeks to make the whole human organism an instrument for realizing the movements out of which music and speech are born. In this sense, eurythmy can awaken us to a fuller consciousness of what we already know. As speakers, we use both physical movements and inner movements of feeling and consciousness to utter language. For example, the vowel 'ah' cannot be spoken with the mouth closed; the sound 't' cannot be spoken without involving the tongue and teeth in particular movements. At the same time, each physical sound embodies a characteristic quality of experience, which gives poets their working material. The eurythmist must transform all this into an exact discipline of movement, just as a musician learns to play his instrument so that it renders faithfully the music he wishes to be heard.

In an artistic performance the movements of eurythmy flow quickly into one another, shaping a continuous stream of movement. In therapeutic eurythmy, individual movements connected, for example, with single vowels or consonants are isolated and intensified through rhythmic repetition so that they can work back on the person performing them. The exercises may aim to change the way a patient relates to the world, to help him concentrate, to free him from crippling emotional responses, etc., or they may aim to influence the physical organism itself through posture and movement; these may even bring changes in the function and structure of specific organs. For example, the person who finds his environment frightening may keep his neck muscles tense, his shoulders hunched, and his breathing shallow. He can then be given eurythmy exercises in which he first experiences more consciously the contracted posture he habitually adopts and the cramped feelings that tend to accompany it. Such an exercise would involve an almost uncomfortable crossing of the arms and legs, and gives rise to an experience of being locked in oneself. This might be followed by an exercise of stretching the arms out in a gesture of wonder. The aim is not just to do the movements but to be open to the type of feeling that can accompany the gestures. In alternating two such exercises not only a physical but also an 'emotional' breathing is encouraged.

Therapeutic eurythmists work with medical doctors. The doctor may prescribe certain exercises for a patient, or doctor and eurythmist may collaborate in a search for exercises suitable for him. However, in the final analysis, given this help from doctor and eurythmist, it is the patient's own activity which has healing value for him.

Art therapies

Therapeutic work in painting, drawing, modelling, sculpture, speech, and music has also been developed from Steiner's indications. Each therapy draws upon different qualities and faculties within the individual, as each art has a different form and rhythm, and works in a different medium. Within any one medium, there is a wide choice of techniques and themes. It rests with the therapist and doctor to determine which can be most helpful in a particular case. For example, in drawing, a particular rhythmic diagonal shading may be used therapeutically. Acquiring this discipline and using it in drawing exercises to balance extreme polarities of darkness and light may be particularly helpful in cases of anxiety, obsessions, and complexes, helping to strengthen and direct the will, and promote clarity in thinking.

Painting therapy centres on the use of colours, to which we respond with our emotions. These, in turn, influence the breathing and circulatory rhythms and consequently the individual's sense of well-being. Water colour paints are used for their luminosity and for the experience of freedom and fluidity of the watery medium itself. Again, a first step will often be to acquire a technique of long, continuous brush strokes, which create a mood of quiet and relaxation. The therapist will then begin to work with specific colour combinations and particular themes. Some individuals needing to come out of themselves and find confidence in their surroundings may be helped through painting clear forms and images. Others, suffering from sclerotic or cancerous conditions, may benefit from more spontaneous exercises, exploring light and dark and movements in pure colours without the use of forms or hard contours.

Modelling and sculpture, using clay, beeswax, and/or plasticine, offer other possibilities. The senses of touch, movement, and balance are awakened in coming to grips with three-dimensional forms. It is particularly valuable to engage in exercises of metamorphosis, transforming one form into another, or making sequences of related forms. These can strengthen imaginative mobility, flexibility and the capacity for change in other aspects of life. Sculpture therapy can be valuable in many psychiatric and psychosomatic disturbances which involve a loss of orientation in space, giddiness, vagueness, disconnected thinking, lack of concentration, and nervousness.

Applications

Although anthroposophical treatment has helped many patients who have not felt helped by conventional medicine, its importance lies less in the statistics of its 'cures' than in the qualities of the healing processes it facilitates, and in its comprehensive approach to the sick human being. However 'human' its practitioners, the reductionist basis of conventional medicine tends to see the patient as an object and illness as an unfortunate breakdown of his physical mechanism. Anthroposophical medicine considers the patient as a developing individual with a meaningful biography, and his illness as a difficult but potentially important episode in his life. This can mean that in some cases, a patient may be challenged to endure certain symptoms longer than if they were treated conventionally, so that a more fundamental improvement, rather than symptomatic relief, may be achieved. However, surgery and other conventional treatments may equally well be prescribed where appropriate. Steiner's insistence that all doctors seeking to extend medicine along anthroposophical lines must be fully qualified widens rather than narrows the scope of their work.

This means that, in principle, an anthroposophical physician can be consulted about any medical problem. While anthroposophical medicine can contribute to the treatment of most illnesses, it has a special value where conventional medicine has little to offer. For example psychosomatic illness, poor vitality and resistance, and functional disorders cannot be adequately understood, let alone treated, by a medicine based essentially on a physiochemical model, whose rational materia medica for such conditions is limited to sedatives, antidepressants, or other symptomatic treatments. Similarly, in treating cancer, conventional medicine must rely on surgery and on destructive treatments which weaken the patient's vitality and general resistance. Here the anthroposophical approach, while not offering miracle cures, has a special contribution to make with specific medicines and other therapies which enhance the patient's vitality and resistance.

Research and development

Steiner saw clearly that science embodies, in effect, a schooling. However, its nature and scope are confined by history and convention to a limited framework, which excludes in advance a full exploration of the phenomena of life, sentience, and human self-awareness. He saw within all human beings the potential for a much wider and deeper schooling. Continuous research is therefore encouraged, but the emphasis is not purely materialistic. It is

'mainly devoted to attempts to understand the relationship between the physical-organic basis and the soul and spiritual aspects of human beings, and their significance in the processes of health and sickness'.[8]

For example, there has been some effort invested in re-examining medical research methodology. In the Department of Clinical Pharmacology at Herdecke Hospital a critical examination of the problems both of animal experiments and of clinical trials has pointed out both the limited value of these trials and the ethical problems arising from the inevitable conflict of interest between giving the best available treatment to each patient, and running the trial so that statistically significant results are obtained.[9]

Research has also concentrated on medicinal plants that are used in the anthroposophical system. There have been clinical and pharmacological studies confirming that mistletoe (*Viscum album*) is a potent immune stimulant, and it can assist in preventing the growth and spread of cancer. Analytical studies suggest that lectins are among the active ingredients. However research is also trying to understand the individualistic way in which some people respond to mistletoe therapy better than others, so as to guide anthropological physicians in the use of the plant.[6] Other plants are also being investigated, sometimes in unconventional ways. For example, surveys of the clinical confidence of anthroposophical doctors in various remedies, together with tests of the physicians level of criticalness, provides a basis for the selection of remedies, without the questionable objectivity of controlled clinical trials. Such surveys have also demonstrated that apart from minor local reactions, such as inflammation at the site of injection of anthroposphical preparations, there are virtually no side-effects.[10]

As the rhythmic processes in life are an essential component of health and healing, basic research has also investigated rhythmic processes, for example in the course of disease or the manifestation of symptoms. Chronobiological research on the heart and on the effect of anthroposophical remedies has been carried out, mostly in Germany.[11]

Types of therapy and availability

A list of practitioners available for consultation is published by the Anthroposophical Medical Association. The length of treatment and the number of consultations depends entirely on the individual case and may vary from one or two consultations to a prolonged course of treatment over many months. The Park Attwood Therapeutic Centre usually suggests a minimum of three weeks' residential treatment to ensure noticeable results.

The cost of treatment depends on the situation. Patients on the list of an anthroposophical NHS general practitioner receive his advice free of charge and can obtain the medicines he prescribes on NHS prescriptions. They will be expected to make some financial contribution if a course of treatment with a specialist anthroposophical therapist is prescribed. A modest fee is normally charged for private consultations with such general practitioners if the patient is not on their NHS list and most private practitioners also charge a modest fee. In recent years patients in various localities have set up funds to support the services of an anthroposophical doctor outside the NHS. The Park Attwood Therapeutic Centre, although independent of the NHS, does not charge fees. Instead, patients are informed of the average costs per patient per week and asked to make a responsible contribution, based on their own financial circumstances in relation to Park Attwood's needs.

References

1. Steiner (1979a). *The philosophy of freedom*. Rudolf Steiner Press, London.
2. Steiner (1979b). *Occult science—an outline*. Rudolf Steiner Press, London.
3. Park Attwood Therapeutic Centre, Trimpley, Bewdley, Worcs. DY12 1RE; Tel: (01299) 861444.

4. Lievegoed, B. (1982). *Phases—crisis and development in the individual*. Rudolf Steiner Press, London.

5. Pelikan, W. (1978). *Healing plants*. Rudolf Steiner Press, London.

6. Luther, P. and Becker, H. (1987). *Die Mistel—botanik, lektine, medizinische Anwendung*. Springer, Berlin. Khwaja, T. A., Dias, C. E., Pentecost, S. (1980). Recent studies on the anticancer activities of mistletoe and its alkaloids, *Oncology*, **43**, 42–50. Bloksma, N., van Dijk, H., Korst, P., and Williers, J. M. (1979). Cellular and humoral adjuvant activity of a mistletoe extract. *Immunobiology*, **156**, 309–19. Kiene, H. (1989). Clinical research on mistletoe therapy in malignant disease. A review. *Therapeutikon*, **3**, 347–53. (In German).

7. Hauschke, M. (1979). *Rhythmical massage*. Rudolf Steiner Press, London.

8. Rosslenbroich, B., Schmidt, S., and Matthiessen, P. F. (1994). Unconventional medicine in Germany. A report on the situation of research as a basis for state research support. *Complementary Therapies in Medicine*, **2**, 61–9.

9. Burkhardt, R. and Kienle, G. (1978). Controlled clinical trials and medical ethics. *Lancet*, i, 1356–9.

10. Evans, M. (1991). On the efficacy of anthropological medicines. *Complementary Medical Research*, **5**, 71–8.

11. Hildebrandt, G. and Hensel, H. (1982). *Biological adaptation*. Thieme, Stuttgart and New York.

9

Ayurveda

Ayurveda, along with its offshoots, Unani and Siddha, is at least as sophisticated as Oriental medicine. It is less popular in the West because it does not have a specific exportable skill, such as acupuncture. Its tenets are also published in Sanskrit. However, there are practitioners in the UK who serve the Asian community, and a wider interest in Ayurveda is developing in the therapeutic community. A number of Western practitioners have now undergone the gruelling and lengthy Ayurvedic training in India.

Ayurveda, or the 'Science of Life', is a section in the last of the Vedas, the *Atherva veda*, written in 2000 BC. However, the main Ayurvedic texts are the *Susruta samhita* and *Charaka samhita*, dating back to the fifth and second centuries BC respectively. It is virtually impossible to give any notion of the thoroughness and erudition of these texts. They set up several branches of medicine and present a practical teaching that covers every aspect of living in great detail. There are ancient texts on surgery which, for example, describe primitive proctoscopes and endoscopes, several different kinds of suturing, and how agents are carried by bodily contact, inhalation, and other channels to cause post-operative infections.[1] These texts were written 2500 years before Semmelweis was persecuted for suggesting that surgeons should wash their hands before operations. Indeed the *Charaka samhita* lists 20 kinds of *krimies* or microscopic pathogenic organisms (in addition to beneficial ones), and describes the body as composed of cells, and was written about 2000 years before the invention of the microscope.

Like other traditional systems, the essence of Ayurveda is balance between all the constituents, qualities, and energies within and without. There are five basic elements (*doshas*): earth (solid components of the body, compactness, structure); water (fluids, soft material, cohesiveness); fire (digestion, metabolism, heat, adaptation); air (sensation, nervous system, animation); and ether (networks, connections, channels). Earth and water are usually combined to give *kapha* (mucus, structural element), fire is *pitta* and *vatha* is air and ether combined as wind or activity. Like Chinese philosophy there are also basic energetic qualities, the *gunas*, namely *sattva* (unifying, wise), *rajas* (active, creating, somewhat like *yang*, and *tamas* (passive resisting, somewhat like *yin*). There are other anatomical and constitutional classifications.

Foods, climates, and all environmental influences and cycles contain the *doshas* and *gunas* to varying degrees. People too are constitutionally of one type or another, and the essence of Ayurvedic self-care knowledge is continually to balance these forces. That implies that not only can foods and environmental influences create harmony and health, they can also affect the state of subtle energy, alertness, activity, and wisdom.

There is probably no dietary system as rich and sophisticated as that embodied within Ayurveda. There is no standard or minimum dietary requirement for everyone, rather each individual would benefit from a specific diet that creates harmony in relation to his constitution and symptoms. For example *pitta* or fire types can benefit from 'cool' spices, such as cardamom, tumeric, or mint, but not 'hot' spices such as cinnamon, fenugreek, ginger, and cloves. For this type, turmeric is a specific to aid liver function, the liver being a *pitta* organ. Each health problem is treatable by a specific dietary regimen for that problem within that constitution. The late Dr Chandra Sharma, a well-known doctor in the UK, described how his mother would examine the climate, the state of health and activity of the family, their digestive energies, their moods and so on, and then cook a meal as a prescription for the occasion. A little of this knowledge has helped to create the complex alchemy of Indian cuisine, in which spices balance each other and the foods they flavour to support health and digestion. For example the water-generating nature of coriander is used to balance the heating quality of chilli. Cardamom reduces the mucous-forming tendencies of dairy foods, and is therefore frequently used to flavour yoghurt and milk sweets. Foods also affect the mind and emotions, and spiritual life. For example one Ayurvedic doctrine suggests that of food or drink, one third is gross and goes to excrement and urine, the middle third goes to flesh and blood, and the most subtle third goes to create mind and spirit.

Ayurvedic diagnosis includes some 32 pulse qualities identifying the condition of the viscera, as well as voice, face, iris, urine, sweat, diagnosis, and detailed personal history including astrological aspects. Complex prescriptions are designed according to the kinds of disease, the patient type, the anatomical site of the condition, the dominance of *dosha* or *guna*, the stage of the disease, the season, the age of the patient and so on. Each is formulated from the 8000 medicines recorded in Ayurveda. Unani medicne uses somewhat similar materials based on a philosophy which owes as much to Greek and Arab sources as the Vedas. Siddha medicine is a variant which has particularly adopted the use of minerals. Typical examples of herbs include *Piper longum* (pippali) used particularly in liver disorders, *Conifer mukul* resin (gogul) in atherosclerosis, *Emblica officinalis* (amalki) in duodenal ulcers and digestive problems, *Azadirachta indica* (neem) against parasites including the malarial parasite, bacteria and as insecticide, *Curcuma longa* (turmeric) for skin infections and liver problems, and *Ocimum sanctum* (tulsi, holy basil) for immune support and viral infections. There are various treatments within Indian traditional medicine, many of them quite unique such as massage and oil baths with medicated oils, special exercises, yogic breathing techniques, surgery, blood-letting, gem therapy, therapy using sounds or mantras, urine therapy, and a multitude of different yogic purification and cleansing procedures. Two new texts provide an excellent guide to these and other Ayurvedic methods.[2]

Research

A very great deal of research is carried out on Indian traditional medicine, although little of it ever reaches the West. A feeling for the research can be gleaned from the *Journal of Research in Indian Medicine*. Much of it is very intriguing. For example there are unusual studies on remedies that assist vitality and longevity known as *Rasayana therapy*. These demonstrate the restoration of more youthful hormonal patterns,[3] and recent studies have confirmed powerful effects on the natural antioxidant defences against free radicals.[4] When I explored Ayurveda in India, while at Benaras Hindu University, I was surprised to see experiments in progress which clearly indicated that certain remedies could induce muscles to regenerate, which is against the conventional assumption that this cannot be done.

Besides the thousands of *in vitro* studies that are carried out in India on Ayurvedic herbs and formulations, there are some recent clinical studies of interest. For example a double-blind, randomized, clinical study with osteo-arthritic patients demonstrated that a classical Indian mixture, which included *Withania somnifera, Boswellia serrata*, turmeric and minerals, produced a highly significant reduction in symptoms compared to placebo.[5] Turmeric also figures in a study on the treatment of 814 people with scabies. Ninety seven per cent were cured within two weeks, and the advantage of the remedy was its cheapness, safety, and availability.[6] The widespread use in the West of garlic as a cholesterol-lowering remedy owes much to Indian medicine. The first clinical and experimental research on garlic as a remedy for atherosclerosis was carried out by Professor Bordia. He was influenced by Ayurvedic knowledge that garlic reduces fat levels in the body. Since that time, other medicinal herbs and spices have been found to have similar properties.[7]

There are many antifertility herbs under study in India, as these herbs are used widely in Indian rural areas. One of them is the classical 'neem' tree, which can block fertility in experimental animals for up to six months after a single application.[8]

Obtaining treatment

Only in India is Ayurveda widely available. There are now some 300 000 Ayurvedic practitioners who belong to the All-India Ayurveda Congress. There are also more than 100 colleges who award a degree after 5 years study. There are a few Ayurvedic practitioners and courses in Western countries. The waters have been muddied by the entry of the Transcendental Meditation movement into Ayurvedic medicine, which resulted in the creation of 'Maharishi Ayur-Veda'. This is a highly commercial venture which employs expensive proprietary mixtures.[9] It should not be confused with real Ayurveda which makes available a choice of thousands of clearly identifiable herbal remedies.

The Ayurvedic and Unani practitioners in the UK are commonly known as *hakims* or *vaids*. They treat largely according to traditional principles, although they will be more Westernized than many. They will have up to 1000 remedies at their disposal. Even so, they can have difficulty in obtaining the best quality materials and also in authenticating plants. There has been a trend towards using ready-made patent mixtures, which deviates from the Ayurvedic tradition of remedies designed and mixed for each patient. One or two of these mixtures, prescribed perhaps by the less qualified of the practitioners, have been found to contain unwholesome amounts of heavy metals.[10] Therefore only properly qualified practitioners should be consulted. However, Indian traditional medicine's usefulness in areas such as rheumatism, arthritis, asthma, metabolic problems, cancer diseases, wound repair, digestive complaints, kidney and gall stones, tuberculosis, obesity, senility, and many other conditions should encourage more Westerners to try Ayurveda.[11]

References

1. Singh, L. M., Deshpande, P. J., and Thakral, K. K. (1970). Sushruta's contribution to the fundamentals of surgery. In *Advances in research in Indian medicine* (ed. K. N. Udupa). College of Medical Sciences, Benares Hindu University.
2. Frawley, D. (1990). *Ayurvedic healing*. Lotus Press, Santa Fe. Svoboda R. E., (1992). *Ayurveda—life, health and longevity*. Arkana/Penguin, London.
3. Varma, M. D., Singh, R. H., and Udupa, K. N. (1973). Physiological endocrine and metabolic studies on the effect of Rasayan therapy in aged persons. *Journal of Research in Indian Medicine*, **8**, 1–10.
4. Singh, B., Sharma, S. P. and Goyal, R. (1994). Evaluation of Geriforte, an herbal geriatric tonic, on antioxidant defense system in Wistar rats. *Annals of the New York Academy of Sciences*, **717**, 170–3.
5. Kulkarni, R. R., Patki, P. S., Jog, V. P., Gandage, S. G., and Patwardhan, B. (1991). Treatment of osteoarthritis with a herbomineral formulation: a double blind placebo-controlled, cross-over study. *Journal of Ethnopharmacology*. **33**, 91–5.
6. Charles, V. and Charles, S. X. (1992). The use and efficacy of Azadirachta indica ADR ('Neem') and Curcuma longa ('Turmeric') in scabies. A pilot study. *Tropical Geographical Medicine*, **44**, 178–81.
7. Jacob, A., Pandey, M., Kapoor, S., and Saroja, R. (1988). Effect of Indian gooseberry (amla) on serum cholesterol levels in men aged 35–55 years. *European Journal of Clinical Nutrition*, **42**, 939–44.
8. Upadhaya, S. N., Kaushic, C., and Talwar, G. P. (1990). Antifertility effects of neem (*Azadirachta indica*) oil by single intrauterine administration: a novel method for contraception. *Proceedings of the Royal Society of London & Biological Sciences* **242**, 175–9.

9. Skolnick, A. A. (1991). Maharishi Ayur-Veda: Guru's marketing scheme promises the world eternal 'perfect health'. *Journal of the American Medical Association*, **266**, 1741–50.

10. Smitherman, J. and Harber, P. (1991). A case of mistaken identity: herbal medicine as a cause of lead toxicity. *American Journal of Industrial Medicine*, **20**, 795–8.

11. Bannerman, R. H., Burton, J., and Wen-Chieh, C. (1983). *Traditional medicine and health care coverage*. World Health Organization, Geneva.

10

Chiropractic

Background

Bonesetting in the nineteenth century enjoyed extensive public support. The bonesetter's methods of treating strains, sprains, fractures, and other musculoskeletal
problems were gentle and instinctive. They were methods that people could
understand. Bonesetters provided stiff competition to surgeons whose techniques
for stretching and reducing joints were both violent and mystifying. Surgeons
and physicians in turn avoided any form of manipulation which they regarded
as unscientific, although some distinguished physicians successfully employed
manipulation in their practices.

Osteopathy and then chiropractic evolved in the USA, during the latter part
of the nineteenth century; both were derived from charismatic and observant lay
bonesetters. Chiropractic—from the Greek *keir* (hand) and *praktikos* (practice)—
was developed by D.D. Palmer in 1895. Palmer was a grocer who also worked as
an osteopath and healer. He realized the potential of spinal adjustments when
he cured one patient who had been deaf for 17 years, and another who had a
history of heart disease, solely by adjusting vertebra in the neck region. He was
so impressed by these achievements that he announced the end of his quest for
the basis of disease: it lay in the spine. Misaligned or maladjusted ('subluxed')
vertebrae restricted nerves; the interference with the proper flow of nervous
impulses prevented the 'innate intelligence' (Palmer's phrase for vital force or
vix medicatrix naturae) from passing through the body. 'A subluxed vertebra
is the cause of 95 per cent of all disease', stated Palmer. 'Luxated bones press
against nerves. By their displacement they elongate the pathway of the nerve
. . . modified impulses cause functions to be performed abnormally.' It followed
that treatment of all diseases could be effected exclusively by manipulation of the
vertebra to realign the joints.

To some extent Palmer's concern with the spine and the nervous system reflected
current medical preoccupations. Earlier in the nineteenth century physicians had
made extensive use of spinal treatments with leeches, cauteries, and so on, in
attempts to treat disease in organs on parallel body segments. During Palmer's

time the nerves were still a focus of scientific investigation. However, Palmer's insistence that virtually all known diseases could be cured by spinal treatments was anathema to the medical establishment, which became implacably opposed to his views. Medical opposition, especially in the USA, has continued, although modern chiropractors no longer hold Palmer's extreme views.

Concepts

The British Chiropractors' Association defines chiropractic as:

. . . an independent branch of medicine concerned with the diagnosis and treatment of mechanical disorders of joints, particularly spinal joints, and their effects on the nervous system. Diagnosis includes the use of X-rays and treatment is done mostly by hand without the use of drugs or surgery.

Chiropractors are therefore spinal specialists who hold that most of the problems relating to the spine stem from misalignments, maladjustments, and excessive strain placed on intervertebral and other joints. They call these problems *subluxations*, or small displacements. When used by doctors this term implies a small physical dislocation. However in chiropractic it is broadened to mean a functional as well as structural defect: 'the alteration of the normal dynamics, anatomical or physiological relationships of contiguous articular structures'. A subluxation may be manifested in physical displacement, or local, or radiating pain; there may be muscle spasm as a result of strain on the joint capsule; restriction or excessive movement of the joint, swelling, or weakening of more distant muscle groups.

Subluxations can be caused by many adverse influences such as strains, accidents, stresses, or innate skeletal distortions. Poor posture is often to blame, particularly where it places uneven or excessive loads on the back joints of the vertebrae. Chiropractors insist, as do many medical authorities, that however caused, defects in the joints will not be restricted to the spine itself, but will affect surrounding muscles, nerves, ligaments, and biochemical function, with which the joints are in intimate relation.

There have been several unsuccessful attempts to understand the subluxation in terms of our current knowledge of the biomechanics of the spine and the functions of the contiguous tissues, particularly where no physical displacements occur or are seen on X-rays. Possible suggestions include a reversible distortion of the cartilage, distension or squeezing of the joint capsule, or stretching of ligaments, all of which could produce the observable symptoms of a subluxation (tenderness, restricted movement, etc.), partly through reflexes triggered off by the nerves around the joint. It is, however, still an under-researched subject. 'The area of spinal mechanics and its implications in neurophysiology has not been explored by orthodox medical science. Chiropractic theories are only just beginning to evolve on a scientific basis from new discoveries and new scientists in the field', wrote the New Zealand Government Commission of Inquiry on chiropractic.[1]

The subluxation might also extend its influence beyond the spine to affect organs and tissues within the relevant body segment. Palmer envisaged this occurring by compression of the nerves as they emerge from the foramina to enervate the viscera. In the light of modern science it is possible to suggest other mechanisms, 15 of which were presented by one senior chiropractic researcher at a US Department of Health Education and Welfare conference on research into chiropractic.[2] For example, persistent irritation of nerves could interfere with the transmission of impulses or the flow of materials along the nerve.

Both chiropractors and osteopaths have observed that certain diseases can occasionally clear up after spinal manipulations, although osteopaths differ in seeking a vascular rather than nervous explanation. Thus dizziness, migraine, or lack of co-ordination can sometimes be associated with a subluxation at the first cervical vertebra in the neck, heart conditions or thoracic pain with one at the second thoracic vertebra. The subluxations are more likely to contribute towards these conditions than actually to cause them. This aspect of chiropractic philosophy has engendered considerable and violent dispute in the past which is still unresolved. There is evidence for the interdependence between the functions of the spine and viscera.[3] (See also Chapter 19). Kunert, an eminent authority in this field stated:[4]

We have no evidence that lesions of the spinal column can cause genuine organic diseases. They are, however, perfectly capable of simulating, accentuating or making a major contribution to such disorders. There can, in fact, be no doubt that the state of the spinal column does have a bearing on the functional status of the internal organs.

Practice

There are several aspects to a chiropractic diagnosis. It begins with a full personal history which would include traumas and injuries going back to childhood, as well as personal health habits. Many chiropractors also use X-rays, in which the spine is photographed segmentally or in its entirety. The use of X-rays is based on the belief that although functional and soft tissue (including intervertebral disc) displacements or damage do not show up, they may be detectable by a careful examination of the alignment of surrounding bony structures. The X-rays also give a powerful indication of the effect of posture on the spine, of any actual displacements of bones, and of medical conditions, such as osteoporosis or cancer, which would modify or prevent manipulative treatment. Palpation of the vertebral column before, during, and after movements is invariably used in diagnosis. For example, the practitioner may feel the play or movements of the vertebra as the patient is passively bent from side to side with his weight supported by the chiropractor. Leg raising and positioning tests are often used to assess pain and the alignment of the pelvis with the vertebral column. Chiropractors also examine posture, measure lengths of the extremities, assess muscle function, and carry out standard neurological and other basic medical tests.

Chiropractic diagnosis aims to discover whether the patient's complaint, usually joint pain, originates from systemic or underlying disease, or from a non-pathological mechanical disorder. The former is referred to orthodox medicine, the latter further investigated for its suitability for treatment by chiropractic. The treatment strategy varies according to whether the complaint is a painful lesion or strain, a disc problem, sciatica, an arthritic condition, and so on. Its main aims will be to restore the proper motion of the joints, to correct distortions or subluxations, to improve posture, and to remove the irritations, interference, or painful stimulation to nerves.

Manipulation is the standard procedure unless contra-indicated. This is accomplished by sudden short thrusts which prevent patient muscular resistance. The manipulation is carried out with considerable precision and control. Indeed, much of the art of chiropractic treatment is in the design and careful execution of manipulations, which are therefore of considerably greater sophistication and power than the manipulation sometimes available from physiotherapists or physicians. For example, a specially built couch is used to position the patient accurately so that each manipulation is most effective.

Other techniques are often used in conjunction with manipulation, in particular soft tissue techniques. These may take the form of sustained pressure on ligaments, or a massage of muscles, in order, for example, to relieve muscle spasm and pain, and prepare the joint for manipulation. Supportive measures are sometimes provided. Occasionally heat treatment or electrogalvanic apparatus is used, and a few chiropractors will also employ a variety of dietary and remedial treatments. Prophylactic advice is often given concerning ergonomics and correct physical activity, and some chiropractors apply a more holistic approach to their patients and will address lifestyle issues that cause the stresses that are built into their physical frame.

Research

The possibilities for research have been severely restricted in the past by the unwillingness of medical researchers to properly examine the therapeutic outcome of manipulation as performed by doctors and physiotherapists, let alone chiropractic. The situation is now changing and much more research is beginning. One boost to research was the US Department of Health, Education, and Welfare conference in 1975 on the basis of spinal manipulation.[2] However, so far little is known about spinal biomechanics and neurophysiology. Studies such as that of Crelin, which failed to find anatomical peculiarities in cadavers at the site of supposed subluxations, only emphasize how difficult it is to even approach the problems.[5] For back problems and back pain, and limitations of movement, are problems of function, and do not necessarily correspond to observable structural and biomechanical disturbances at the site of joints.

There have, however, been a number of serious studies of the success of manipulation in general and chiropractic manipulation in particular for various kinds of musculoskeletal problems (see also Chapter 19). The best known clinical trial of chiropractic was carried out by the Medical Research Council at their Medical Care Unit in Northwick Park Hospital. It was a response to the Cochrane Committee on Back Pain's recommendation that chiropractic be properly tested, echoed in Parliamentary debates. The researchers chose a 'pragmatic' assessment comparing the overall treatment of chiropractors with overall treatment at a hospital out-patients' department. This was more meaningful to the public than the other option, a 'fastidious' trial comparing specific treatment techniques. The importance of the trial was in its large numbers, 741 patients, and the long time, 2 years, in which cure was assessed by freedom from pain and by mobility. The results were that 'patients treated by chiropractors were not only no worse off than those treated in hospital but certainly fared considerably better, and that they maintained their improvement for at least 2 years.' The improvement was greater for those patients who had a more severe problem and a history of back pain.[6] This study is certainly the clearest vindication of chiropractic yet, although it drew a not unexpected flurry of critical comments from the medical community, from the simple anger—'physiotherapy has been given a stab in the back'—to the justified comment that to compare the unhurried, private treatment of a chiropractor to that of a rushed, impersonal, and understaffed NHS physiotherapy clinic would weight the scales towards chiropractic whatever the treatment given.[7]

Moreover, as the treatment given in the physiotherapy departments was predominantly medical manipulation ('Maitland' or 'Cyriax' techniques), the trial was actually a comparison of chiropractic versus conventional manipulation. Manipulation itself, of either kind, has been proven to be more effective than conventional passive treatments, usually consisting of rest and a painkiller, and/or diathermy or massage by the physiotherapist. For example a careful randomized controlled study on 256 patients with persistent neck and back problems, in which a placebo was used (detuned diathermy or ultrasound) demonstrated a clear advantage of manipulation which was noticeable immediately, and also persisted over some time.[8] When measures of normal function are used to assess outcomes, the results are more favourable for manipulation versus conventional massage and passive treatments than if only the symptoms are assessed.[9] It is also of interest that manipulation seems to be clearly preferable to other treatments if the problem is more severe—for example if there is sciatica and limited mobility as well as back pain.[10] However it is also true that non-specific or placebo effects do play a large part in outcomes. Thirty-five randomized trials were recently critically reviewed, and though manipulation stands the test against passive or conservative treatments, quite a few studies were unable to show a clear advantage of manipulation, probably because of the small number of patients involved, and the difficulty of designing a genuine placebo.[11] Patients, of course, cannot be fooled by a false and ineffective manipulation. These trials do in fact demonstrate the powerful influence of these non-specific, 'placebo', effects in treatment, which can overshadow the precise technique used, whether by physiotherapists or chiropractors.[12] This should encourage chiropractors to work more holistically and to develop themselves as healers so as to make use of these effects.

Workmen's Compensation Commissions have provided an opportunity to compare the efficiency of chiropractic and medical treatment in occupational terms. For example, the medical director of the Oregon Workmen's Compensation Board found that 82 per cent of the claimants with certain injuries treated by chiropractors could return to work within one week, twice as many as those with similar injuries who were treated by doctors.[13]

These comparative studies have concerned themselves only with musculoskeletal problems. However chiropractors have always claimed that some other organic conditions are treatable by chiropractic manipulation. This has raised the hackles of the medical profession, although it must be said that such claims are controversial even within the chiropractic community. The situation is complex because it is obvious that tension in the musculoskeletal system could spread to other areas of the body and cause or exacerbate a variety of organic symptoms in some patients. However, this does not necessarily mean that it is a suitable treatment for all or even the majority of cases. Headaches, for example, may arise from lack of or excessive mobility in the neck vertebra; patients who have fixations in these vertebra which show up on X-rays often report headaches. A recent review of a number of uncontrolled quantitative studies has suggested that manipulation can help about two thirds of such headaches that are traceable to muscle problems in the neck.[14] However this may not apply to migraine headaches. A group at the University of New South Wales has carried out a randomized controlled trial to assess the value of chiropractic in the treatment of migraine. Migraine patients were selected on the basis of their expectations from treatment, as well as other factors, and were well matched. It turned out that the patients who had been treated with manipulation by chiropractors had around 40 per cent reduction in migraine headaches, but the patients who were simply helped by physiotherapists to move their neck and shoulders also reduced the severity of their migraines by 34 per cent giving comparable results. The authors conclude that a proportion of patients could be helped by physical methods, but there was no real advantage in chiropractic.[15] This proportion is almost the expected proportion of patients who will get better by the placebo effect alone, and manipulation, involving touching and individualized attention, must be a fairly strong placebo. Chiropractic may be helping some patients in this way, but claims must be limited, and it is not necessarily the actual manipulation that is doing the trick.

A similar result has been found in a trial comparing proper manipulation with sham manipulation in 40 women with dysmenorrhoea. The full manipulation did reduce the perceived menstrual stress and plasma levels of prostaglandin F2a. However the sham manipulation did likewise. Since the sham manipulation was as intensive as the proper manipulation, but at an incorrect site, it is likely that the results were due to the placebo effect. In other areas such as high blood pressure,[17] and even hyperactivity of children,[18] studies have failed to support the specific use of chiropractic, and until there are serious studies in which the outcomes of chiropractic and the known effective therapies for such conditions, one can only agree with the conclusion of a recent review, that claims for treating non-musculoskeletal conditions are unfounded.[19]

Uses and risks

Around 80 per cent of the population experience back problems at some time or another, with 12–30 per cent suffering at any one time. This leads to at least 32 million working days lost per year in the UK alone, and the cost of back problems in the USA is a staggering $26–56 billion. Despite improvements in diagnosis, disability from low back pain is getting rapidly worse, and has been increasing in the USA during the last few years 14 times faster than the population growth.[20] According to Dr Mikheev, medical director of the World Health Organization, traditional management based on bed rest and passive care, including corsets, can be counterproductive. A more active management is needed including a recognition of physical and psychosocial influences.[20]

Most common musculoskeletal problems are treatable by chiropractic. These include arthritic and rheumatic conditions which may respond well to manipulation, for the extent of joint deterioration (spondylitis) may not be as irreversible as has been supposed. Sciatica, lumbago, neuralgia, slipped disc, non-specific back pain, strains, dislocations, and so on are the major cases seen by chiropractors. However, some musculoskeletal conditions, in particular systemic rheumatism, gout, osteoarthritic hips, bone malignancy, infections, and prolapsed (i.e. ruptured) spinal discs, are referred elsewhere for treatment, usually to doctors or conventional medical specialists.

Less than 10 per cent of chiropractic cases are seen because of an organic disease. Chest pain, migraine and headache, asthma, digestive disorders, and neurological disorders are organic conditions occasionally treated, and sometimes respond well if the chiropractor concerned uses various methods in an holistic manner. In some cases the patient and even the patient's doctor will assume an organic disease which is, in reality, pain radiating out from a problem in the vertebral column; these cases respond well to classical chiropractic treatment.

Chiropractic manipulation is safe. Responsible chiropractors ensure that in sensitive cases pressure techniques are used. The risks of treatment are rare. Some cases of neck damage and even paralysis have been reported, and also damage to blood vessels[21] but their frequency is less than virtually all known medical treatments.

The chiropractic treatment available in the UK is predominantly from graduates of the Anglo-European College of Chiropractic. There are also chiropractors from the McTimony school who treat the whole spine (rather than simply the subluxations) at every session, using massage and gentle manipulation to adjust its overall alignment.

References

1. Report of the Commission of Inquiry (1979). *Chiropractic in New Zealand.* New Zealand Government Printer.
2. National Institute of Neurological Communicable Disorders and Stroke (1975). *The research status of spinal manipulative therapy.* Department of Health, Education and Welfare, NIH, Washington D.C.
3. Kunert, W. (1963). *The vertebral column, autonomic nervous system and internal organs.* Enke, Stuttgart.
4. Kunert, W. (1965). Functional disorders of internal organs due to vertebral lesions. *CIBA Symposium*, **13**, 85–110.
5. Crelin, E. S. (1973). A scientific test of chiropractic theory. *American Scientist*, **61**, 574–81.
6. Meade, T. W., Dyer, S., Browne, W., Townsend, J., and Frank, A. O. (1990). Low back pain of mechanical origin: randomised comparison of chiropractic and hospital outpatient treatment. *British Medical Journal*, **300**, 1431–7.
7. Edgar, M. A. (1990). Letter. *British Medical Journal*, **300**, 1648.
8. Koes, B. W., Bouter, L. M., van Mameren, H. et al, (1992). A blinded randomised clinical trial of manual therapy and physiotherapy for chronic back and neck complaints: physical outcome measures. *Journal of Manipulative and Physiological Therapeutics*, **15**, 16–23. Mierau, D., Cassidy, J. D., McGregor, M., and Kirkaldy-Willis, W. H. (1987). A comparison of the effectiveness of spinal manipulative therapy for low back patients with and without spondylolisthesis. *Journal of Manipulative and Physiological Therapeutics*, **10**, 49–55. Cassidy, J. D., Lopes, A. A. and Yong-Hing, K. (1992). The immediate effect of manipulation versus mobilization on pain and range of motion in the cervical spine: a randomized controlled trial. *Journal of Manipulative and Physiological Therapeutics*, **15**, 570–5.
9. Hsieh, C.-Y. J., Phillips, R. B., Adams, A. H., and Pope, M. H. (1992). Functional outcomes of low back pain: comparison of four treatment groups in a randomized controlled trial. *Journal of Manipulative and Physiological Therapeutics*, **15**, 4–9.
10. Mathews, J. A. and Mills, F. et al. (1987). Back pain and sciatica: controlled trials of manipulation, traction, sclerosant and epidural injections. *British Journal of Rheumatology*, **26**, 416–23.
11. Koes, B. W., Assendelft, W. J. J., van der Heijden, G. J. M. G., Bouter, L. M. and Knipschild, P. G. (1991). Spinal manipulation and mobilisation for back and neck pain: a blinded review. *British Medical Journal*, **303**, 1298–303.
12. Koes, B. W. et al. (1992). Effectiveness of manual therapy, physiotherapy and treatment by GP for non-specific back and neck complaints. A randomised clinical trial. *Spine*, **17**, 28–35.
13. Martin, R. A. (1975). A study of time loss back claims: Workmen's Compensation Boards (Medical Director's Report, State of Oregon). *Archives of the California Chiropractor's Association*, **4**, 83–97.
14. Vernon, H. (1991). Spinal manipulation and headaches of cervical origin. *Journal of Manual Medicine*, **6**, 73–9.
15. Parker, G. B., Tupling, H., and Pryor, D. (1978). A controlled trial of cervical manipulation for migraine. *Australia and New Zealand Journal of Medicine*, **8**, 589–93.

16. Kokjohn, K. Schmid, D. M., Triano, J. J. and Brennan, P. C. (1992). The effect of spinal manipulation on pain and prostaglandin levels in women with primary dysmenorrhoea. *Journal of Manipulative and Physiological Therapueutics*, **15**, 279–85.

17. Yates, R. G., Lamping, D. L. and Abram, N. L. (1988). Effects of chiropractic treatment on blood pressure and anxiety: a randomized controlled trial. *Journal of Manipulative and Physiological Therapeutics*, **11**, 484–8.

18. Giesen, J. M., Center, D. B. and Leach, R. A. (1989). An evaluation of chiropractic manipulation as a treatment of hyperactivity in children. *Journal of Manipulative and Physiological Therapeutics*, **12**, 353–63.

19. Brown, P. (1994). Chiropractic: a medical perspective. *Minnesota Medicine (NBY)*, **77**, 21–5.

20. Kliger, B. N. (1994). World chiropractic congress 1993: occupational back pain. *Complementary Therapies in Medicine*, **2**, 45–7. Chapman-Smith, D. (ed.) (1993). *The chiropractic report*. World Federation of Chiropractic.

21. Mueller, S. and Sachs, A. L. (1976). Brain stem dysfunction related to cervical manipulation. *Neurology*, **26**, 247. Terrett, A. G. J. (1987). Vascular accidents from cervical spine manipulation. Report on 107 cases. *Journal of Australian Chiropractor's Association*, **17**, 15–24. Terrett, A. G. and Kleynhams, A. M. (1992). Complications arising from manipulation of the low back. *Chiropractic Journal of Australia*, **22**, 129–39.

11

Creative and sensory therapies

Creative therapies

The creative therapies, that is art and music therapy, are unusual in that they
integrate mind, body, and spirit in a manner familiar to complementary medicine
yet are also an accepted part of conventional medicine. These therapies are
supplementary to conventional psychiatry and psychology. They are also used
in various contexts of rehabilitation, nursing and geriatric homes, and centres for
the mentally disabled and chronically ill.[1] Art and music therapy can be used more
psychotherapeutically, as tools for self-discovery, in holistic and complementary
health centres which focus on cancer and mind-body diseases.

Creative therapies are to a large extent beyond the scope of this book, because
their concern is with mental rather than physical handicap, and they are often
part of, rather than complementary to, conventional medicine. Nevertheless their
approach emphasizes wholeness.[2] They use the same media but an entirely
different philosophy to anthroposophical medicine. So we will present a brief
overview only in this chapter. An indication of their rationale can be gained
from the following quotations: 'We act as a bridge, not only between a client's
inner and outer world, while he may not yet be able to do so for himself,
but also between himself and his outer social world . . . a connecting link but
not a betraying one.' 'The art therapy department in a psychiatric hospital
is often an asylum within an asylum . . . It provides people with space to
express inconvenient or unspeakable feelings. The relationship between an
Art Therapist and the hospital that employs him is often abrasive. It can
scarcely be otherwise since . . . the pictures often get worse as the patient gets
better'.[3]

This latter quotation hints at the difficult position that an art therapist often
finds him or herself in, arising from the fact that art therapists are the only
psychotherapists registered by the State and employed by the NHS. There is
sometimes a deep conflict between systems; between the holistic, subjective,
individual-centred view of healing of an art therapist, and the reductionist,
objective stand of the psychiatrists who refer patients to them. For example,

should an art therapist willingly accept a doctor's request to use the paintings of a patient as a guide for his drug treatment?

Within art therapy itself there are a number of different ways of working, and a dynamic dialogue between various groups. Traditional art therapy was begun by artists who worked in hospitals. Here the patient and his picture, and the inner dialogue of the patient and himself, is paramount. It is non-directed. The therapist stays in the background, and lets the creative process provide its own healing. Interpretation of the art by the therapist is treated with suspicion, for it pressures the patient to find meaning or understanding instead of allowing unselfconscious and spontaneous expression which is beyond words.[4] However many art therapists have felt that a more directly therapeutic approach is needed. Indeed, some have come from psychotherapy backgrounds within which art is used as a non-verbal therapeutic dialogue with the therapist. Here art itself is not central—the therapeutic relationship with the therapist is central: 'art may be of secondary importance because it is a means to an end, i.e. an additional way of coming to understand the transference . . . '.[5] This new trend became known as Art Psychotherapy, rather than Art Therapy. The two trends were locked in heated debates in 1991 which resulted in two streams within the art therapy movement, and the creation of a new association.[6] In addition there is a third stream which one might call Analytical Art Psychotherapy. This uses image and archetype, to identify unconscious forces in a Jungian manner. For example hidden and protected emotions might be revealed in symbol within the picture. As the patient changes, the images change: there is a dialogue with image and imagination.[7]

Music therapy is a rich and ancient therapy, used extensively in ancient Greek and Egyptian medicine, and throughout history. In modern times it is used very widely within similar contexts as described above for art therapy, for example in rehabilitation and geriatrics.[8] In many cases, however, it is used in an ill-defined and poorly targeted way, and though of proven benefit, it goes unnoticed as therapy. An example might be the use of relaxing music in a hospital setting to counter the stress and anxiety of medical procedures.[9]

Music therapy might be active, in which a patient or group of patients play musical instruments or sing. The music is usually improvised, according to the needs of the patient, perhaps beginning with the simplest of rhythmic instruments. Active music therapy is often used as an aid to socialization and expression, and can help the infirm to keep moving, listening, and thinking.[10] It is particularly valuable in countering the isolation of patients who cannot communicate through speech, for example because of dementia. David Aldridge has made a powerful case for the direct and intentional use of active music therapy in Alzheimer's patients. He points out that the basic elements of language itself are musical, and deeper than the semantic function, and that Alzheimer's patients seem to be helped by the use of rhythm and intentional playing and repeating of melodic phrases together with a therapist.[11] In addition, the playing of music can stimulate awareness and mind – body integration and co-ordination. The healing power of playing is also used in drama therapy, another of the creative therapies, although this requires more verbal communication skills.[12]

Passive music therapy, in which music is played to patients who relax and listen, has somewhat different goals. The music can be chosen according to the needs of the patient, perhaps being more or less stimulating, and eliciting different kinds of emotions. Passive music therapy is often used in cases of anxiety, mental disturbance, and psychosis; in coronary or cancer units; in the therapy of children, especially disturbed, autistic, and otherwise mentally handicapped children. It is intended to gradually improve mood, lift depression and anxiety, and heal the emotions.[13] In this context, its approach is truly holistic, emphasizing well-being and integration.[10]

Research in music therapy is fragmented, largely because of a lack of consensus as to what is being measured and how to evaluate outcomes. This is the point made in an excellent recent review of music therapy research by David Aldridge.[14] There has been a relatively long history of research on the way in which music effects blood pressure, heart rhythm, and breathing, with mixed results. It is possible to demonstrate some entrainment of cardiac and respiratory patterns to the rhythms of music, but it depends on the interest and involvement of the subjects.[15] Many studies have demonstrated that music relaxes patients, for example in Intensive Care Units, and they report feeling in a better mood and more at ease.[16] A number of similar studies, all relatively anecdotal and unstructured, suggest that music can aid patients during pre-surgical stress and in cancer care.[17] Again, better results were obtained when the patients were more absorbed and involved, for example, live music was more effective than taped music. Research on outcome has been very difficult, and most is impressionistic. Besides the positive changes seen in the elderly, mentioned above, there are studies with mentally handicapped adults and children, for whom much of modern music therapy has been designed.[18] Autistic and handicapped children appear to relate to music more than other forms of contact, and music has become important in their treatment and rehabilitation.[19] However real assessment of benefit requires new research models, which, perhaps, might be commonly applied to all research in the creative therapies.[20]

There is more interest today in introducing art and music into NHS hospitals for long stay patients, as part of the interior landscape. This is not a use of art as therapy, more as an attempt to humanize the hospital environment. There is a growing intention to integrate art, architecture, interior design, and exterior landscaping in new NHS hospitals. In general the staff feel that including art in the environment improves the ability of the staff to give care and the patients to receive it.[21] Its main use may be in hospitals for the mentally handicapped, and here it has been shown to aid the quality of life of residents, creating an environment which is more 'pleasing, stimulating and yet calming' as one resident put it, than the usual bleak institutional structures.[21]

Colour and sound therapies

As the creative therapies are on the fringe of conventional medicine so colour and sound therapies are on the fringe of complementary medicine. They are of an ancient vintage: colour and sound were used in therapy by the Greeks, and are still used by traditional Ayurvedic Indian practitioners. The theory behind these therapies is uncertain: it is a mixture of psychological, sensory, and parapsychological. On the psychological level it is well known that colours affect mood quite profoundly; blue is appealing, and relaxing, red is alarming and arousing. There are published studies showing how contemplation of blue light will lower blood pressure while red light will raise it.[22] Our language is full of colour–mood connections, such as green with jealousy or yellow as fear.

Yet the theory of colour therapy goes beyond this. It asserts that colour contains energy of a particular vibrational character which can complement or interfere with the energy of the function of the body.[23] It sees the body, or its organs, in illness as lacking one or other colour types, and aims to harmonize and balance body energy by the application of missing colours.[24] Colour therapists diagnose by reading the colours of the skin or perhaps of the aura, to assess which is missing. Colours are given by means of food of particular colours, liquids that have been bathed in coloured lights or sunlight, the environment and clothes, or special colour-emitting lamps. In India gems are used to focus coloured light on specific parts of the body. Meditation on different colours, as in Kabbalistic practice, is a common aspect of the therapy.

Sound therapy is also taken at a number of different levels. On the one hand practitioners point to the well known prosaic action of sound on the human organism—for example the ability of ultrasonics to shatter kidney stones or stimulate healing when used in physiotherapy. The power of music is conventionally accepted. On the other hand there could be a healing power of sound when used at a more subtle level, for example the mantric seed syllables used in meditation. In a similar manner to colour therapists, sound therapists believe each tissue resonates at a particular frequency and the frequency is changed by illness. Therapists treat illness by applying what they believe is a vibration of exactly the correct frequency to the outside of the body so that the vibrations penetrate to the desired spot. The mix of frequencies is specific to the organ and its condition.

Sound therapy is most frequently used in rheumatic complaints which seem to respond to the vibrations. Colour therapists, like healers, do not claim a specific effect on disease conditions, rather on the energetic state and resistance of the individual. In recent years electronic apparatus has been developed both for the practitioner, and for the patient's use at home. For example, there are sophisticated units which 'inject' colour into acupuncture points as part of electro-acupuncture treatment. There is as yet little accumulated experience or research exploration of these therapies.

References

1. Dalley, T. (1994). *Art as therapy*. Routledge, London.
2. Case, C. and Dalley, T. (1992). *The handbook of art therapy*. Routledge, London.

3. Gulliver, P. and Holton, R. (1986). In: *Ideas in art therapy* (eds. D. Waller and A. Gilroy). British Association of Art Therapists, London.

4. Dalley, T. (ed.) (1984). *Art as therapy: an introduction to the use of art as therapeutic technique.* Tavistock, London.

5. Shaverien, J. (1994). Analytical art psychotherapy. *Inscape*, 2, 47–57.

6. Waller, D. and Gilroy, A, (1991). *Art therapy, a handbook.* Oxford University Press. Oxford.

7. McNiff, S. (1992). *Art as medicine: creating a therapy of the imagination.* Shambala, Boston & New York.

8. Bunt, L. (1994). *Music therapy. An art beyond words.* Routledge, London.

9. Anon. (1993). The music of the body: music therapy in medical settings. *Advances*, 9, 17–35.

10. Halpern, S. and Savary, S. (1985). *Sound health: music and sounds that make us whole.* Harper & Row, New York.

11. Aldridge, D. (1994). Alzheimer's disease: rhythm, timing and music as therapy. *Biomedicine* and *Pharmacotherapeutics* 48, 275–81.

12. Jennings, S. (1992). *Drama therapy, theory and practice.* Routledge. London.

13. Aldridge, D. (1989). Music, communication and medicine: discussion paper. *Journal of the Royal Society of Medicine*, 82, 743–6.

14. Aldridge, D. (1994). An overview of music therapy research. *Complementary Therapies in Medicine*, 2, 204–16.

15. Haas, F., Distenfeld, S., and Axen, K. (1986). Effects of perceived musical rhythm on respiratory pattern. *Journal of Applied Physiology*, 61, 1185–91.

16. Updike, P. (1990). Music therapy results for ICU patients. *Dimensions of Critical Care Nursing*, 9, 39–45.

17. Bonny, H. and McCarron, N. (1984). Music as an adjunct to anaesthesia in operative procedures. *Journal of the American Association of Nurses*, Feb, 55–7. Bailey, L. (1985). Music's soothing charms. *American Journal of Nursing*, 85, 1280.

18. Wesecky, A. (1986). Music therapy for children with Rett syndrome. *American Journal of Medical Genetics*, 1 (Suppl), 253–7.

19. Grimm, D. and Pefley, P. (1990). Opening doors for the child 'inside'. *Paediatric Nursing*, 16, 368–9.

20. Aldridge, D., Brandt, G., and Wohler, D. (1989). Towards a common language among the creative art therapies. *The Arts in Psychotherapy*, 17, 189–95.

21. Miles, M. F. R. (1994). Art in hospitals: does it work? A survey of evaluation of arts projects in the NHS. *Journal of the Royal Society of Medicine*, 87, 161–3.

22. Birren, F. (1950). *Colour psychology and colour therapy: a factual study of the influence of colour on human life.* McGraw-Hill, New York.

23. Zantac, A. (1993). *Catching the light.* Bantam, New York.

24. Clark, Linda A. (1975). *Ancient art of colour therapy.* Devin-Adair, Old Greenwich, Connecticut. Gimbel, T. (1994). *The book of colour healing.* Gaia Books, Devon.

12
Healing

Background

Spiritual healing can be described as the re-creation of the flow of life energy between body, soul, and consciousness so that the whole person may return to balance and harmony. Healing can be given by anybody who restores energy and attitude in another person. However, it usually implies an active transmission of therapeutic energy by a healer, or group of healers, to a patient.

Healing involves experiences that are sublime yet awe-inspiring. They do not lend themselves to easy interpretation, and are difficult to grasp by people who do not themselves share these altered states of consciousness. Analyses of healing reflect as much the view of the commentator as the phenomenon he is describing. Thus some people see it anthropologically as beneficial social ritual, others as a form of hypnosis; some try and subvert it to rational physiological explanations,[1] while others visualize it as a miracle of divine intervention. Today, in our post-atomic era, there is a current of explanation which makes use of the notion of 'energy'. This may be a helpful model, yet it is still a gross concept describing subtle and inexplicable processes.

The primitive roots of healing are in shamanism and magic. Elaborate rituals are used to create attunement between the shaman, his guiding influences or spirits, and the patient. The shaman enters a trance state by means of drugs, breathing, dancing, or music. Power is invoked by supplication, and then focused towards the patient.[2]

The magical nature of healing has, since medieval times, strained its relationship with organized religion in the West, although not in the East. While the great spiritual teachers could usually heal, the religious institutions that bear their names have kept this activity at arm's length. The 'gifts of the Spirit' in Corinthians, 12, was confused with the Old Testament warning that 'Thou shalt not confer with familiar spirits', so that all true intuitive communication was considered heretical. While it is possible to accept that some individuals have exercised their powers in a negative way, most healing has been beneficial to the recipients. Nevertheless, healing groups within Christianity (e.g. Christian

Scientists, Pentecostalists), Islam (e.g. Sufis), and Judaism (e.g. Hasidim) are still on the fringe.

Fundamental concepts

It is useful to distinguish faith healing from psychic or spiritual healing.[3] The first involves an interaction between the psyche and physiology of the patient, and is essentially a marshalling of the will and energy of the patient to release his self-healing capacities. It is based on trust in the ability, authority, and personality of the healer, or direct hypnosis. This sort of healing is also involved in the placebo effect. It operates through the power of suggestion. Its mechanisms are discussed in Chapter 15.

The second type of healing concerns us here. This is the transmission of some form of energy, as yet unknown, from the healer to the patient. The energies involved are similar to those manifest in other paranormal phenomena, particularly psychokinesis. In this kind of healing, energy acts directly on the patient's body and spirit, and although the receptivity of the patient and a belief in healing is useful, it is not necessary. Indeed, as seen in the section on research, this kind of energy can heal animals and affect isolated cells and tissues. Of course, there is a good deal of overlap between faith and psychic healing; a healer may transmit energy through touch, for example, and healing may occur also through the patient's faith in this act as a symbol.

Psychic healing is predominantly a gift or a 'grace'. It comes to some people naturally when they have attained a refined and pure state of consciousness. Contemplatives and ascetics see the arrival of healing abilities as one of the *siddhis* or psychic powers indicating progress on the spiritual path. Occasionally people discover that they have this gift without self-development. For example, two well-known healers, Oscar Estebany and Bruce McManaway, both discovered it while fighting in the army. Perhaps the stress and demand of battle crystallized this potential within them.

Healing is also taught. This teaching used to be part of an initiation given by word of mouth to those who had reached the required stage in their overall spiritual development. The secret doctrine was considered to be of such potency that years of patient study and devotion were necessary in order to prepare for the privilege of service to mankind. Today there is a tendency to teach healing as an uncovering, expressing a form of energy that exists to some extent in most of us though obscured by thought forms and conditioning.

One general prerequisite for healing is a strong desire to do so. As one well known healer put it:

the healing gift is born of the feelings of inner compassion and sympathy for the sick. This is expressed through a deep inner yearning to help take away pain, suffering and sickness . . . It follows that many nurses and doctors possess the healing potential even though they may not be aware of it.[4]

The healer is a channel, and the desire to offer healing enables him to open the mind towards the receipt of these energies and their controlling influences. As the healer becomes more receptive, so the purity of his channel is increased. Pure white light is often seen as a tangible representation of the divine energy and all healers wish to be able to convey this. White light is of course made up of all colours, each at a correct and balanced level. However, the healer who has not progressed very far will block much of the healing spectrum because of his own impurity.

Healers have different beliefs concerning the source of this channel of energy. Many healers talk of discarnate entities which they allow to work through them whilst others prefer to feel that all healing comes from their own being. One group links with the source of light, whilst others focus on God. Those that make use of discarnate entities sometimes recognize them to have been doctors or healers when alive. They state that it is reasonable that someone who has spent his earthly life in helping others should wish to continue to do so after death. The effectiveness of that help will be in accord with the knowledge and understanding of the intelligence directing it.

There may be two levels to a healer's energy. On one level it reaches a patient's physical body. This is sometimes known as magnetic healing[5] and it can be done by many people, the mother for her child, a visitor to the sick, or the doctor or nurse for their patient. It is a more physical energy which, when given, will often leave the healer feeling sapped or exhausted. The healer has effectively given out some of his own energies and unless certain simple techniques are used for their replacement, he may suffer. The second level is at the energy prototype of the physical body (sometimes known as the etheric). This contains all the disharmony of the inherited character, the anxiety of negative thoughts and situations, as well as the flow of life energy. Healing of the etheric stems from the souls of the patient and the healer and may well not be felt by either healer or patient. However, it may be possible for an intuitive healer to 'watch' the energies being transferred by means of clairvoyant sight. This is seen as changing colours radiating towards the patient and harmonizing tones.[6] The greater the self-purification of the healer the more refined and powerful are the energies which he can transmit.

Despite a vast literature on healing energy in particular and psychic energy in general, very little is actually known concerning what it is or how it affects the body. Reich's 'orgone energy', Hall's 'animal magnetism', Herder's 'universal force', von Reichenbach's 'odic force', not to mention the Eastern concepts of *prana*, *Qi' shen*, and so on, are all descriptive systems depicting the same vital energy. Yet it is seen by its effects; its nature is a mystery. This remains the case despite some fascinating studies. For example, during healing the hands of a healer emit flares visible in Kirlian photographs, with simultaneous changes in the photograph of the recipient,[7] a healed person sometimes experiences considerable heat; psychic phenomena are prevented in a positively charged ionic atmosphere.[8] Modern physics has been encouraging in its revelation that not only is energy an emanation of matter, but matter itself is actually a form of energy. It is then suggested that the state of energy permeating our physical body will inevitably affect its organization and renewal. However, this raises other imponderables.

Diagnosis and treatment

Since disease or disharmony is caused by incorrect flow of life energy it follows that the deficiency must be isolated before a cure can be found. Diagnosis in psychic healing is therefore a two-stage process; first locating the physical seat of the problem, the disease, and then determining its origin in the etheric. It is felt that the physiological processes and cellular replication give off radiations which can be 'seen' through a sixth sense. Disharmonies are reflected in this aura. Therefore those who are sensitive and experienced can spot diseases through the aura at their very earliest stages.

The use of parapsychological faculties in diagnosis has certainly increased since the time of Edgar Cayce whose phenomenal abilities astounded the world but who was regarded as something of a freak. Now a large number of therapists and trainee therapists are learning to develop this insight. The more relaxed climate of opinion towards the supernatural helps them to keep an assured and balanced mind, an essential prerequisite to the development and use of these faculties. The technique may vary from observation of the colours of an aura or corona around individuals, to visualizing patches of light or shade on their bodies, or to sensing heat or tingling from diseased areas.

Just as there are different channels whereby the healer gains access to his energy, there are different practices whereby this energy is transferred on to the patient. Many healers lay their hands on a person or on a diseased part. This is particularly the case with therapists, such as osteopaths or nurses who have used hands to ease discomfort manually and then discovered a healing ability which is effective with the hand above as well as on the body. The hands may also be used to 'stroke' the space around a person in a form of psychic massage. This is sometimes called 'Therapeutic Touch' when used today by nurses, and health professionals, especially in the United States. However, in all cases the hands are only focusing instruments for the healer's energy. Many healers heal without hands, and without even the presence of the patient. This is known as absent healing, and is carried out by many of the healing groups in the UK.

The most common form of healing is prayer. This can be done either through a direct request for divine intervention to bring about some change, or by the focusing of creative thought which surrounds the patient with the energies needed to assist in reharmonization. Personal prayer is a powerful and effective method, especially when it is accompanied by the recognition that some change in attitude and lifestyle may well be necessary to re-create balance and harmony. It can take time to work because the body may well be already depleted of energy and unable to respond quickly enough for the patient to feel the difference. Thus he may become dispirited and wonder if the effort is worthwhile.

Perhaps the best method of healing is the use of the technique of visualization of the problem, together with the provision of those energies which will bring about a change. This can be effective when used to help a patient who does not know that it is happening but a speedier result will be achieved if co-operation is possible. If the patient knows that healing will be transmitted at a certain time of the day, he can then relax, open his mind, and visualize the energies surrounding and healing. This disciplined schedule and the knowledge that someone is helping can be very effective.

The visualization method can be illustrated by an incident related by the well-known healer Matthew Manning.[10] He described a vision he had while treating an autistic child. He felt himself travelling through her mind which appeared to him as a vast dark network. He moved about it as an aircraft moved over a dark city at night. As he moved he saw areas light up. The process continued until there was a sudden almost audible explosion of light at which point the girl's eyes focused for the first time.

Healers generally fall into two main classes. The vast majority are those who have developed their abilities and use them to provide a service to the public whilst continuing with a full time occupation. The strain required to do this is sometimes considerable. These healers do not charge fees for they believe that 'you cannot serve God and Mammon'. Furthermore, a stated fee might well prevent someone receiving healing because of restricted means. The second class of healer is the one who has had outstanding success and the demand for help has meant that healing has become a full-time occupation. As healers in this category rely on fees from patients they are obliged to state the minimum which they require. Some organizations run a referral service to both full- and part-time healers.

Healing is often combined with counselling. This enables the patients to look at their own attitudes in depth and discover unhelpful traits which they can then put right for themselves. Thus the thought processes are realigned towards harmony and the reactions are modified accordingly, so that after healing the physical body is not left in a stressed condition under which the disease will return.

Research

Many researchers, fascinated by the potential of applying science to the unknown world of spiritual powers, have carried out research on healing. There is a huge amount of this research that has accumulated over the years. It has been excellently reviewed and analysed in an exhaustive four-volume compendium written by Dr Daniel Benor.[11] When examining this research it rapidly becomes clear that even the best research is often shipwrecked on the rocks of unrepeatability, inconsistency, and mystery. Even very small changes in research protocol can result in radically different conclusions. This happens with research on plants or animals, in which there is no apparent placebo effect. With clinical studies, not only are there the usual problems of all research in complementary medicine, but also some other problems; that healing is so subtle that small changes in conditions have powerful effects on the intervention; that healing does not have a specific measurable outcome, but can affect living beings or tissues in unpredictable ways, depending on the needs of the moment; that healing happens beyond the sphere of rational thought and intentions so that even the best-laid plans go awry, for example it is never possible to say that healing does not happen in placebo situations, and it is never foolproof, and so on.

There are a large number of anecdotal human studies[12] which will not be reviewed here. A double-blind controlled randomized trial with 393 cardiac patients at San Francisco General Hospital investigated whether intensive Christian prayer healing could assist the recovery of patients. The results were very clear: those patients prayed for had significantly fewer complications, needed less antibiotics and other drugs, and less ventilatory assistance. None of the prayer group needed intubation compared with 12 of the controls, and 3 of the prayer group had a cardiopulmonary arrest, compared with 14 of the other patients.[13] There have been studies with patients with high blood pressure. A double-blind study of absent healing found that there was a significant improvement in systolic blood pressure in hypertensive patients, but not in diastolic blood pressure.[14] However a very sophisticated study carried out at the University of Utrecht by Dr Jaap Buetler and colleagues on hypertensive patients failed to find any difference between groups that were healed by laying on of hands, groups that were healed in absence and without their knowledge, and controls without any healing, although more of the patients who were healed by laying on of hands reported feeling better. Interestingly, all the groups lowered their blood pressure considerably and to a similar extent throughout the trial over 15 weeks.[15] Just being part of the trial seemed to cure their problem. The placebo was everywhere; healing occurred just through contact with people involved in the trial.

It could be argued that blood pressure is too complex a symptom to use as a yardstick for healing energy. There have been some interesting recent studies on a simpler measure—wound healing. Volunteers were given a punch biopsy and then given healing (therapeutic touch) under double-blind conditions. That is, through technical means the patients did not know they were being healed, nor did the experimenters know which patients were healed. There was a highly significant improvement in the rate of scar formation and rate of closure by epithelial tissue of the wounds in those who were healed.[16] However, as with all healing research, only sometimes was the experiment repeatable.

Therapeutic touch, carried out by nurses in Intensive Care Units and with post-operative patients clearly reduces patient anxiety. In a number of studies of healing it proved to be considerably better than placebo.[17] The placebo in these cases was usually someone going through the motions of healing but actually thinking of other things, or untrained people. It must be said that such a placebo may not be realistic, as people can often, consciously or unconsciously, see through the act, while if the actor is very good, healing may occur, in either case confounding the placebo. Similar studies on tension headache[18] and post-operative pain[19] showed highly significant positive results. In the latter case, Reiki healing was used on patients who had operations to remove two molars, one with and one without healing using a randomized crossover design so that each patient was their own control.

Laboratory studies have tended to be more consistent. This is despite the fact that laboratory conditions often lack the peace and tranquillity required for marshalling these energies, and so are not ideal for most healers.[20] A classical series of experiments carried out at McGill University in the 1960s showed that wounded mice healed much faster when a healer held his hands over them for 15 minutes twice a day. The controls in this case were a group of wounded mice who were similarly treated by a person who was not a healer, and an untreated group.[21] Similar kinds of experiments have shown that the growth of plants or fungi can be significantly affected by healing.[22] Recent research in biophysics laboratories in Eastern Europe, where healing energy is traditionally regarded as a form of physical and even electromagnetic energy, has confirmed these earlier studies, showing, for example, significant increases in seed germination after healing compared with controls.[23]

Human cells cultured in the laboratory have been used in such studies. In one case a healer induced cancer cells to drop off the glass tube to which they had adhered but this did not happen when the tube was handled without switching on the healing intention. In another case Matthew Manning was able to prolong the life of red blood cells within a weak salt solution (in which they normally burst) by up to four times. The chance of this happening normally was, according to the experimenters, about 100000 to 1.[24]

Experiments have been carried out with pure enzymes (biological catalysts) in the test tube. Under controlled conditions, a healer was asked to hold flasks of the enzyme trypsin. Other flasks of similar enzymes were either left untouched or exposed to a strong electromagnetic field. Time and again the effect of the healer's hands was found to be similar to that of the magnetic field. The activity of the enzymes was increased although the healer was not emanating any measurable electromagnetic energy.[25]

There have also been failures. Many noted healers dry up in a laboratory setting, and others fail for reasons that are quite inexplicable to them. Matthew Manning, in reviewing his past record of 32 psychic experiments, stated that 17 were deemed successful by the experimenters. These were invariably with animals or biological materials, rarely with physical targets such as electrical gadgetry. He argues that naive or sceptical experimenters almost never obtain significant results in their controlled experiments. The identical tightly controlled experiment performed within a positive milieu will generate positive results. The experimenter, he concludes, 'has to conduct his tasks not as an Inquisitor, but as a partner.'[26]

It is also necessary for the experimenter to use his insight in order to disentangle a complex interaction within healing situations. For example, consider the phenomena of psychic surgery. In Brazil and the Philippines healers have traditionally used a technique in which they appear to extract diseased tissue, kidney stones, or tumours from patients who are then remarkably cured.[27] However, when the tissue is analysed, it has been found to be derived from an animal and not from the patient at all, a discovery that has been used in attempts to discredit these healers.[28] More dogged investigators have learnt that the healers do not really claim to have extracted the tissue, but use it for the display and theatre that attunes the patient to the healer. For as Westerners believe in surgery, the healer appears to accomplish it for their benefit. It certainly is not all trickery. Lyall Watson reports that after submitting to a psychic injection blood appeared on his arm under several layers of plastic sheet which was not punctured.[29] These controversies do not disprove the healers' undoubted powers.

Another fruitful line of research has been the analysis of brain wave patterns. Max Cade has demonstrated with electroencephalographic brain wave monitoring devices that healers, clairvoyants, and yogis show similar brain wave patterns when utilizing their concentrative abilities. The brain wave patterns of some patients alter simultaneously with the receipt of healing, sometimes even with absent healing when the patient was not told when the healer intended to begin.[30] Some similar studies have shown that healers at a distance can alter the Galvanic Skin Response (GSR) measured by biofeedback devices. This measures stress as skin resistance. There was a greater effect with subjects who had a high GSR and were under stress.[31]

Uses and risks

Healing is potentially applicable to any kind of condition; however, it is especially useful in the treatment of chronic conditions which are not too deeply set, but where the patient has insufficient energy and vitality for his own natural immune and self-healing abilities to operate. It is also very useful in a preventive role, restoring wholeness and resistance in an individual who is at risk, before a full blown disease develops.

The famous miraculous instant cures of long-term and otherwise incurable diseases are a rarity in healing. Often a patient may lose his pain immediately and seem to be better— the 'throwing away of crutches'. However, the condition is still there and the symptoms soon return. It has, for example, had better results with depression and chronic problems like ME in which a general return of vitality is part of the cure, than with asthma which is a chronic over-reaction of the body.[32] Healing is, rather, a gradual process of removal of the problem and repair of the energies, which may take a considerable time. In addition, since patients may have incurred their disease through in some way living contrary to basic laws of natural good health, changes may be needed in their attitudes and lifestyle before the problem can be permanently overcome.

Healers report cases where cancer sufferers have overcome the disease with their help. The majority of cancer cases do not consider healing until they have been told that their situation is terminal. At this stage, the physical body will often be weakened but it is never too late to begin work.[33] Where the disease does not regress the healer is very often capable of relieving the pain and distress.[34]

There are no direct risks involved. Occasionally there may be a transient worsening of the symptoms after healing. This is usually a good sign, indicating that the body is throwing off the condition. The only risk is that, as with other therapies, a patient may delay other treatment that he needs while he is being healed. For this reason, if a patient has symptoms he should consult a relevant practitioner first as a matter of course. Healing can then be given in addition to or after other kinds of treatment, and it is obviously beneficial if the healer and doctor or other practitioner work together.

References

1. Sargant, W. W. (1973). *The mind possessed: a physiology of possession, mysticism and faith healing.* Heinemann, London.
2. Eliade, M. (1964). *Shamanism: archaic techniques of ecstasy.* Princeton University Press, Princeton. Chesi, G. (1980). *Voodoo.* Perlinger, Worgl, Austria.
3. Csordas, T. J. (1994). *The sacred self: a cultural phenomenology of charismatic healing.* University of California Press, Berkeley, California. Calestro, K. M. (1972). Psychotherapy, faith healing and suggestion. *International Journal of Psychiatry,* 10, 83–113. Haynes, R. (1977). Faith healing and psychic healing. Are they the same? *Parapsychology Review,* July, 10–13.
4. Bloomfield, B. (1984). *The mystique of healing.* Skilton and Shaw, Edinburgh.
5. Taylor, A. (1992). *The healing hands.* Macdonald Optima, London. De Saussure, R. (1969). The magnetic cure. *British Journal of Medical Psychology,* 42, 141–63.
6. Regush, N. M. (ed.) (1974). *The human aura.* Berkeley Medallion, New York.
7. Gennaro, L., Guzzon, Fl, and Marsigli, P. (1987). *Kirlian photography.* East West Publications, London. Moss, T. (1981). *The body electric.* Granada, St Albans.
8. Puharich, G. (1977). *Beyond Telepathy,* Granada, St Albans.
9. Krieger, D. (1979). *The therapeutic touch: how to use your hands to help or heal.* Prentice Hall, Englewood Cliffs, New Jersey.
10. Manning, M. (1981). *Wrekin Trust lecture.* Loughborough University, Loughborough.
11. Benor, D. (1993). *Healing research. Volumes 1–4.* Helix, Munich, Oxford.
12. Le Shan, L. (1985). *From Newton to esp.* Viking, New York.
13. Byrd, R. C. (1988). Positive therapeutic effects of intercessory prayer in a coronary care unit population. *Southern Medical Journal,* 81, 826–9.
14. Miller, R. N. (1982) Study of remote mental healing. *Medical Hypotheses,* 8, 481–90.
15. Beutler, J. J., Attevelt, J. T. M., Schouten, S. A., Faber, J. A. J., Mees, E. J. D. and Geijskes, G. G. (1988). Paranormal healing and hypertension. *British Medical Journal,* 296, 1491–4.
16. Wirth, D. P., Brenlan, D. R., Levine, R. J., and Rodriguez, C. M. (1993). Full thickness dermal wounds treated with non-contact therapeutic touch: a replica and extension. *Complementary Therapies in Medicine,* 1, 127–32. With, D. P., Barrett, M. J. and Eidelman, W. S. (1994). Non-contact therapeutic touch and wound reepithelialization: an extension of previous research. *Complementary Therapies in Medicine* 2, 187–92.
17. Heidt, P. (1991). Helping patients to rest: clinical studies in therapeutic touch. *Holistic Nursing Practitioner,* 5, 57–66. Quinn, J. (1984). Therapeutic touch as energy exchange: testing the theory. *Advances in Nursing Science,* 6, 42–9.
18. Keller, E. and Bzdek, V. M. (1986). Effects of therapeutic touch on tension headaches. *Nursing Research,* 30, 101–6.
19. Wirth, D. P., Brenlan, D. R., Levine, R. J., and Rodriguez, C. M. (1993). The effect of complementary healing therapy on postoperative pain after surgical removal of impacted third molar teeth. *Complementary Therapies in Medicine,* 1, 133–8.

20. Laboratory studies have been well reviewed in: Benor, D. (1990). Survey of spiritual healing research. *Complementary Medical Research*, 4, 9–33.
21. Grad, B. (1965). Some biological effects of laying on of hands—a review of experiments with animals and plants. *Journal of the American Society for Psychical Research*, 59, 95–126.
22. Barry, J. (1968). General and comparative study of the psychokinetic effect on a fungus culture. *Journal of Parapsychology*, 32, 237–43.
23. Jerman, I., Kustor, V., and Kurincic-Tomsic, M. (1994). Biotherapy—one of the most common methods of unconventional healing in Slovenia. *First COST Conference*, London.
24. Braud, W., Davis, G., and Wood, R. (1979). Experiments with Matthew Manning. *Journal of the Society for Psychical Research*, 50, 199–223. Braud, W. (1989). Distant mental influence on the rate of haemolysis of human red blood cells. *Research on Parapsychology*, 1988, 1–6.
25. Smith, M. J. (1972). Paranormal effects on enzyme activity. *Human Dimensions*, 1, 15–19.
26. Manning, M. (1979). Why experimenters upset results. *Alpha*, November, 11.
27. Valentine, T. (1975). *Psychic surgery*. Pocket Books, New York.
28. Granada Television (1975) '*World in Action*' (4 April 1975).
29. Watson, L. (1982). *Supernature*. Hodder & Stoughton, London.
30. Cade, M. and Coxhead, N. (1987). *The awakened mind: biofeedback and heightened states of awareness*. Element Books, Shaftesbury, Dorset.
31. Schlitz, M. J. and Braud, W. G. (1985). Reiki plus natural healing: an ethnographic/experimental study. *Psi Research*, 4, 100–23.
32. Robertson, J. (1991). Spiritual healing in general practice. *Journal of Alternative and Complementary Medicine*, May 1991, 21–3.
33. Magaray, C. (1981). Healing and meditation in medical practice. *Medical Journal of Australia*, 338, 340–1.
34. Cadwell, D. (1986). Healing. *Health Visitor*, 59, 347.

13

Herbalism

Background

The use of plant materials for the treatment of illness is as old as civilization. Records containing lists of plants going back some 5000 years have survived from both ancient Egypt and China, with plants differentiated according to specific disease conditions for which they could be used.

There is certainly no form of human society known which, having access to flora in the locality, does not exhibit a profound understanding of the potential use of these plants. They are used for foods, medicines, and dyestuffs as well as for arrow poisons and antidotes, in religious rituals as hallucinogens, and for cosmetics. Indeed, such understanding seems to match directly the extent to which that society is integrated with its natural surroundings; the onset of civilization has often tended to diminish rather than enhance this fund of knowledge.[1]

Herbal knowledge is gathered through trial and error over long periods. Large numbers of plants are collected for various conditions and purposes, from food preparation and household maintenance at the one extreme to ritual practices at the other. Another source of herbal knowledge is intuitive revelations. Healers have often trained for years to amplify their sensitivity, observation, and intuition. They may detect effective substances by trying them out on themselves, or by receiving information while in ceremonial or altered states of consciousness. Most folk cultures will tell how plants appeared to their witch doctor in his dreams and told him of their powers. The Emperor Shen Nung, the 'heavenly husbandman', originator of Chinese herbal medicine, is said to have had a 'grace' which allowed him, on one occasion, to discover 70 new remedies in one single day. It is interesting to speculate that perhaps remedies discovered in this way are mild, adjustive, and preventive, just those remedies which cannot be detected by trying them out on sick people.[2]

From time to time in human history the evolution of a prosperous, creative civilization has been accompanied by attempts to formalize the available health care systems, most notably during the Greek and Islamic eras in the West, and as a continuous process in China and India in the East. However, at the level of village society, even today, primary health care is still largely herbal, and in the hands of an untrained, most often female, member of the group, who has maintained her direct intuitive link with local plants.[3] The herbal practitioner still trusts in experience and intuition rather than in works of scholarship. This has meant that herbal medicine has escaped literate attention and in its essential form has played little part in the social affairs of man in the West.

The use made of plants as medicines has always conformed to the whole view of the human organism in its universe. In China and India the cosmology has emphasized the integration of existence. This has produced vitalistic concepts in which the qualities of herbs are matched to the qualities or disharmonies which have caused disease. For example, according to Chinese medicine, the tastes of plants are an indication of their likely effects on disturbed organ systems. The early traditions of the West, particularly Greece, led to an inclination to see the world analytically, producing a symptomatic cause-and-effect manner of using plants (see p. 11). This way of using plant medicines has tended to dominate in the West and has shaped, during the nineteenth century, the methods of drug use of modern medicine.[1]

During medieval times the use of herbs was laden with superstition, incantation, and ritual. A sick person taking a certain herb might have to walk seven times round a tomb reciting a Latin phrase to ensure efficacy. When European herbals were being written in the sixteenth and seventeenth centuries, a large part of the information came from ancient Greek (Dioscorides and Galen) and Islamic (Avicenna) sources; these were combined with scatterings of folklore to create the patchy accounts for each remedy that have marked popular books on herbalism ever since.[4] Traditional herbalists still practised relatively efficiently at the village level but in urban areas the stage was occupied by practitioners pursuing symptomatic medicine.[5] These found herbal remedies unsuitable for their purposes and turned more and more to inorganic remedies and surgery. Violent arguments raged between the herbal 'Galenicists' and the 'Chymists'. The power and purity of the Chymists' compounds were so attractive to a rapidly growing technological age that herbal remedies were gradually discredited. With the arrival of scientific medicine this process continued—not because the herbal remedies were demonstrably ineffective, but because they did not fit into the system. 'Many of the plants used as medicines can no longer be considered within the pale of rational therapeutics', explains a pharmacology textbook.[6] The plants were dropped from the pharmacopoeia during the first part of this century despite the fact that plants were and still are used as starting materials for the manufacture of drugs. Of 1.5 billion prescriptions dispensed in the USA annually 25 per cent contained active constituents obtained from plants but only 2.5 per cent contained crude plant material. More serious, the knowledge of how best to use these plants was also threatened with extinction.

The survival of modern herbalism owes a good deal to widespread emigration from Europe to North America in the eighteenth and nineteenth centuries. In this period thousands of emigrants were distributed over the huge continent with a minimum of standard European health care. They brought with them the memories of common herbal treatment in rural areas of their native country and often the actual medicinal plants themselves. They also encountered the considerable medical intelligence of the North American Indian, based very largely on herbs. It was in many other ways of course a destructive meeting, but in medicine the combination of necessity, disenchantment with European sophistication, and a raw enterprise resulted in the brief flowering of many new developments. Osteopathy and chiropractic have survived to this day, but there were also several short-lived schools of herbal medicine. Several times around the turn of the century the new herbal medicine was re-imported back to the UK where it hybridized well with the herbal traditions still surviving there. Today, the largest body of herbal practitioners in the UK sees itself as the heir to the North American experiment.

In the UK medical herbalism has for centuries been practised mainly in country districts and, after the Industrial Revolution, in the new working-class cities. It has survived to the present day and a combination of a successful move to protect the definition 'medical herbalist' under the terms of the 1968 Medicines Act, and the emergence of a new generation of practitioner seeking an alternative to allopathic practice, has now transformed the profession.

Fundamental concepts

Because of the primitive and diffuse origins of herbal medicine, in the West, there has never been any 'school' determining basic philosophy nor even any universally accepted fundamental concepts. Because it has been *the* medical system for most people most of the time, it has tended to be all things to all people. However, the main assumption in herbal medicine is that there is a vitality in the human frame that stands apart from the therapeutic endeavours of the practitioner. This vital force can be seen as a purposeful, self-correcting, resistant force transcending the abrasions of life. For example, the astonishingly exact maintenance of body temperature through a wide range of situations is to the modern herbalist a clear manifestation of an ability that no man-made therapy can augment. The aim of herbal medicine is to support the action of this vital adaptive energy wherever it appears to be weakening.

Modern Western herbalists use much the same terminology and concepts as current orthodoxy but they are interested in detecting and restoring normal function rather than acting to stop a pathology. The symptom is seen as a sign, if read correctly, pointing to the seat of the disorder. For example an infection may point in the first place to 'stagnation' of the affected tissues. Healthy tissues, like running water, cannot suffer colonization by bacteria; such an invasion can only occur in the histological equivalent of the brackish pond. Treatment of infections then demands that the tissue be 'cleansed' and brought back into the vital circulation. Antibiotics would only be necessary in this scheme if the colonization was so excessive that there was real doubt as to the host's ability to overcome it from vital resources, and then appropriate only if underlying stagnation were treated as well. Using antibiotics alone is seen as being as productive as pouring disinfectant into a brackish puddle and pronouncing it 'clean'.

The same concern with underlying causes marks the herbal practitioner's approach to other conditions. A spasmodic condition like asthma or colitis speaks first of an irritant factor combined with a tendency to over-react. An inflammatory condition like skin disease or arthritis speaks of a healthy but insufficient attempt to eliminate toxic accumulations. Similarly, in dealing with migraine or the autoimmune conditions a primary aim is to search for the source of toxicity, perhaps in defective digestive or liver function or in inadequate elimination.

Victorian herbalism divided herbs into classes according to their effect on discrete physiological processes—diuretics to cause urination, alteratives to adjust the metabolism, purgatives to clean out toxic materials from the digestive system, and so on. Modern herbalism is much more sophisticated, but it has developed these adjustive concepts, largely through an awareness of modern medical and biochemical science, rather than displaced them.

What are the essential therapeutic features of the herbal remedy? They can be classified in three ways.[7]

1. Herbal remedies have challenging qualities which tend to provoke a number of protective responses from the body. In particular they make excellent local applications in damage to skin and stomach lining. Mucilaginous components, such as marshmallow root, soothe and provide physical protection and relief from irritation and pain; tannins and other astringent factors, such as witch hazel, form tough antiseptic coats over exposed tissue or mucosal surfaces. Both these properties generate useful reactions in the stomach, reducing spasm and colic. Other herbs trigger helpful physiological reactions. For example the anthraquinone glycosides of senna work by gently irritating the bowels to produce elimination, the acrid glycosides in chilli, ginger, and mustard stimulate the blood vessels to increase the flow through the tissues, and the bitter herbs, such as gentian, stimulate a range of digestive reflexes (flow of bile, movement of gastrointestinal muscles, gastric secretions, appetite, etc.) when held in the mouth. Other examples include the production of expectoration (cough) reflexes or diuresis in the urinary system. These kinds of agents rely on the presence of the reactions in the body which the plant triggers.

2. Herbal remedies can adjust body processes. They exhibit a normalizing, supportive action on organs and tissues, acting almost like foods rather than medicines. For example, the effect of oat extracts on chronically poor vitality, nervous exhaustion, or 'neurasthenia' is likely to be due to the balance of minerals and other nutrients supplied as well as to the dynamic action of saponins and alkaloids; a similar relationship is likely to hold for the dandelion root and the liver, coltsfoot and the lungs, or couch grass root (*Triticum repens*) and the kidneys. A balanced action can be demonstrated for other remedies. By simultaneously increasing coronary blood flow and yet slowing the heart rate,

the hawthorn (*Crataegus oxyacantha*) finds application in cases where the heart is under strain.[7] In another variation, the action of the ginseng root improves the ability of the adrenal cortex to respond optimally to stress. The fruit of the chasteberry tree (*Vitex agnus castus*) is thought to influence a wide range of gynaecological problems by acting on the pituitary to 'balance' the secretions of progesterone and oestrogen. In other cases the presence of a number of constituents in the same plant helps to explain paradoxical actions. The isolated cardiac glycosides of the lily-of-the-valley plant (*Convallaria Spp.*) are not as powerful as those of the foxglove (*Digitalis purpurea*) yet in the context of the whole plant it is a most useful and relatively safe cardiac remedy for it has a graded effect and is also a diuretic. In all these cases much of the benefit arises from the whole remedy being used, the many often uncounted constituents having total effects greater than the sum of their parts.

3. In a great number of ways herbal remedies are eliminatory. They are particularly good at improving the action of the eliminatory organs, the bowels, kidneys, lungs, and sweat glands, and at improving circulation ('heat'). This results in increased nourishment as well as drainage, both to tissues at large and to particular organs. Herbal remedies also work at improving the ability of the digestive system to handle and detoxify potentially dangerous substances in the diet and particularly at enhancing the ability of the liver to convert and excrete the whole range of metabolites. The herbalist feels justified in claiming to be able to 'clean out' the body to a degree that other therapies do not attempt to match.

There are also a considerable number of herbs, derived from folk medicine and used today as household remedies, which have effects on specific symptoms outside the above categories. Examples include aloe vera (wound healing, antibacterial, and anti-inflammatory), garlic (antibacterial, antifungal), valerian (sedative), or wormwood (antihelminthic).

Diagnostic and therapeutic practices

The modern Western herbalist most often uses the diagnostic methods and tools of the good general practitioner in Britain, although he will place more emphasis on finding out why the disease occurred at this particular time. There are also some practitioners who use Chinese diagnostic methods (see Chapter 6) or radionics, iridology, and some intuitive methods. Generally, the herbalist will determine the patient's medical history, the nature of current stresses, dietary habits and lifestyle, and performance of the main functions of the body: digestion, respiratory system, genito-urinary systems, circulation, and nervous and emotional functions. This is combined with such clinical assessments as are considered useful: blood pressure, pulse taking, physical examination, microscopic assessment of urine and blood smears, etc. The terms of the diagnosis may only partly include the name of a disease state or pathology and it usually includes functional terms such as 'vascular spasm', 'hypersensitivity', 'hyperacidity', 'chronic inflammation', 'nervous debility', and so on, the better to reflect the therapeutic direction of the treatment.

Treatment is selected according to what aspect of health is judged most in need of support. An attempt will be made to deduce what is likely to be the 'primary lesion' and this treated first; this might present some difficulties in those advanced pathologies where layers of secondary effects and tissue damage have to be taken into account. Advice is given concerning environmental stresses and diet, the consensus opinion being that where possible diet should be as primitive as is practicable, using whole foods, fresh fruits, and vegetables. Nervous tension, both obvious and otherwise, is treated less by herbal 'tranquillizers' (such as Passiflora) than by use of 'relaxants', such as camomile or hops, that reduce the effect of such tension on the viscera. Where there are debilitated conditions these will be treated with restoratives, trigger remedies may be given to arouse normal function, and temporary protection will be provided where practicable by the use of mucilaginous and other such agents. The overall aim is to lead to sufficient correction of body functions that normal homeostatic regulation may take over; in other words treatment is as short as possible and discontinued as early as conditions allow. Any extended treatment is seen as something of a failure and generally denotes either an advanced pathology or else incorrigible environmental stresses.

For example, in the treatment of rheumatoid arthritis a dietary regime may first be organized, usually with vitamin supplementation and instructions on avoiding certain foods. Internal remedies may include angelica to increase diuresis and sweating and *Apium* where there is depression. *Cimifuga* is used where sciatica and neuralgia exist; this is combined with *Phytolacca dec.* especially where the condition is chronic, and *Galium aparine* which aids in effects on lymph. *Dioscorea vill.* is used for rheumatism and rheumatoid arthritis, acting through the hormones, and *Filipendula* against acidity. External applications of *Symphytum* will reduce inflammation, rosemary is used against pain, and it also, like mint and cayenne pepper, aids the circulation.

Preparations may contain a complex mixture of constituents: a dozen would not be unusual. The remedies will usually be provided by the practitioner rather than through a third party. Sometimes they are provided 'off the shelf' by retail herbalists although this is now rare. They will most often be in the form of tinctures (concentrated extracts of the herbs in water/alcohol solvent) for ease of dispensing. If bulk is not a problem the herbs may be provided in capsule or tablet form. However, these are inappropriate in many cases due to the large quantities of herbs often needed; a tincture remains the most compact way of administering herbs.

Uses and risks

Medical herbalists generally feel confident in treating most conditions that they might encounter.[7,8] There are one or two legal limitations in the UK, notably venereal disease, and acute and dangerous conditions are referred to accident and emergency departments or doctors. Moreover most practitioners avoid interfering with vital allopathic treatment already under way, such as insulin, antithrombotic drugs, and so on because of the risks involved. Herbalists will often refer patients or work together with other practitioners. In particular, manipulative work will be referred elsewhere for appropriate treatment, and psychiatry or emotional disorders are often passed on as well. Epilepsy, schizophrenia, and neurological diseases prove particularly resistant to treatment, and no false claims are made when there is other established tissue damage to contend with.

Herbal medicine comes into its own where there are physiological tasks to be done and where there are accumulations to clear. It is thus useful in organic problems of any sort, for chronic infective conditions anywhere in the body, and for restoring debilitated organs or functions. It also has a largely undervalued role in external applications where there is no suitable alternative therapy. There are few risks with professional herbal treatment provided it is monitored by a competent herbalist. However, as material dosages of plant medicines are used minor side-effects, such as irritations from the stimulating trigger remedies, might occasionally be encountered. Herbs, when used by the herbalist to restore function, do not have the toxic effects of the more pharmacologically incisive conventional drugs.

There have been some rare cases of toxic effects of herbs used in self-medication, sometimes from contaminants in Chinese herbs.[9] Comfrey root (but not leaf), chaparral, and coltsfoot are examples of traditional, widely used herbs that have been banned from open sale because they contain potentially toxic pyrrolizidine alkaloids. But this must be put into proper perspective. The consumption of the whole plants are known to be completely safe.[10] In the last 15 years only four cases of possible comfrey poisoning were found; all of them cases in which other medicines and treatments including steroids were being taken.[11] These were widely reported in the medical literature. But this appears to be a good example of publication bias, in which these few adverse effects are welcome in the major medical literature but not the multitude of reports of successful herbal treatments, whereas with modern drugs the reverse is true. The National Poisons Unit in the UK carried out a survey of all poisoning by herbs from 1983–1991, and found less than 1 case per year, apart from 24 cases of drowsiness caused by people trying (and failing needless to say) to commit suicide with herbal tranquillizers.[12] Considering that some 10 million people take alternative medicines per year in the UK,[13] then only about 1 in a 10 million people report toxic reactions to herbs per year. By comparison, toxic reactions to non-steroid anti-inflammatory drugs that are hugely prescribed and freely available for sale in pharmacies, can be 1 in 200, causing around 1000 deaths per year in the UK, without being taken off the shelves.[14] The National Poisons Center in the USA reported that Toxicity from *all plants* was only 1 per cent that of a single category of modern drugs, antidepressants. Toxicity from plants was never from herbal remedies, but only from toxic home and garden ornamentals.[15] Another example of the way adverse effects are political rather than public health issues concerns the sweet tasting plant

Stevia rabaudiana which was banned from importation because of a laboratory study hypothesizing adverse effects. Yet it has had extensive traditional use and is currently licensed and widely sold as a sweetener in several countries such as Brazil and Japan without any reports of adverse effects. Meanwhile, 80 per cent of all complaints to the FDA of adverse reactions to food concerns one substance—the artificial sweetener aspartame.[16]

Research

There is an enormous amount of research on plants and plant products that is being carried on at present, especially in countries that have not abandoned their interest and use of plant medicines, for example Germany, India, China, Japan, and Eastern Europe. Hundreds of new papers are published monthly and there are many specialist journals and databases on plant medicine and phytochemistry.[17] The author has 1000 references on garlic alone and 2000 on ginseng. There are some authoritative new texts which summarize the pharmacological and clinical aspects of this research, including Professor Varro Tyler's *Herbs of choice*, Dr Douglas Kinghorn and Manuel Balandrin's *Human medicinal agents from plants*, and Professor Hilbert Wagner and colleagues' *Economic and medicinal plant research*, Vols 1–5.[18] The standard text on pharmacognosy (identification and phytochemistry) is *Trease and Evans' Pharmacognosy*.[19] The main pharmacopoeia is the *British herbal pharmacopoeia*, which has an invaluable associated reference work, *The British herbal compendium*, which also authoritatively reviews research, chemistry, registration, adverse effects, dosages, etc.[20]

In the last few years, pharmaceutical companies have woken up to the potential of new drugs derived from plants.[21] At least half of the major multinationals now have research programmes to look for such medicines, for example in the sea, in Amazonian rainforests, or among Chinese herbs, and there is now some government research funding. Around 120 pharmaceuticals contain plant-based compounds. Early examples include the anticancer substances vinblastine and vincristine from periwinkle; the blood pressure lowering and antitussive reserpine from the *Rauwolfia*, the Indian insanity herb; steroid hormones from the yam (*Dioscorea spp.*). A recent example is the antileukaemia drug taxol, obtained from the Pacific yew (*Taxus breviofolia*).[22] However the approach here is essentially the opposite of that of herbal medicine which employs the balance and safety of all the constituents in their original natural vehicle, the whole plant, rather than a single, targeted, strong, and usually toxic isolated constituent.

It is impossible to do justice to this extensive research here, so a few topical examples will be selected as illustrations. Garlic is the top-selling cardiovascular remedy in Europe. Some 30 clinical studies have been published showing that around 1 clove per day, or equivalent in dried garlic tablets, can reduce cholesterol levels by 10–15 per cent.[23] These studies have been confirmed in some recent authoritative meta-analyses of the literature.[24] Garlic also lowers blood fat and reduces the risk of thromboses.[25] The active principles are known to be allicin and other sulphur compounds.[26] Studies have shown that liquorice root is more effective at healing gastric ulcers than any current conventional drug, provided it is taken on an empty stomach.[27] Silymarin is an extract of the milk thistle (*Silybum marianum*). It is widely used in Europe and the USA as a remedy for all chronic liver problems, especially those arising from drugs, alchohol, chemicals, and pollutants. It has considerable pharmacological and clinical research support.[28] Echinacea is also widely used on both sides of the Atlantic as a support for the immune system. There are many clinical and other studies indicating that it aids immunological function, interferon production, resistance to viral and other infections, recovery from flu, colds, and chronic infections.[29] A large number of hallucinogenic and traditional ritual remedies—datura, iboga, yage, peyote, cannabis, psilocybe, coca, etc.—have all been shown to contain psychoactive substances of great interest.[30]

Ginger is a safe antinausea and antivomiting remedy. It has been used since ancient times to aid digestion and absorption, and also as an important component in herbal mixtures, helping to warm the body and improve circulation.[31] Recently, a spate of new clinical trials has demonstrated that it is as effective as conventional tranquillizers used to prevent nausea and vomiting after surgery, and that it is highly effective against travel sickness and morning sickness.[32] As it works on the stomach, not the central nervous system it is without the side-effects of conventional drugs. Aloe vera has been demonstrated to improve skin blood supply, reduce inflammation, and hasten wound healing and cell growth.[33] In the last few years the leaves of the Chinese tree, *Gingko biloba* have become one of the most widely sold of all remedies in European pharmacies, with sales of around $300 million per year. It is used to improve the peripheral blood supply, especially in the brain and limbs, and has become a key treatment for age-related loss of memory and mental function, strokes, and peripheral vascular disease. There is a great deal of pharmacological and clinical work; a recent meta-analysis of 40 clinical trials found the results overwhelmingly positive.[34]

Yet it is very clear that published research has only scratched the surface. There are half a million plants on this planet, and only about five per cent have been scientifically investigated. Even in these cases they have only been tested against certain diseases.[35] Researchers can, however, greatly increase the chance of demonstrating medicinal activity in plants by working with the traditional practitioners that use them.[36] There is no lack of opportunity.

Types of therapist

The most common types of herbal therapists now practising in the UK can be classified into five groups:

1. The retail herbalists, still occasionally found in the Midlands and North, supplying across-the-counter medicines in a near-symptomatic fashion. Until 20

years ago, this was the only significant body of herbal practitioners in this country, but is now diminishing in number. Health shops are taking their place in the supply of herbs to the public. Retail herbalists often possess an uncanny knack of hitting the nail on the head but also provide a refuge for incompetent practitioners.

2. Therapists practising various kinds of indigenous medicine. There are now a few Oriental practitioners of Oriental and Tibetan herbal medicine, often working within the Oriental community. There are also many European acupuncturists and others who prescribe Oriental herbs. This is discussed in Chapter 6. Hakims, the name give to herbal practitioners in Islam and the Indian sub-continent, practise in immigrant areas administering the various Indian medical systems to immigrant patients.

3. The professional medical herbalists, applying Western herbal medicines in the confines of the consulting room. Usually members of the National Institute of Medical Herbalists, these practitioners have increased in number recently. They tend to hold a sophisticated view of their therapy and provide a total primary care medical system. A few are medical practitioners.

4. A miscellaneous group who use herbal medicine secondarily to other modes of diagnosis or treatment. It is almost impossible to generalize about them. Some use healing, dowsing, radionics, or iris diagnosis; others are also osteopaths or naturopaths or even homeopaths primarily, using herbs as a supporting therapy. Many use herbs as part of modern naturopathy in which diet and dietary supplements are the main treatment.

5. Aromatherapists use herbs in the form of distilled essential oils. These oils are concentrated, and often used as an adjunct to massage (see Chapter 16). However the more experienced aromatherapists also carefully prescribe essential oils internally in doses of a drop or two, for example to relieve symptoms such as intestinal cramps and pain in the case of peppermint oil or lift mood in the case of basil oil, or relieve headaches and congestion with rosemary oil.[37]

References

1. Griggs, B. (1991). *Green pharmacy: a history of herbal medicine*. Healing Arts Press, Rochester, Vermont. Jill Norman, London.
2. Fulder, S. (1993). *The book of ginseng, and other Chinese herbs for vitality*. Healing Arts Press, Rochester, Vermont.
3. Bannerman, R. H., Burton, J., and Wen-Chieh, C. (1983). *Traditional medicine and health care coverage*. World Health Organization, Geneva. Doyal, L. (1987). Health, underdevelopment and traditional medicine. *Holistic Medicine*, 2, 27–40. Anderson, E. F. (1993). *Plants and people of the Golden Triangle: ethnobotany of the hill tribes of Northern Thailand*. Dioscorides, Portland Oregon.
4. Culpeper, N. (1987). *Culpeper's complete herbal*. Foulsham, Slough, Middlesex;

Meyerbooks, Glenwood, USA. Grieve, M. (1982). *A modern herbal.* Peregrine Books, Harmondsworth, Middlesex. This title is the best traditional-style herbal available. Wren, R. W. (1988). *Potters new cyclopaedia of botanical drugs and preparations.* Health Science Press, Holsworthy.

5. Ruppere, V. (1981). The survival of traditional medicine in lay medical views. *Medical History,* 25, 411–14. Whorton, J. C. (1987). Traditions of folk medicine in America. *Journal of the American Medical Association,* 257, 1632–5.

6. Melmon, K. L. and Morrelli, H. F. (eds) (1990). *Clinical pharmacology.* Macmillan, New York.

7. Mills, S. (1991). *Out of the earth: the essential book of herbal medicine.* Viking Arkana, London, New York. Ody, P. (1993). *The complete medicinal herbal.* Dorling Kindersley, London, New York, Stuttgart. Wichtl, M. (1994). *Herbal drugs and phytopharmaceuticals: a handbook for practice on a scientific basis* (trans. and edited by Bisset, N. G.). CRC Press, Baton Rouge, Florida.

8. Tyler, V. E. (1994). *Herbs of choice. The therapeutic use of phytopharmaceuticals.* Haworth Press, Binghampton, New York. Weiss, R. F. (1985). *Herbal medicine.* Beaconsfield Press, Beaconsfield, UK.

9. De Smet, P. A. G. M., Keller, K., Hamsel, R., and Chandler, R. F. (1992). *Adverse effects of herbal drugs, Vol. 2.* Springer Verlag, New York. Mills, S. (1991). Are herbs safe? *British Journal of Phytotherapy,* 2, 76–83.

10. Duke, J. (1985). *CRC Handbook of medicinal herbs.* CRC Press, Baton Rouge, Florida.

11. Awang, D. V. C. (1991). Comfrey update. *Herbalgram,* No. 25, Summer 1991, 20–3. Weston, C., Cooper, B. *et al.* (1987). Veno-occlusive disease of the liver secondary to ingestion of comfrey. *British Medical Journal,* 295, 183.

12. Perharic, L. (1994). Toxicological problems resulting from exposure to traditional remedies and food supplements. *Drug Safety,* 11, 284–94.

13. Mintel Ltd. (1993). *Alternative medicines: Mintel Market Intelligence report,* Mintel, Long Lane, London.

14. *The Independent* (1992). 9 September 1992. *Chemical Marketing Reporter* (1989). 2 January 1989.

15. Litovitz, T. L. *et al.* (1990). 1989 annual report of the American Association of Poison Control Centers national data collection system. *Emergency Medicine,* 8, 394.

16. McCaleb, R. S. (1992). Food ingredient safety evaluation. *Food and Drug Law Journal,* 47, 657–63.

17. Important journals in English include: *Lloydia, Planta Medica, Journal of Ethnopharmacology, Herbalgram, British Journal of Phytotherapy, International Journal of Pharmacognosy, European Phytotelegram, Phytomedicine, Chemical and Pharmaceutical Bulletin, Fitoterapia, Economy Botany,* etc. The most important international database is 'NAPRALERT' a WHO centre at the Department of Pharmacy, University of Illinois, Chicago. For other databases, CD-ROM sources, journals, etc. see: Hoffman, D. (1994). *The information sourcebook of herbal medicine,* Crossing Press, Freedom, California. For phytochemistry, good surveys of the chemical constituents of medicinal herbs include: Chadwick, D. J. and Marsh, J. (eds) (1990). *Bioactive compounds from plants.* John Wiley, London and New York. Duke, J. (1992). *Handbook of biologically active phytochemicals and their activities.* CRC Press, Baton Rouge, Florida. Harborne, J. B. and Baxter, H. (eds) (1993). *Phytochemical dictionary: a handbook of bioactive compounds from plants.* Taylor and Francis, Bristol, Pennsylvania.

18. Kinghorn, A. D. and Balandrin, M. F. (1993). *Human medicinal agents from plants.* American Chemical Society, Washington, D. C. Tyler, V. E. (1994). *Herbs of choice.*

Haworth Press, New York, London. Wagner, H. and Farnsworth, N. R. (eds) (1991). *Economic and medicinal plant research*. Academic Press, San Diego, London.

19. Evans, W. C. (1989). *Trease and Evans' Pharmacognosy*, 13th edition. Baillière Tindall, London, Philadelphia.

20. Bradley, P. (ed.) (1992). *The British herbal compendium, Volume 1. A handbook of scientific information on widely used plant drugs*. The British Herbal Medicine Association, Dorset.

21. Editorial (1994). Pharmaceuticals from plants: great potential, few funds. *Lancet*, **343**, 1513–14. Grindley, J. (1993). The natural approach to pharmaceuticals. *Scrip Magazine*, **December 1993**, 30–3. Akerele, D. (1993). Nature's medicinal bounty: don't throw it away. *World Health Forum*, **14**, 390–5.

22. Huang, P. L., Huang, P. L., Huang, P. Huang, H. I., and Lee-Huang, S. (1992). Developing drugs from traditional medicinal plants. *Chemistry and Industry*, **20th April 1993**, 290–3.

23. Fulder, S. and Blackwood, J. (1991). *Garlic: nature's original remedy*. Healing Arts Press, Rochester, Vermont. Jain, A. K., Vargas, R., Gotzkowsky, S., and McMahon, F. G. (1993). Can garlic reduce levels of serum lipids? A controlled clinical study. *American Journal of Medicine*, **94**, 632–5. De A Santos, O.S. and Grünwald, J. (1993). Effect of garlic powder tablets on blood lipids and blood pressure—a six month placebo controlled double blind study. *British Journal of Clinical Research*, **4**, 37–44. Mansell, P. and Reckless, J. P. D. (1991). Garlic: effects on serum lipids, blood pressure, coagulation, platelet aggregation, and vasodilation. *British Medical Journal*, **303**, 379.

24. Silagy, C. and Neil, A. (1994). Garlic as a lipid lowering agent—a meta-analysis. *Journal of the Royal College of Physicians*, **28**, 39–45. Warshavsky, S., Kamer, R. S., and Sivak, S. L. (1993). Effect of garlic on total serum cholesterol. A meta-analysis. *Annals of Internal Medicine*, **119**, 599–605.

25. Kiesewetter, H., Jung, F., Mrowietz, C., Pindur, G., Heiden, M., and Wenzel, E. (1990). Effects of garlic on blood fluidity and fibrinolytic activity: a randomised, placebo-controlled, double-blind study. *British Journal of Clinical Practice*, **Supplement 69**, 24–9. Lawson, L. D., Ransom, D. K., and Hughes, B. G. (1992). Inhibition of whole blood platelet-aggregation by compounds in garlic clove extracts and commercial garlic products. *Thrombosis Research*, **65**, 141–56.

26. Lawson, L. D. (1993). Bioactive organosulfur compounds of garlic and garlic products, and their role in reducing blood lipids. In: *Human medicinal agents from plants* (ed. A. D. Kinghorn and M. F. Balandrin), pp. 1–25, American Chemical Society, Washington, D. C. Block, E. (1985). The chemistry of garlic and onions. *Scientific American*, **252**, 94–9. Yeh, Y-Y. and Yeh, S-M. (1994). Garlic reduces plasma lipids by inhibiting hepatic cholesterol and triacylglycerol synthesis. *Lipids*, **29**, 189–93.

27. Turpie, A. G. G., Runcie, J., and Thompson, T. J. (1969). Clinical trial of deglycyrrhizinated liquorice in gastric ulcer. *Gut*, **10**, 299–305. Tewari, S. N. and Wilson, A. K. (1972). Deglycyrrhizinated liquorice in duodenal ulcer. *Practitioner*, **210**, 820–3. Kassir, Z. A. (1985). Endoscopic controlled trial of four drug regimens in the treatment of chronic duodenal ulceration. *Irish Medical Journal*, **78**, 153–8.

28. Morazzoni, P. and Bombardelli, E. (1995). Silybum marianum. A review. *Fitoterapia*, **65**, 3–42.

29. Hobbs, C. (1994). Echinacea: a literature review. *Herbalgram*, No. **30**, Winter 1994, 33–48. Foster, S. (1991). *Echinacea, Nature's immune enhancer*. Healing Arts Press, Rochester, Vermont. Schumacher, A. and Frieberg, K. D. (1993). The effect of Echinacea angustifolia on non-specific cellular immunity in the mouse. *Drug Research*, **41**, 141–7.

30. Schultes, R. E. (1969). Hallucinogens of plant origins. *Science*, **163**, 245–54.

31. Fulder, S. J. (1993). *Ginger, the ultimate home remedy*. Souvenir, London.
32. Bone, M. E., Wilkinson, D. J., Young, J. R., McNeil, J., and Charlton, S. (1990). Ginger root—a new antiemetic. The effect of ginger root on postoperative nausea and vomiting after major gynecological surgery. *Anesthesia*, 45, 669–71. Mowrey, D. B. and Clayson, D. E. (1982). Motion sickness, ginger and psychophysics. *Lancet*, 1, 655–7. Fischer-Rasmussen, W., Kjaer, S. K., Dahl, C., and Asping, U. (1990). Ginger treatment of hyperemesis gravidarum. *European Journal of Obstetrics and Gynaecology and Reproductive Biology*, 38, 19–24.
33. Zawahry, M., Hegazy, M. R., and Helal, M. (1973). Use of aloes in treating leg ulcers and dermatoses. *International Journal of Dermatology*, 12, 68. Cere, S. *et al.* (1980). The therapeutic efficacy of aloe vera cream in thermal injuries. *Journal of the American Animal Hospital Association*, 16, 768.
34. Funfgeld, E. W. (1988). *Rökan: gingko biloba, recent results in pharmacology and clinic*. Springer, Berlin, London. Kleijnen, J. and Knipschild, P. (1992). *Gingko biloba* for cerebral insufficiency. *British Journal of Clinical Pharmacology*, 34, 352–8. Bauer, U. (1984). 6-month double-blind randomised clinical trial of *Gingko biloba* extract versus placebo in two parallel groups in patients suffering from peripheral arterial insufficiency. *Drug Research*, 34, 716–20.
35. Farnsworth, N. (1993). Ethnopharmacology and future drug development: the North American experience. *Journal of Ethnopharmacology*, 34, 145–52.
36. Farnsworth, N.R. and Kaas, C.J. (1981). An approach utilising information from traditional medicine to identify tumour inhibiting plants. *Journal of Ethnopharmacology*, 3, 85–99.
37. Dew, M., Evans, B. J. and Rhodes, J. (1984). Peppermint oil for irritable bowel syndrome: a multicentre trial. *British Journal of Clinical Practice*, 38, 11–21. Aqel, M. B. (1991). Relaxant effect of volatile oil of rosemary on tracheal smooth muscle. *Journal of Ethnopharmacology*, 33, 57–62.

14

Homeopathy

Background

Homeopathy is a system of treatment developed from the natural law of *similia similibus curantur*—'like is cured by like'. That is, a substance or preparation which can cause groups of symptoms, whether physical, emotional, or behavioural, in the healthy, can cure similar groups of symptoms when they appear as a deviation from normal in the sick. This principle was recognized by both Hippocrates and Paracelsus but was only developed as a practical method of healing by Dr Samuel Hahnemann who published his *Homeopathic Materia Medica* in 1811.[1] Hahnemann first noticed this principle in action in observing the effect of Peruvian bark, the standard treatment for malaria at the time; it produced 'malarial' fevers when he ingested it.

Through careful observation of the effect of remedies upon himself and others over a period of years, Hahnemann was able to define the effect of very many substances. He called this system 'the proving of remedies'. The conditions for this self-testing procedure were stringent. Only healthy and balanced individuals could test the remedies. Any deviations from usual function and patterns of behaviour, however small, were noted. In some cases Hahnemann mentions up to 4000 symptoms.

Although Hahnemann was most successful with his form of selecting remedies, he was aware that in using significant dosages he often added to the symptoms caused by the disease. Because he was always concerned that medicine should cure without harm, he attempted to give small dosages of his remedies to patients. But these had reduced therapeutic effects. It was then that he made a curious and astonishing discovery. When he shook the preparations violently during dilution, he retained their potency despite a considerably reduced dose. This process, described as 'potentization' has become a key element of homeopathy. In some ways it has wrongly eclipsed the other aspects of Hahnemann's system, for 'homeopathy' has crept into common language as a word for a minute dosage.

Hahnemann went on to discover that although the homeopathically indicated remedy cured the patients' acute conditions with ease, it did not seem to stop more than temporarily the degeneration of health we call chronic disease. He spent some 12 years in research and observation to find out why. Finally, he deduced that there were general influences, inherited and acquired, which affect the whole of our health processes. These chronic disease tendencies, which he called 'miasms', are the soil in which the weeds of disease can grow. They are not what we call disease but without them there could be no disease. This theory has provoked controversy among homeopaths and others ever since it was formulated in the *Theory of chronic diseases* published in 1828.[1]

Hahnemann died in 1846, leaving behind a reasonably complete system for curing the sick. Since then, many homeopaths have added to the store of knowledge, not the least of whom was Constantine Hering, who formulated what was known as the Law of Cure, an observation about the progression of symptoms in the disease process and the healing process. He observed that if the patient was being cured then the symptoms moved from the vital internal organs to the less vital organs, and finally to the skin; symptoms also disappeared downwards and in the reverse order of their development. Observation by other homeopaths over the past 120 years has verified this law, which has the value of revealing if the patient is being cured or the condition suppressed.

Fundamental concepts

The therapeutic system known as homeopathy works because of certain generally unacknowledged characteristics of human and other organisms. These characteristics are defined as follows:

1. The organism is in a constant state of self-repair, and all organs and parts are constantly renewing themselves. This means that there is a considerable capacity for overcoming the cause of disease, if that capacity can be stimulated into activity.

2. The cure can only be achieved by the organism through its own devices. This means that the homeopathic definition of cure may be different to more common uses of the word.

3. The organism becomes sensitive to that which will stimulate cure: i.e. that which is *homeopathic* to the patient. The extreme degree of sensitivity of the organism to the unique (homeopathic) stimulant is appreciated by those who are familiar with the amount of dilution involved with most homeopathic remedies.

Homeopathy employs an essentially 'vitalistic' model of the body. As Hahnemann stated:

'In the healthy condition of man the spiritual, vital force, the dynamism that animates the material body (organism), rules with unbounded sway and retains all parts of the organism in admirable harmonious vital operation . . . when a person falls ill . . . it is only the vital force, deranged from such an abnormal state, that can furnish the organism with its disagreeable sensations, and incline it to the irregular process we call disease.'

Disease therefore occurs when the vital principle is unable to cope with changes occurring to the organism. It becomes overwhelmed, demonstrating that fact by the production of symptoms in the body.

In homeopathy, disease is regarded as a process not a 'thing'. It can be detected as close to its origin as the training and sensitivity of the observer or patient allows. The conventional usage of the word disease describes only the final stage of its development, the pathological stage where the *structure* of the physical body begins to lose its integrity and there is tissue damage. However, there are several other stages previous to this where there is a loss of integrity of *function*. A characteristic of these previous stages is a sense of malaise, of dis-ease, within the person, the 'I don't feel well' stage which may precede development of the pathological stage by days, weeks, months, or even years. These previous stages are accessible to the homeopathic practitioner. Cure can therefore be accomplished further 'upstream', before a serious condition develops.

The homeopath does not regard the symptoms as being the disease, rather as an expression of the body in its reaction to the underlying problem. He therefore reads the symptom picture of the body in order to define the sort of curative efforts the body is making of itself. He will then work for the remedy that will stimulate self-healing. The correct remedy is the one which produces an identical pattern of symptoms when given to healthy people in material dosages. The art of the homeopath is, to a large extent, the interpretation and matching of the symptom picture of the patient with the correct drug picture of a remedy.[2] For example, arsenic poisoning produces symptoms so close to those of cholera that it is hard to tell them apart without tests. Therefore, highly diluted arsenic trioxide is a remedy for cholera or gastroenteritis. The process is like that of finding two patterns which interlock exactly, or two vibrational frequencies which will resonate together. For that reason a single remedy, the *simillimum*, the most similar, is sought. A remedy that duplicates three-quarters of the symptoms of the patient, even if combined with another which duplicates the other quarter, will be useless.

The matching of symptoms defines homeopathy: 'the determination as to whether or not a remedy is homeopathic is derived neither from its amount nor from its form, but solely from its relation to the disease' is a classic definition put forward by the German national homeopathic organization in 1836. However, it is based on empirical observation going back to Greek medicine. The reason for it is still mysterious, although a recent bold attempt to derive a 'unified field theory' of homeopathy has suggested that there are archetypes in nature (from which remedies are derived) and human archetypes (expressed as characteristic sets of symptoms). If the archetypes match, they cancel each other out, like the self-annihilation of two equal but opposite vibrations.[3]

Conventional medicine could accept a small segment of homeopathic teaching, largely in the field of immunology. Hahnemann in fact referred to Jenner's cowpox vaccine as homeopathic. There are treatments which are comparable, though unrelated to, homeopathy. Today's 'attenuated' vaccines are viruses which are so highly diluted that they stimulate body defences without producing the disease itself. In pharmacology some metabolic and anticoagulant remedies work on a like cures like principle,[4] and it is very well known that remedies which have toxic effects at higher dosages are stimulatory or beneficial at low dosages. A good example is strychnine, from *Nux vomica*, which is highly toxic but used in both conventional and homeopathic medicine in small doses.

It is this question of dose which has caused the greatest controversy. Not so much that the patient is sensitive to the minute doses of the exact remedy that will cure him, but that the doses involved are sometimes so minute that it seems inconceivable that any of the original material is left at all. For if something is diluted beyond Avogadro's Constant (6×10^{23}) there should no longer be a single molecule of the original left. Many homeopathic remedies are diluted well above this, and these high dilutions are regarded by experienced homeopaths as their most potent. They are often used in more chronic and difficult conditions. To some extent homeopathy regards this as a conundrum only for scientists, and a reliable everyday reality for practitioners. However, much of the research on homeopathy has been directed towards this 'magic of the minimum dose'.[5] This research tends to show a remarkable phenomenon, that when poisons stimulate biological processes at the lowest invisible dosages, there are 'peaks' and 'troughs' of maximal and minimal activation. Mercuric chloride has been found, for example, to activate an enzyme, diastase, maximally at 10^{-15}, 10^{-25}, 10^{-45}, 10^{-65}, 10^{-75}, and 10^{-110}, and minimally at 10^{-20}, 10^{-55}, 10^{-85}, and 10^{-105}. However this activation only happened with dilutions prepared with vigorous shaking. An ingenious proposal has been put forward by two American physicists, who attempt to explain this not in terms of chemicals but of information. They suggest that a dissolved substance leaves an imprint of itself after high dilution. That is, the energy of shaking aids the substance to act as a template, producing matching configurations within the water, which are then replicated within the body. Homeopathic remedies do not transmit chemicals but information. The homeopathic physician matches 'the pure quantised informational content of particular chemicals to the informational needs of his patient'.[7] This is discussed further in the research section below.

On the other hand physical explanations may be missing the point. These high potencies may be acting at a subtle level on the subtle energy body rather than the physical body. It may be that at high potencies homeopathy takes off into this realm of healing, whether the homeopath recognizes it or not.

Diagnosis and treatment

Diagnosis involves finding out what changes from the normal the patient has experienced. These changes may be registered by the patient or observed by the homeopath and may be physical, sensory, emotional, mental, or even moral. The aim of 'taking the case' is to describe the abnormal, which we call symptoms, as completely as possible. A pain may be noted by the patient, but the homeopath will ask what time of day the pain occurs, whether the pain is intermittent or continuous, how the patient feels under different weather or temperature conditions, and so on. The peculiar or abnormal symptoms (e.g. 'pain in wrists when lying down') are the most important in a hierarchy of significance; how they vary under changing conditions is next. The psychological profile of the patient is also significant, while general habits and preferences such as liking for sweet or sour foods, are added on to give a constitutional picture. There is usually a physical examination.

Diagnosis in homeopathy is expressed not in the name of a disease, nor even in a description of a symptom picture, but in the name of the remedy which corresponds to it. A good description of this is given by Vithoulkas[8] who lists various kinds of influenza experienced during an epidemic (influenza being one of the most straight forward cases). A *Gelsemium semper virens* influenza is characterized by lethargy, dullness with a paradoxical tendency to insomnia, the face is flushed, the lips and skin dusky, there is an unstable heat reaction to the fever, the skin hot and sticky, the lips very dry, there is a throbbing congestive headache with dizziness, and so on. *Bryonia Alba* patients have some of these symptoms, but are also irritable and depressed. During their influenza they experience thirst with generalized aching pain, they are restless, and always moving about. There are many other types of influenza each with a somewhat different set of symptoms.

In acute cases the remedy may be any one of hundreds and the homeopath is guided to it by the individual version of disease produced by the patient. In chronic cases the remedy will usually be what is called the 'constitutional', since it is indicated by the individuality of the *patient* and not the individuality of the disease. The *constitution* of an individual is more or less fixed and the remedy which stimulates the recuperative ability will usually stay the same throughout life, although with the increased pace, pressure, and complexity of our lives, and the increasing power of symptom-modifying orthodox drugs, the clarity of the constitutional picture is sometimes much obscured. One talks, for example, about a *Nux vomica* type, a *Sulphur* or *Pulsatilla* type. These types arise empirically during provings where it is noticed that certain kinds of constitutions react strongly to certain remedies. However the same remedies can also be used for acute conditions. *Pulsatilla* is often indicated in the symptom grouping of measles. Some remedies are also chosen on the basis of affinity to the affected part. Thus *Sepia* (squid ink) corresponds to the female reproductive organs.

Only one remedy needs to be given at a time, except where the patient has had previous suppressive therapy in which case this is usually treated first. The homeopath will observe the changes in the patient produced by this remedy. A temporary aggravation of the symptoms indicates that a curative process has been stimulated in the body and is a good sign. Similarly, if symptoms move outwards, for example, if skin eruptions occur in an asthma patient, a curative process has been stimulated. When there is no result the homeopath will try to match another remedy, or re-question the patient to establish what symptoms were omitted previously. The more experienced homeopaths use high potencies which are more subtle and yet powerful. However, less experienced homeopaths usually use remedies at a lower potency, such as 6x, which is 1×10^6. First aid remedies available to the public are generally at a low potency. In the cases where several chronic disease tendencies (miasms) are involved then treatment may be prolonged, involving peeling off 'the layers of the onion' one at a time. This process is the re-creation of lost health and not merely a conquering of disease as we normally think of it.

Remedies are prepared by grinding plant materials in alcohol and leaving them for two weeks before filtering to give a 'mother tincture'. This, as with all homeopathic remedies, should be stored away from chemical influences such as strong smells. Minerals and insoluble materials are very finely ground with lactose. Dilutions are then prepared by mixing with solvent and dropping the bottle onto a hard rubber slab or by trituration with more lactose. 1:10 dilutions are described as 1 x 2 x . . .; 1:100 as 1c, 2c . . .; and 1:1000 as 1M, 2M . . . x dilutions are meant to be more powerful than c dilutions. The remedies are presented in the homeopathic pharmacopoeia of various countries, which are currently being unified. There are about 3000 remedies: plant, mineral, and occasionally animal. Only some 500 are in regular use.[9]

Research

Homeopathy has been extensively researched for most of this century, the earlier work being in Germany, and the more recent research coming from the large homeopathic establishment in France, as well as India, the UK, and the USA. Most of this research is reported in the national homeopathic journals; however some is now appearing in the conventional medical literature.

As far as mechanism is concerned, despite a great deal of effort and thought, all one can say is that: 'something is happening, but we don't know what it is'. Techniques such as nuclear magnetic resonance, change in electrical storage capacity, or alterations in the intensity and wavelength of light passed through the solution have all shown certain differences between highly diluted shaken and unshaken solutions.[10] But this is a long way from describing a 'template' that may have been left in the solution by the solute even after it has been diluted to nothing. Modern concepts of fractal patterns which have different biophysical effects depending on the starting conditions, may be a useful line of research. Perhaps the leading biophysicist involved in this research, Fritz Popp, suggests that we should look at stable coherent states, as in lasers, for models.[11] However this work is still at the level of speculation and hypothesis.

There is no doubt that biological systems can respond to, and amplify, a single molecule which acts as a trigger, for example a pheromone. Biological effects at very high dilutions are no longer considered absurd in science. Some of the most successful homeopathic studies have demonstrated effects of extraordinarily high dilutions on animals or animal cells. One classical model uses arsenic, metals, or other poisons which were first given in toxic doses. When this is followed by homeopathic doses of the same material it resulted in an immediate washing out of the poison from the body. A great many of these studies have been carried out, some with large numbers of animals (700 rats in one case) in blind conditions. Similar 'hair of the dog' research has shown that animals that were made diabetic could be partly cured by homeopathic doses of diabetogenic material.[12] Or small doses of radiation can protect against radiation.[13] Actually, it is not only the homeopaths who have discovered this effect. It was also found, and labelled 'hormesis' at the National Environmental Research Centre in Plymouth, UK. Dr Stebbing has shown that minute doses of metals or poisons will stimulate, in a cyclic oscillating pattern depending on dilutions, growth of previously poisoned cells or organisms. He has observed stimulatory effects at doses as low as 1 part in 10 million with copper sulphate and other poisons.[14] Biochemically, it is likely that these minute doses of poisons stimulate or induce enzymic repair processes.

The most powerful demonstration of the biological effects of homeopathic dilutions has been that of Professor Benviste at INSERM, the French government's medical research institute. It created a furore in medical circles because the research was so good that it could not be dismissed, and it was published in *Nature* with an impolite editorial reservation that 'there is no physical basis for such an activity.' The French team showed that certain white blood cells, basophils, which dump their stocks of histamine when challenged by antibody, still did so when the antibody had been diluted with shaking in the homeopathic way, down to 1×10^{120}. At this dilution there cannot be any molecules of the antibody left. As the other experiments described above, the release happened most in peaks at certain dilutions on the way. The experiments were repeated many different times at 6 different centres, and the release always tended to happen at the same dilutions. By using filters and resins, they also showed that the active agency in the solutions was not a physical molecule of antibody size, that it absolutely required strong homeopathic shaking, and that it was destroyed at temperatures above 70°C.[15] The studies have been repeated by different laboratories using different cellular models such as immune responses created with homeopathic doses of interferon.[16] The fact that such homeopathic doses do have biological effects is no longer in doubt. The question is how? Generally it is thought that information is left after the molecules have been diluted away. One view is that we have been trapped by a dualistic thinking about material and non-material phenomena. Instead of regarding the placebo effect and psychic phenomena as non-material, while remedies are real chemicals, we could see a continual gradation, in which chemical specificity declines on dilution and informational specificity increases.[11]

In the last few years there have been a number of clinical trials of homeopathy, and much discussion of methodology. A major critical review has been published in the *British Medical Journal*. Eighty-one out of 105 clinical trials showed significant positive results compared with placebo. Though there were methodological problems with many studies, and there could have been publication bias in which only the positive studies see the light of day, the authors state that 'The amount of positive evidence even among the best studies came as a surprise to us. Based on this evidence we would be ready to accept that homeopathy can be efficacious, if only the mechanism of action were more plausible.'[17] This is a powerful confirmation of homeopathy but also expresses science's paralysis when faced with alternative paradigms. Of all the therapies, homeopathy has been most subject to the ignominious attitude of medical science, that if it does not fit into the system it cannot be true. However at long last it is changing, and as an example of this, in the same review, the authors ask rhetorically: 'Are the results of randomised double blind trials convincing only if there is a plausible mechanism of action?'

As with other therapies, it is often only possible to carry out a full double-blind trial if the therapy is compromised on its basic principles. A series of trials at Glasgow Royal Infirmary tested homeopathic immunotherapy, in double-blind studies in which a high potency (diluted 30c) mixed grass pollen or other antigen is given symptomatically against hay fever and asthma. The trials all showed improvements in breathing and other symptoms compared with placebo, and more to the point, were repeatable.[18] One can imagine that there may have been even better results if the full power of homeopathy had been employed.

This has clearly emerged in a series of British trials with rheumatoid arthritis. The first was a large study in which complete homeopathy over a year was compared with aspirin. The results were strongly in favour of homeopathy in that nearly half the homeopath's patients stopped all other medication, while all the placebo group dropped out of the trial.[19] But this was criticized in that it was unfair to compare all of homeopathy with just one conventional drug (aspirin). So several repeats were carried out, one of them where one homeopathic remedy (*Rhus tox.*) was compared with one conventional remedy (fenoprofen) in osteoarthritis patients. In this case homeopathy failed,[20] and now the homeopaths rightly complained that what was tested was not homeopathy, but a remedy used as if it were a modern drug. A way out was found in a recent trial with fibrositis patients in which the homeopath first diagnosed and reviewed patients, only selecting for the trial those for whom *Rhus tox* was appropriate. The results were good, and at least a quarter of the patients received a highly significant reduction in symptoms, and this over only one month.[21]

To some extent, the ice has broken. Clinical research on a variety of health problems is being carried out.[22] Though the debate on testability will continue, trials can be carried out if compromises are made between rigour and realism.[23]

Uses

In homeopathy it is axiomatic that there are no incurable diseases. There are however incurable people. It is the vitality of the individual which determines what can be expected. A normally serious condition in someone with high recuperative power is not so serious as a normally mild condition in somone of low recuperative power. Therefore patients who respond best are those who have had a simple, ordered, stress-free life, living on wholesome, energy-full foods, and plenty of contact with nature. Where the natural healing resources of the body have been interfered with by destructive habits or by electroconvulsive therapy, cortisone, prolonged drug treatments, radiation, etc., cure is more difficult.

Homeopathy can be successful in all diseases though not all patients. It is especially applicable in acute conditions where the patient does have the vital energy to effect a cure, but relief is needed for distressing symptoms; in chronic cases such as gastric ulcer, digestive problems, gall stones, haemorrhoids, liver complaints, migraines, allergies, skin conditions, angina, psychogenic diseases, and rheumatoid conditions; for convalescents, children, and those who are sensitive to allopathic drugs. Cases which homeopathic practitioners refer to medical or other practitioners include emergencies, musculoskeletal injuries, or serious infectious diseases which the patient is failing to overcome, or chronic diseases such as cancer. However, in these cases there may be a role for the adjunctive use of homeopathic remedies.

Risks

Since homeopathy stimulates the organism to the natural activity we call healing, there are no risks involved. There are cases where over-stimulation by too high a potency or too frequent a repetition may take place. This over-stimulation is rare, but is possible in cases with severe morbid pathology or in the moribund patient. The means of preparation of the remedies eliminates any risk of toxic side-effects. There is sometimes an initial aggravation, which is short-lived, lasting from a few minutes to a few days, depending on the condition of the patient. Bearing in mind Hering's 'Law of Cure', old symptoms will sometimes reappear for a short time. By the same laws the externalization of the disease will sometimes produce discharges such as catarrh, diarrhoea, colds, skin eruptions, boils, flu-like symptoms, etc. These are also short-lived and are a process of health, not a disease process.

Types of therapy

Homeopaths, in general, practise according to the rules laid down by Hahnemann: only a single remedy is required; the minimum dose needed to produce reaction, usually a single dose, should be given; both prescriber and patient are to wait until the patient's curative response to the remedy has stopped before another dose is given. This is known as classical homeopathy. There are modern variants of this traditional practice; some homeopaths use potentized substances in other ways, namely:

1. Certain remedies specifically for particular diseases.

2. Remedies for parts or organs instead of for the whole patient.

3. Combinations of remedies for specific diseases or even specific symptoms.

4. Homeopathic remedies derived from pathogenic organisms or disease-causing agents—'isopathy'.

More medically oriented homeopaths would tend to restrict homeopathy to the kinds of conditions which do not respond to conventional medicine, such as rheumatoid arthritis or allergies. They would not use it in many acute infections or in tuberculosis. The more classical homeopaths will treat a much wider range of problems, without necessarily differentiating them into conventional disease categories. They may also pay attention to diet and general lifestyle.

Simple homeopathy is very widely used in the UK by other practitioners—naturopaths, chiropractors, osteopaths, and therapeutic masseurs—as a supplement to their techniques. It is a common form of complementary medical household first aid.

A variant of homeopathy was developed by a renowned physician and homeopath Dr Edward Bach. He eliminated certain classes of remedies, restricting his sources of homeopathic materials to flowers and twigs. By means of a gentle serial dilution he obtained potentized solutions or extracts which he felt captured the essences of the flowers more effectively than the more violent classical methods of succussion. His remedies are used, on diagnosis, as treatment for subtle psychological roots of disease.[24]

References

1. Hahnemann, S. (1983). *The organon of medicine*, 6th edition. (translated by Kunzli, J., Nande, A., and Pendleton, P.). Gollancz, London. Hahnemann, S. (1981). *The chronic diseases, their peculiar nature and their homeopathic cure.* Jain, New Delhi, India. (Translated by Tafel, L. from the 1835 edition.)
2. Good general guides to homeopathy include: Vithoulkas, G. (1980). *The science of homeopathy.* Grove Press, New York. Grossinger, R. (1993). *Homeopathy: an introduction for sceptics and beginners.* North Atlantic Books, Berkeley, California. Blackie, M. (1986). *Classical homeopathy.* Beaconsfield Library, Beaconsfield.
3. Whitmore, E. (1981). *Psyche and substance.* North Atlantic Books, Richmond, Cal. (Highly recommended to those interested in the metaphysics of homeopathy.)
4. Guttentag, O.E. (1966). Homeopathy in the light of modern pharmacology. *Journal of Clinical Pharmacological Therapy*, 7, 425–8.
5. Shepherd, D. (1990). *The magic of minimum dose.* Health Science Press, Saffron Walden, Essex.
6. Boyd, W. E. (1954). Biochemical and biophysical evidence of the activity of high potencies. *British Homeopathic Journal*, 44, 7–44. Herkovits, J. and Perez-Coll, C. S. (1993). Dose—response relationship within the potentized microdoses phenomenon. *Complementary Therapies in Medicine*, 1, 6–8.
7. Barnard, G. P. and Stephenson, J. H. (1967). The microdose paradox: a new biophysical concept. *Journal of the American Institute of Homeopathy*, 60, 277–86. (Evidence is presented that many physical characteristics of highly dilute solutions change on shaking.)
9. Vithoulkas, G. (1989). *Homeopathy—medicine of the new man.* Arco Press, New York. (Perhaps the best short introduction available.)

10. Endler, P. and Schulte, J. (eds.) (1994). *Ultra high dilution physiology and physics.* Kluwer Academic, Dordrecht, Netherlands.
11. Popp, F. (1990). Some elements of homeopathy. *British Homeopathic Journal,* 79, 161–6. Resh, G. and Gutman, V. (1987). *The scientific foundations of homeopathy.* Bartel and Bartel, Berg Am Starnberger See, West Germany.
12. Cazin, J. C., Cazin, M., and Goborit, J.L. (1987). A study of the effect of decimal and centesimal dilutions of arsenic on the retention and mobilization of arsenic in the rat. *Human Toxicology,* 6, 315–20. Fisher, P., House J., Belon, P. *et al.* (1987). The influence of the homeopathic remedy Plumbum metallicum on the excretion kinetics of lead in the rat. *Human Toxicology,* 6, 321–4. Righetti, M. (1991). Characteristics and selected results of research in homeopathy. *Berlin Journal of Research in Homeopathy,* 1, 195–203.
13. Macklis, R. M. and Beresford, B. (1991). Radiation hormesis. *Journal of Nuclear Medicine,* 32, 350–9.
14. Stebbing, A. R. D. (1982). Hormesis. The stimulation of growth by low levels of inhibitors. *The Science of the Total Environment,* 2, 213–34.
15. Davenas, E., Beauvais, F., Amara, J., Oberbaum, M., Robinzon, B., Miadonna, A. *et al.* (1988). Human basophil degranulation triggered by very dilute antiserum against IgE. *Nature,* 333, 816–18.
16. Bastide, M., Daurat, V., Doucet-Jaboeuf, M., Pèlegrin, A., and Dorfman, P. (1987). Immunomodulator activity of very low doses of thymulin in mice. *International Journal of Immunotherapy,* 3, 191–200. Daurat, V., Dorfman, P., and Bastide, M. (1988). Immunomodulatory activity of low doses of interferon in mice. *Biomedicine and Pharmacotherapy,* 42, 197–206.
17. Kleijnen, J., Knipschild, P., and ter Riet, G. (1991). Clinical trials of homeopathy. *British Medical Journal,* 302, 316–23.
18. Reilly, D., Taylor, M., McSharry, C., and Hitchinson, T. (1986). Is homeopathy a placebo response? Controlled trial of homeopathic potency, with pollen in hayfever as model. *Lancet,* 2, 881–6. Reilly, D., Taylor, M. A., Beattie, N. G. M., Campbell, J. H., McSharry, C., Aitchison, T. C., and Carter, R. (1994). Is evidence for homeopathy reproducible? *Lancet,* 344, 1601–6.
19. Gibson, R. G., Gibson, S. L. M., MacNeill, A. D., Gray, G. H., Dick, W. C., and Buchanan W. (1978). Salicylates and homeopathy in rheumatoid arthritis: preliminary observations. *British Journal of Clinical Pharmacology,* 6, 391–5. Gibson, S. L. M., McNeill, A. D., and Buchanan, W. W. (1980). Homeopathic therapy in rheumatoid arthritis: evaluation by double-blind clinical therapeutic trial. *British Journal of Clinical Pharmacology,* 9, 453–9.
20. Shipley, M., Berry, H., Broster, G., Jenkins, M., Clover, A., and Williams, I. (1983). Controlled trial of homeopathic treatment of osteoarthritis. *Lancet,* 1, 97–8.
21. Fisher, P., Greenwood, A., Huskisson, E. C., Turner, P., and Belon, P. (1989). Effect of homeopathic treatment on fibrositis (primary fibromyalgia). *British Medical Journal,* 299, 365–6.
22. Sudan, B. J. (1993). Abrogation of facial seborrhoeic dermatitis with high dilutions of tobacco: a new visible model of Beneviste's theory of memory of water. *Medical Hypotheses,* 41, 440–4.
23. Buckman, R. and Lewith, G. (1994). What does homeopathy do—and how? *British Medical Journal,* 309, 103–6. Wallach, H. (1994). Is homeopathy accessible to research? *Schweizer Rundschau Med. Praxis,* 83, 51–2.
24. Weeks, N. (1979). *Medical discoveries of Edward Bach, physician.* Keats Publishers, New Canaan, Conneticut.

15

Hypnotherapy

Background

In the course of a trance, a person becomes extraordinarily receptive to suggestion. Primitive healers use this receptivity to implant suggestions for self-cure, and have done so from ancient times. Healing trances include the various kinds of exorcism and convulsive catharsis so frequently recorded in medieval Europe. Hypnosis is also a form of trance but it is passively receptive rather than convulsively explosive. Indeed the word was coined by the Scottish surgeon James Braid since he first erroneously thought of it as an induced sleep.

Franz Anton Mesmer is regarded as the founder of hypnotism. He was a charismatic therapist who successfully treated a large number of people by inducing deep trances. He too discovered that convulsions were not necessary for success. Healing could also be accomplished by means of a deeply relaxed and somnambulistic state. His demonstrations were extraordinary and unequivocal. However, he roused considerable antagonism by wearing flowing robes and using magicotheatrical stage settings. The trance state was anyway in disrepute; scientists saw it as medieval and the Church saw it as a mystical heresy. Despite frequent convincing demonstrations of therapeutic successes, conventional medicine retained its hostility to hypnosis even when new neurophysiological theories were developed by James Braid. During the last century hypnosis was quite widely used in France for neuroses, 'hysterical' (i.e. psychosomatic), and mental disorders. However, in the UK, medical opinion insisted that hypnotic phenomena were mimicry, the hypnotic state was one of collusion, and the mind could not influence organic diseases.

During the 1950s doctors began to accept that certain restricted conditions of the body could be generated by the psyche. These psychogenic or psychosomatic conditions were at first regarded as peripheral illnesses that were hard to treat and risky to explore. However, it gradually became clear that the mind had great powers over health or illness. Experiments were carried out in which hypnosis was shown to relieve skin disease and cause warts to disappear. A British

Medical Association committee eventually approved it for certain psychogenic and behavioural problems.[1]

Concepts and theory

Hypnosis can be loosely defined as 'a state of mind in which suggestions are not only more readily accepted than in the waking state, but are also acted upon much more powerfully'.[2] However, the boundaries of the hypnotic state are much wider than this. Indeed, any state in which (a) the cognitive controls over the mind are loosened or dissociated; and (b) the person is not asleep and can receive and act on messages, is a hypnotic or partly hypnotic state. While the hypnotic state can be brought on by a repetitive inductive process of one sort or another, it can also occur spontaneously, for example in situations of great fear, tension, space disorientation, starvation, sleeplessness, or when confronted with repeated stimuli such as evenly spaced trees while driving down a road. In fact, it may be that accidental self-hypnosis is an unwitting cause of illness. Debilitating anxieties may be produced in people if they accept suggestions about themselves such as 'I am a failure' while in states of heightened emotion or confusion. 'If the mind is concentrated as the result of any incident or idea of sufficient emotional importance then it is in a condition of hypnosis. Any idea which is then introduced will act in the same way as a hypnotic command.'[3]

Extraordinary potentialities are available to a person in the hypnotic state; feats of strength or of memory, the belief in illusory ideas and perceptions (demonstrated in stage hypnosis by, for example, making the hypnotized individual climb an imaginary barrier), the relinquishing of will and ego, the control over involuntary body processes, and the cure of diseases. In curative hypnosis, a therapist induces a hypnotic state as a means of passing by the conscious mind, and not an end in itself.

Hypnosis usually begins by lulling and distracting the conscious mind through repetitive sensations. Parallel commands to follow the hypnotist's instructions are given. The individual is, at least at the beginning, quite aware of the proceedings, and where instructions are given, feels that they will happen to him rather than by him. The electroencephalogram gives a reading halfway between sleeping and waking, the person relaxes more deeply and muscular action of all kinds, including speech and facial expression, tends to cease. Eventually catalepsy—rigid holding of position—occurs. This is often demonstrated in stage hypnosis by the hypnotist supporting a person solely by chairs under the head and feet.

Many subdivisions of trance states have been proposed, although none can claim to be more than cuts in a length of string. Therapists often find it useful to distinguish three levels:

1. *Light trance*: the eyes are closed, the person deeply relaxed, general psychological and ego-strengthening suggestions are accepted.

2. *Medium trance*: the person is fully hypnotized, physiological processes slow down, the person will be partially insensible to pain, allergic reactions will cease and it is in this state that most therapy is effected.

3. *Deep trance*: the person is in a somnambulist state, in which eyes can be open, but total anaesthesia is possible, along with special powers, age regression, removal of warts, and some of the 'virtuoso' manifestations of hypnosis.

It is said that 9 out of 10 people can be hypnotized by any skilled hypnotist, while the other 10 per cent can be hypnotized by finding a method particular to them. However, it appears that 90 per cent of the population cannot readily enter deep trance states. In some cases this may be because an individual experiences flashbacks or realizations which act as a barrier to entry into deeper states, in other cases it may be a general lack of concentrative ability. Deeper states sometimes become possible to these patients after repeated entry into lighter trances with the therapist assisting in overcoming barriers on the way. In general, the best subjects are those who can be easily absorbed in what they are doing, while the worst are those with restless, active, questioning, and analytical minds. Often women are more easily hypnotized than men.

The question of susceptibility to hypnosis has been a prime research consideration for a number of years. Various scales, particularly the Stamford Hypnotic Suggestibility Scales, have been designed to measure hypnotizability and then applied to studies in which hypnotherapy occurs. Two bodies of opinion have arisen from these studies. One states that an individual's suggestibility is the major factor in healing and the particular method of inducing the state of heightened suggestibility is not relevant: that is, a suggestible person will tend to be healed whether hypnosis or some other form of implanting suggestions, that is, the placebo effect, is used. This downgrades the value of the hypnotic state as such.[4] The opposite view holds that the hypnotic state is one in which a person is maximally disposed to absorb effective therapeutic suggestions, that it is necessary for therapy, and that clinical successes can be obtained with everybody whatever their level of suggestibility.[5] There are many studies which will support both views. For example, it is known that hypnotizability is a stable personality trait which is correlated with suggestibility of people when awake. The occasional dramatic cures of migraine, warts, and allergies are related to hypnotizability. On the other hand, alleviations are produced under stringent experimental conditions in people of different hypnotic susceptibilities, provided the hypnotherapist uses appropriate methods. In the end the hypnotizability question is not very relevant in a clinical situation where the will and co-operation of the patient, the rapport with the therapist, the expectations on both sides, the type of method used, the focus attained in each session, the adjunctive use of drugs or other treatments, and other factors will all influence the outcome with each patient whatever his innate suggestibility.

It is important to realize that the effectiveness of hypnosis as a therapy lies in the extent to which a patient retains a suggestion in his waking state. The hypnotic state is used as a vehicle to implant a post-hypnotic suggestion. The simple post-hypnotic suggestion of the stage hypnotist, such as 'when the clock strikes you will stand up and blow your nose' will usually work after a single session because there are no contrary habits or psychological formations. However, in therapy the hypnotist is at the very least attempting to alter ingrained patterns of behaviour, and often he is attempting to root out destructive mental conditionings, moods, and neuroses, replacing them with positive self-esteem, new awareness, and capacities. The post-hypnotic suggestions here have to be inserted gradually, strengthened and maintained by the patient as well as the therapist.

Use is often made in therapy of autohypnosis where the therapist trains the patient to hypnotize himself, using the hypnotic state to introduce instructions which will make this easier. In this way the patient can continually reinforce the therapist's suggestions. For example, autohypnosis can be invaluable for relief of pain since the patient can instruct himself to reduce pain whenever attacks occur. Naturally the question arises as to how a person can use his conscious mind to by-pass his conscious mind. In fact for autohypnosis the person must enter an in-between state of relaxed uncritical awareness called the 'hypnoidal' state. In this bridging situation it is possible to formulate instructions and insert suggestions, including those of the manner of waking from self-hypnosis.

Method

The induction of hypnosis follows a basic pattern. The therapist will talk in a slow, relaxing, controlled, and confident way, drawing the patient's mind into a concentrated and detached state. This may involve depiction of an image, such as a walk down a country lane, or successions of colours, or repetition of a monotonous series of statements. Visual concentration can also be trapped and held by means of lights or wheels, a pendulum, or a pencil held at the upper limit of vision. The therapist then encourages heaviness and closing of eyes, followed by other simple test instructions, such as raising an arm. At this stage, usually after about 15 minutes, the person is already in a light trance. Deeper levels are attained by the therapist counting to the patient from 1 to 10, or asking the patient to imagine descent in a lift. The patient is continually exhorted to let everything go bar the instructions of the therapist, and it is at this stage that some trust in the therapist will assist the patient to surrender and go deeper. The whole process can happen very much more quickly in people already 'primed' by states of shock, injury, or distress. This is of considerable use to army medical hypnotists who can often hypnotize wounded soldiers more or less by the pass of a hand. Milton Erikson pioneered a subtle method in which hypnosis is introduced during an apparently normal conversation. In all cases the hypnotist will usually plant a post-hypnotic suggestion which enables the subject to enter a trance much more quickly on subsequent occasions.

Some hypnotists then simply plant the suggestion that the symptom is going—'your migraine is going'—combined with general suggestions of positivity, health, and self-confidence. This may sometimes work, but is generally frowned upon. As the symptoms are usually manifestations of a deeper disturbance at the psychological or physical level, the hypnotist ought to work psychotherapeutically. This is certainly true when hypnotherapy is used to treat chronic pain which, if it is to be of long-term use, must involve a re-education of the patient so as to change his attitude to his suffering. Pain-blocking suggestions are given, for example that another feeling, say tingling, is substituted for the pain, or that the patient alters the meaning of and tolerance to, his pain. However these should usually be combined with work which bares the inner fear, anxiety, guilt, anger, or feelings of hopelessness of the patient. These can then be gradually replaced by positive suggestions such as that the patient is after all glad and successful in that he is alive, that he should have confidence and be aware of the transience of his pain, or that he has suffered enough. It is necessary to teach the patient self-hypnosis so that the therapy can be incorporated into daily life.

Hypnosis can be valuable in psychotherapy because it facilitates the considerable recall of past events. Therefore, the hypnotherapist can get to the roots of a destructive behaviour pattern such as overeating or a psychosomatic condition such as asthma much more quickly than with lengthy verbal fencing with the conscious mind. Old experiences are dredged up, relived, and cathartically removed. The patient can go right back to childhood and beyond. In deep hypnosis patients can experience their birth, and sometimes even talk with the voice of their own childhood.

A very useful uncovering technique is that of ideomotor questioning, developed by Le Cron.[6] Patients are asked to respond to questions by movements, such as a raised finger, rather than words. Therapists who use it find that it allows greater access to hidden subconscious material than if the patient had to use verbal processes in order to answer the questions. Ideomotor questioning is also of great value in communicating with patients who are unconscious, say after an accident.

A thorough hypnotherapeutic course of treatments might go through the following stages:[3]

1. History taking and general diagnosis.

2. Training of the patient to develop his ability to relax, to go deeper into hypnosis to develop re-induction of hypnosis when the therapist suggests it, and to hypnotize himself.

3. A diagnostic exploration under hypnosis in which the patient is questioned so as to dig up deeply rooted causes of his current condition.

4. Analytic procedures to relieve, expose, and remove the emotional content from early experiences.

5. A final synthesis phase to check the level of insight gained, and to re-educate and encourage the patient.

Research

There is now a great deal of published research on the possibilities of hypnosis and its relationship with other states of mind.[7] However like other research on altered states of mind, it lacks context, that is it is often based on experimental and cognitive psychology which minimizes cultural, social, and situational factors. Research on hypnotherapy, like medical research generally, has been limited by a lack of interest in the patient's subjective experience, and perhaps because of this, very little is known of the mechanism by which hypnotic suggestions cause the cure or regression of disease. One pioneering study was begun in the UK by Black, who reported his ability to relieve asthma and allergic conditions by hypnosis in the 1950s. He went on from there to show that after a successful treatment of allergy, the patient's hypersensitive skin reactions to challenge by antigens had stopped even though the patient still had circulating antibodies to this antigen. Black concluded that hypnosis had prevented the uncomfortable inflammatory results (liberation of histamine) of challenge by antigen but not the underlying immunological situation.[8] Several kinds of controlled experiments have now been able to demonstrate that under hypnosis subjects can control blood supply, sensitivity to damage or burning, and pain tolerance in their limbs.[9]

Some preliminary research has attempted to compare other psychological strategies of controlling pain or blood supply to hypnosis. In general, hypnosis has been found more effective than biofeedback in enabling an individual to control the blood supply to his limbs. Although it should be remembered that biofeedback is a self-learned procedure that lacks the therapeutic benefit of the presence of a therapist.[10] An interesting controlled experiment compared hypnosis, acupuncture at true loci, and acupuncture at false loci, with drugs—namely morphine, a benzodiazepine tranquillizer, aspirin, and placebo—for the relief of experimentally induced pain. Each procedure was carried out at its optimum time before the administration of the pain. Results of pain ratings show that hypnosis was much better than any of the other procedures ($P > 0.001$). Acupuncture (at appropriate loci only) was next best and shared second place with morphine.[11]

It is not clear to what extent the hypnotherapy technique itself is responsible for these results; it is difficult to disentangle the effects of hypnotherapy from those of relaxation and therapeutic contact with the therapists. Very often hypnotic induction can be substituted by visualization or states of deep relaxation and meditation in which suggestions can be fully absorbed. For example, in one study students were told that they were being touched by poison ivy leaves although the leaves were actually harmless. More of the subjects produced contact dermatitis in the local area as a result of prior non-hypnotic relaxation than prior hypnosis. Two groups of women were then hypnotized and given suggestions for breast enlargement. The group which practised autosuggestion, did better than the group with hypnosis alone. In these cases the authors showed that the blood supply was increased at the site of these effects.[12]

Clinical research is still limited, although more is appearing in mainstream journals. Hypnosis is being tried in the treatment of various kinds of gastrointestinal disease, particularly duodenal and peptic ulcer and refractory irritable bowel syndrome (IBS) which is widespread and notoriously difficult to treat. Dr P. J. Whorwell and colleagues at the Department of Medicine of the University Hospital of South Manchester have reported a remarkable 80 per cent cure rate with IBS cases that were incurable by any other method. Unlike classical hypnotherapy which attempts holistically to reduce stress and general unconscious disease-causing patterns, they use a limited method of directly relating to gastrointestinal symptoms. Patients are given information on how their intestine functions, and hypnosis is directly targeted at removing intestinal symptoms. The patients are also taught to use imagery, such as the steady flow of a river through their intestines. The treatment takes three months.[13] As it helps to reduce the relapse rate, hypnotherapy could also be a useful adjunct to other forms of treatment.[14] Asthma also has a clear psychogenic component, and should be helped by hypnotherapy. At least one clinical study has shown impressive results, with a considerable reduction in drug requirement and hospital admissions.[15] However, one of the main areas of clinical use and research is to reduce symptoms during painful medical procedures and in pain associated with serious conditions such as cancer. Newton reports a long-term evaluation of the use of hypnosis in 283 cancer patients. He found improvements in their general condition, tolerance to chemotherapy, and life expectancy.[16] There have been several controlled studies showing that hypnosis, as well as deep relaxation and imagery, can reduce the nausea and discomfort resulting from chemotherapy.[17] Pain, bleeding, and the general level of stress and anxiety are considerably reduced.[18] These studies have led to routine use of hypnosis in some American oncology departments, which moved Ashley Conway to mourn that 'What is remarkable and apalling is that this kind of support is not widely available to patients in this country. Mainstream oncologists should be aware that hypnosis has an important part to play in the treatment of their patients'.[19] It is obvious that hypnosis is moving away from 'wart-magic' towards a more truly complementary role, however it is still limited by a lack of holism in the approach of most conventional doctors and some alternative therapists.

Uses and risks

The public have generally associated hypnosis with the cure of obsessive habits, in particular, smoking and over-eating. Indeed, together with sexual problems, these are the stock in trade cases of lay hypnotherapists. However, today hypnosis is becoming better known as a genuine mind-body treatment, which overlaps with relaxation and imagery. Many kinds of problems are now treated including phobias, allergies, amnesia, gastric ulcer, stress, asthma, anxiety, inhibitions, insomnia, menstrual disorders, migraine and tension headaches, psoriasis, eczema, tremor, tinnitus, and pain. Hypnosis can be used in any situation where a particular mental stance will promote healing or relieve discomfort. This includes the increasingly important application of the relief of the suffering and depression of people in the terminal stages of their illness, or undergoing severe medical treatment. In these cases hypnosis can not only reduce symptoms, but also anxiety and fear. In terminal illnesses hypnosis can prepare the patient for the possibility of dying, improve the quality of life, and aid in the relationship with those looking after the patient.[20]

Expectations of success vary enormously. Hypnotherapists generally feel that anxiety, phobias, and habitual behaviours respond best. Asthma, allergies, and psychosomatic conditions respond well but take time, and often benefit from a combined holistic aproach in which hypnosis is combined with counselling, and other complementary therapies such as herbalism or naturopathy. Pain treatment can often be very successful. For example, one British consultant reports that 90 per cent of minor fractures can be reduced in a casualty department without anaesthesia if hypnosis is used.[21] A similar success can be achieved when hypnosis is used during childbirth.

Hypnosis is very safe. Evidence of significant adverse effects has not surfaced, despite many years of wide use all over the world. However, one can imagine three kinds of possible risks. The first is through the careless use of post-hypnotic suggestion without proper familiarity with the case. A few cases where death occurred as an indirect result of the use of hypnosis have been reported. For example, a woman was told that she would have no fear of crossing a road, and she was promptly run over. A second kind of risk is that by superficial removal of symptoms or uncovering of unconscious traumas a more serious condition, physical or psychological, is precipitated. This is possible, and is sometimes used by practitioners to uncover deeper psychophysical problems during diagnosis, for example of psychogenic cardiac problems that would not surface in a normal physical diagnosis.[22] It is recommended that all hypnotists have some training in psychotherapy so as to be able to respond appropriately to any problems which surface during hypnosis. The third kind of risk is that of manipulation by the hypnotist. A hypnotist probably can make people do things against their will, provided he has time gradually to establish his control and bring the subject into deep hypnosis. However, the situation here is similar to psychotherapy where transference can have a similar result. There is usually no time for this in stage performances. Controlled studies of experimental hypnosis have failed to pick up side-effects. Generally the hypnotized subjects have felt better, less anxious, and more relaxed in daily life. Indeed, the deeper the hypnosis the better they felt afterwards.[23]

Obtaining treatment

There is a variety of approaches in hypnotism, used by both medical and lay hypnotherapists. It is better to go to hypnotherapists who are fully qualified, who do not advertise that they can aid in overcoming smoking or over-eating, and who use a psychotherapeutic approach to treatment. There is often someone in hospital who has been trained in hypnosis whom a patient can call for assistance. It is worth noting that many doctors have been trained in hypnosis but lack the opportunity and confidence to use it.

References

1. Asher, R. (1956). Respectable hypnosis. *British Medical Journal*, 1, 309–13.
2. Hartland, John (1971). *Medical and dental hypnosis*. Balliére and Tindall, London. Udolf, R. (1986). *Handbook of hypnosis for professionals*. Van Nostrand, New York.
3. Hartman, B. J. (1977). The treatment of psychogenic heart syndrome by hypnotherapy. *Journal of the National Medical Association*, 69, 63–5.
4. Hilgard, E. R. and Hilgard, J. R. (1984). *Hypnosis in the relief of pain*. William Kaufmann, Los Altos, California. Diamon, M. (1977). Issues and methods for modifying responsivity to hypnosis. *Annals of the New York Academy of Sciences*, 296, 119–28.
5. Barber, T. X., Spanos, N. P., and Chaves, J. F. (1986). *Hypnosis, imagination and human potentialities*. Pergamon Press, Oxford and New York.
6. Le Cron, L. M. (1954). A hypnotic technique for uncovering unconscious material. *Journal of Clinical and Experimental Hypnosis*, 2, 76–9.
7. Burrows, G. D. and Dennerstein, L. (eds.) (1980). *Handbook of hypnosis and psychosomatic medicine*. Elsevier, North-Holland, Amsterdam. Fellows, B. J. (1990). Current theories of hypnosis: a critical overview. *British Journal of Experimental and Clinical Hypnosis*, 7, 81–92.
8. Black, S. (1963). Inhibition of immediate-type hypersensitivity response by direct suggestion under hypnosis. *British Medical Journal*, 1, 925–9.
9. Chapman, L. F., Goodell, H., and Wolff, H. G. (1959). Changes in tissue vulnerability induced during hypnotic suggestion. *Journal of Psychosomatic Research*, 4, 99–105. Maslach, C., Marshall, G., and Zimbardo, P. G. (1972). Hypnotic control of peripheral skin temperature: a case report. *Psychophysiology*, 9, 600–5.
10. Barabsz, A. K. and McGeorge, C. M. (1978). Biofeedback, mediated biofeedback and hypnosis in peripheral vasodilator training. *American Journal of Clinical Hypnosis*, 21, 28–37.
11. Stern, J. A., Brown, M., Ulett, G. H., and Stetten, I. (1977). A comparison of hypnosis, acupuncture, morphine, valium, aspirin and placebo in the management of experimentally induced pain. *Annals of the New York Academy of Sciences*, 296, 175–93.
12. Conway, A. V. (1986). Cancer and the mind; a role for hypnosis. *Holistic Medicine*, 1, 43–55.
13. Whorwell, P. J. (1991). Use of hypnotherapy in gastrointestinal disease. *British Journal of Hospital Medicine*, 45, 27–9. Taylor, E. E. and Whorwell, P. J. (1993). Cost effective provision of hypnotherapy in a hospital setting: a practical solution. *British Journal of Medical Economics*, 6, 75–79.
14. Colgan, S. M., Faragher, E. B., and Whorwell, P. J. (1988). Controlled trial of hypnotherapy in relapse prevention of duodenal ulceration. *Lancet*, 2, 1299–300.
15. Morrison, J. B. (1988). Chronic asthma and improvement with relaxation induced by hypnotherapy. *Journal of the Royal Society of Medicine*, 81, 701–4.
16. Newton, B. (1982). The use of hypnosis in the treatment of cancer patients. *American Journal of Clinical Hypnosis*, 25, 104–13.

17. Redd, W. H., Rosenberger, P. H., and Hendler, C. S. (1983). Controlling chemo-therapy side effects. *American Journal of Clinical Hypnosis*, **25**, 161–72. Mastenbrock, I. and McGovern, L. (1991). The effectiveness of relaxation techniques in controlling chemotherapy induced nausea—a literature review. *Australian Occupational Therapy Journal*, **38**, 137–42.

18. Zeltzr, L. and LeBaron, S. (1982). Hypnosis and non-hypnotic techniques for reduction of pain and anxiety during painful procedures in children and adolescents with cancer. *Journal of Paediatrics*, **101**, 1032–5. Ament, P. (1982). Concepts in the use of hypnosis for pain relief in cancer. *Journal of Medicine*, **13**, 233–40. Kohen, D. (1986). Applications of relaxation mental imagery (self-hypnosis) in paediatric emergencies. *International Journal of Clinical and Experimental Hypnosis*, **34**, 283–94.

19. Conway, A. (1989). Review of paper by Walker, L. G. *et al.* In: *Complementary Medical Research*, **3**, 43.

20. Dempster, C. R., Batson, P., and Whalen, B. Y. (1976). Supportive hypnotherapy during the radical treatment of malignancies. *International Journal of Clinical and Experimental Hypnosis*, **24**, 1–9.

21. Jameson, R. M. (1963). Hypnosis for minor surgical procedures. *British Journal of Anaesthesia*, **35**, 269–71.

22. Conway, A. (1989). Hypnosis and research into mind/body relationships. *Complementary Medical Research*, **3**, 9–11.

23. Coe, W. C. and Ryken, K. (1979). Hypnosis and risks to human subjects. *American Psychologist*, **34**, 673–81.

16

Manual therapies including reflexology and aromatherapy

Remedial massage

Although remedial massage has its own techniques and disciplines, it is based on the strongly human instinct to hold or rub a place which hurts. Thus the simplest form of massage may well go back to primitive man. As a minor and instinctive form of therapy, the history of its usage is largely unwritten. We do not know of its systematic use until spas and watering-places became popular during the last century and massage was used in conjunction with hydrotherapy.[1]

Interest in massage is currently undergoing something of a revival. Its value has been newly recognized and re-assessed, and the instinct to use the hands as instruments to assist healing has been formalized into set patterns and types of movement to bring about a desired effect.[2]

Massage is applied to the soft tissues of the body—the muscles and ligaments— but this has a resulting beneficial effect on the nervous and circulatory systems. Techniques are designed to relax, or strengthen and stimulate; both may happen at the same time. Massage eases tensions and knotted tissue, increases the circulation of the blood, and stimulates the lymphatic system, which helps to eliminate waste material. Massage helps to break down adhesions and restore strength and mobility after injury. It is obviously useful in maintaining muscular tone and blood circulation for people confined to bed or wheelchairs for long periods of time. Massage is often used in conjunction with osteopathy or chiropractic in re-establishing and maintaining the postural integrity of the body. In addition, massage also has an undoubted psychological effect, inducing a sense of ease and well-being.

The most commonly used form of massage treatment is Swedish massage, which may be broken down into four main movements.

1. *Effleurage*: a stroking movement which soothes the patient and relaxes the superficial muscles in preparation for stronger movements. Effleurage may be stimulating if used vigorously.

2. *Pettrisage*: involves kneading, rolling, and squeezing the tissues, much as one kneads bread.

3. *Friction*: used deeply with small circular movements against the bone, with the intention of releasing specific areas of tension and blockage.

4. *Tapotement*: movements are stimulating and designed to tone and strengthen the muscles. Cupping, hacking, flicking, and clapping should be followed by further effleurage movements.

In recent years the basic forms of massage have been extended and added to by a number of special techniques. For example, polarity therapy, developed by Dr Randolph Stone, involves concentrated pressure on specific body points in order to re-align posture, and encourage the flow of energy ('Qi' or 'prana') around the body.[3] Reflexology, structural integration, shiatzu, and kinesiology, are described later in the chapter. These extensions to basic massage recognize the psychological and emotional aspects of being, and aim to restore well-being on all levels.[4]

Massage has a wide area of application but there are a number of contra-indications. Massage should not be used in the acute inflammatory stage of arthritis, or any other condition where there is high temperature or inflammation, although its use may be very helpful once the inflammation has dispersed. Restoring strength and mobility after a sprain, or in fibrositis, are obvious examples. Massage should not be used in serious heart disease, or in phlebitis, where a blood clot might be disturbed. Neither should massage treatment be given where there is an infective skin condition.

Massage and touch are now seen as one of the main tools that are available to nurses in hospital to humanize the caring and to develop the role of nurses to become therapists in their own right.[5] Certain situations have been identified in which massage could be of immense value. For example, in the case of institutionalized elderly patients, a recent study has found that massage significantly reduced anxiety, tension, and heart rate, and was much appreciated. Massage was more effective than conversation, which in turn was more effective than doing nothing.[6] Such studies are short-term, and do not address the obvious long-term benefits that might come from adding contact and life to institutional existence.

Recent studies have looked at massage in the case of cancer patients. A study carried out at the Institute of Cancer Research, the Royal Marsden Hospital, evaluated the effect of massage in a real life situation of a cancer ward. The nurses concluded that the experience 'was an overwhelmingly positive one, and appeared to have made a great contribution to making peoples lives with cancer better, and in helping the patient to feel cared for and accepted. This effect was even more profound where a patient's cancer or treatment had left visible scars or physical changes.' The patients reported relaxation and a release of tensions, aches, and pains: half stated that it improved their physical symptoms. The effects lasted for several days after each massage.[7] In a similar study with cancer patients who were experiencing pain, 60 per cent reported a reduction in pain after a half an hour massage, and again physiological tests showed relaxation and a reduction in anxiety.[8]

Massage can not only help with the distress of disease, but also that of modern medicine itself, which is often impersonal and unfamiliar. A review of the use of massage in Intensive Care Units determined that it could be profoundly beneficial to a patient's general mood and level of anxiety. Concerns that it may overstimulate the heart in cardiac patients were found not to be the case, although in some critically ill patients, even the minor stimulation of a massage might be unwise.[9] Massage has also been studied in premature babies in the hospital neonatal intensive care units. It has been found to stimulate the development of the sympathetic nervous system; and 70 per cent of babies gained weight rapidly compared with 40 per cent of those who did not receive massage. The babies who had complications benefited most from massage.[10]

Many of the benefits of massage have been widely assumed but never tested, and indeed as one of the main points of a massage is the subjective experience, there has been little incentive to check the claims objectively. However research investigating the physiological results of massage does exist but was not widely known. Obviously there is a reduction in anxiety, which can sometimes be determined physiologically, for example by lower cortisone hormone levels.[11] The issue of improved blood flow is another assumption which is now confirmed. After massage, the surface blood vessels dilate, and there is more return of venous blood to the heart. The improved blood flow lasts for at least an hour after a massage.[12] Blood supply to one limb is improved even by massage to the other one.[12] Connective tissue massage, which is much deeper, can also improve blood supply to deep-seated organs. Massage seems to be better for this purpose than some other physiotherapeutic techniques such as ultrasound or short wave diathermy.[13] The healing effects of massage are also due to return of fluid via the lymph to the heart, which allows the drainage of swollen tissues.[14] There are many studies confirming pain relief produced by massage, which not only reduces subjective effects of pain, relieves spasm, and causes a release of endorphins.[15]

Reflexology

Reflexology is a form of ancient Chinese medicine involving treatment by massage of pressure points in the feet. Research has shown that reflexology was also known to some early African tribes, the American Indians, and the early Egyptians. It was rediscovered in the early 1920s by an American ear, nose, and throat consultant, Dr William Fitzgerald, who found that by applying pressure to a certain area of the foot he was able to anaesthetize the ear; this enabled him to perform minor ear operations. His findings attracted the attention of other medical practitioners and the main pioneer in the field was a nurse, Eunice Ingham, who toured the USA lecturing, treating, and training students. One of her students was the late Doreen Bayly who returned to England and introduced the method there in the early 1960s.[16]

There are reflexes in the feet for all parts of the body and these are arranged in such a way as to form a map of the body in the feet. The right foot represents the right side of the body and the left foot represents the left side of the body. The reflexes are found mainly on the soles of the feet but also on the top and sides of the feet. An imaginary line drawn across halfway down the foot corresponds to the waistline in the body. Hence, the big toes represent the head and brain, the little toes represent the sinuses, and the heart reflex is found only in the left foot above the waistline. By massaging a specific area of the foot, an effect can be brought about in a part of the body or a zone quite distant from the foot. By working on these reflexes, the circulation of blood to the corresponding part of the body is improved and a reduction in the nervous tension in the area occurs. This can be of considerable benefit since many disorders are due to tension in parts of the body. It is also able to stimulate the healing forces present in the body and thus increase the body's ability to heal itself.[17]

Similar reflexes are found in the hands. However, the feet are normally used for treatment since the reflex areas are larger and the feet are more sensitive to massage since they are protected in socks and shoes. The hands, though, can be most useful for self-treatment. Another set of reflexes, called cross reflexes, are also employed by the reflexologist; these are links between the shoulder and hip, elbow and knee, and wrist and ankle on the same side of the body. It has been found that a tender area in, for example, the hip will have a similar tender area in the shoulder.

When giving reflexology treatment, the hands, and particularly the thumbs, are used. The thumb is bent and the side and end of the thumb pressed firmly onto the reflex point. To release the pressure, the thumb is pulled back with a slight circular movement. To move from one reflex to the next, a forward creeping movement is used so that the thumbs are kept in contact with the foot as much as possible. Each reflex is about the size of a pin's head so the massage must be precise. If the area being worked on is out of balance, a tenderness will be felt in the foot. This tenderness can be likened to a piece of glass being pressed into the foot; it can feel extremely sharp and often the practitioner may be accused of sticking his finger-nail into the foot. The degree of tenderness felt will depend on how out of balance the corresponding part of the body is and the method can therefore be used as a means of diagnosis. At some of the reflexes, it is sometimes possible to feel little granules beneath the skin. By massaging the areas, these granules can be dispersed so that they are re-absorbed by the circulatory system and excreted from the body. In different cases, different amounts of pressure are required; although as there will probably be tender areas in the feet, the pressure should not be such that it causes agony to the patient since this will not allow him to relax.

During a treatment, all the reflexes in both feet are massaged so that the body is treated as a whole. Each treatment lasts about three-quarters to one hour. Areas which appear tender are given massage and normally these areas will become less tender after a few minutes. However, it is not possible to remove all tender areas with one treatment. It is difficult to predict how many treatments are required to correct the imbalances but, in general, results should become evident after about three treatments and a course of six to eight treatments is usually recommended. Those conditions of long standing will probably require more treatments than those of a shorter duration. Children, in particular, seem to respond to the treatment quickly.

A wide range of disorders can be treated using reflexology and it is fair to say that most conditions will benefit to some extent from a course of treatment. Conditions such as migraine, sinus trouble, back problems, poor peripheral circulation, and stiffness and tension can all be helped.[18]

Following treatment, no unpleasant side-effects are experienced. Some people feel revitalized and have a sense of well-being, whilst others may feel tired. In some cases, a form of healing crisis, such as a cold, worsening of a skin rash, or the need to pass water more frequently, may occur. All of these reactions are, however, short-term effects as the body fights to rid itself of toxins. As well as being used to treat disorders, reflexology treatment at regular intervals can help maintain the body in a state of good health. It is always advisable to receive treatment from a trained practitioner. There are certain instances, including heart trouble, thrombosis, shingles, or pregnancy, when treatment should not be given or when extra care is required.

There has been little research on reflexology, perhaps because, again, it has been hard for medical researchers to digest a model in which such specific and non-anatomical points in the feet have distant influences throughout the body. While the model has not been explored, clinical studies on reflexology have begun. In one case women with Premenstrual Syndrome received reflexology treatment to foot, ear, and hand over an eight-week period. This was compared with placebo reflexology in which inappropriate points were treated in incorrect though convincing ways. Although all participants felt good during treatment, those receiving true reflexology had much less somatic and psychological PMS symptoms, and the difference was noticeable for two months after the treatment had finished.[19] In another, smaller study, reflexology was found to be as effective as flunarizine in the treatment of headaches, and was very helpful in restoring urinary system function after gynaecological surgery.[20] Nurses are considering reflexology as a useful tool for patient care, and it will probably be nursing groups who break new ground in research.[18]

Structural integration—rolfing

In common with most specific manual therapies structural integration was developed by one inspired teacher, Ida Rolf. She treated people by a special deep form of massage for 30 years before her technique gained recognition and acclaim. It is based on the premise that the shape and contour of our body is a dramatization of our experience. Life events and stresses impose distortions on the body which, over time, are set into the connective tissues. For example, a head forward posture, associated with states such as agitation or timidity, could encourage an opposite bend in the spine and hunched shoulders to re-create an upright posture. However, this misalignment is only maintained as a result of expenditure of energy, continuous muscular tension, and eventually stresses locked into the structure of the body.[21]

Rolfing is a deep and powerful massage designed to soften the collagenous fascias of the body. The masseur applies his weight through fingers, knuckles, and often elbows, reaching into body areas to loosen and realign the musculature and its supports. Misalignment is corrected session by session. In fact clinical research has demonstrated that rolfing is able to noticeably restore the pelvic inclination in young men who have an anteriorly tilted pelvis.[22]

The standard treatment consists of 10 one hour sessions, each of which is devoted to one particular body area. The final sessions reintegrate the newly flexible tissues. It is a drastic and painful treatment. Yet people emerge from it measurably taller, as from Alexander Training. Posture, chronic musculoskeletal pains and tensions, voice, sensitivity, breath control, attitude to self, and mood can all be affected by this massage. However for a more permanent beneficial effect rolfing should be combined with self-care. It should not, however, be used in cases of organic disease.

Shiatzu—Japanese pressure point massage

Shiatzu is a massage technique which combines massage with finger pressure to acupuncture points and meridians. In Oriental medicine fingers were and are often used instead of acupuncture needles, for example in young children where very mild treatment is indicated, when an individual wishes to treat himself, or for use in emergencies such as snakebite, haemorrhage, or shock where no acupuncturist is to hand. Oriental medicine acknowledges that deep pressure applied to certain points will have a similar effect to puncture with needles, although it is milder and less tightly controlled and the points may differ from the needle points. Because it does not need as much precision and knowledge as acupuncture, and is even safer, it has been taken up as a family and folk self-treatment method, especially in Japan. There are still tens of thousands of shiatzu practitioners in Japan. Some of them are blind, for it used to be one of the classical professions of the blind.

Shiatzu has specific and general applications. It is used in the treatment of specific chronic diseases. The shiatzu practitioner may sometimes diagnose visually in the same way as an acupuncturist and he may be especially expert at interpreting the feel of the body, the painful, hot, or knotted areas. Treatment is then given on several points on the required meridians, as well as by general kneading massage, in order to promote the flows of energy in the required directions. It is particularly effective in the long-term treatment of rheumatic, sexual, and circulatory problems. However extensive training in shiatzu is required to use it as a specific therapy in this way. Instead, many people are finding that points can be used for self-treatment and first aid in daily life. For example, a point on the eyebrows can give relief from headaches, other points on the face will anaesthetize the gums in dentistry, certain points will affect mood and energy, others, such as the 'revival' point on the perineum, can be used in emergency.[23]

The general use of shiatzu is in whole-body prevention and self-care. A shiatzu massage of this kind will cover all the meridians, paying particular attention to those meridians which need (or 'ask for') attention. The masseur works in a particular sequence, moving down the meridians and opening them to greater flow of energy on the way.[24] It is also an intuitive practice in which the touch of the masseur transmits his healing energy. For this reason shiatzu practitioners must keep themselves in properly balanced health. A kind of do-it-yourself shiatzu, combined with Japanese limbering and tonifying exercises, forms a health practice called Do-In.

As shiatzu employs a great deal of acupressure, research on acupressure is relevant to shiatzu. Some of this research is described in Chapter 6. Here we discuss research in which acupressure is self-administered or within a context of traditional massage. Pain is obviously one of the main symptoms that have been studied. In one large trial employing over 500 patients with headache, self-administered acupressure enabled a large proportion to dispense with conventional pain medication.[25] Acupressure on the limbs has been shown to be effective in temperomandibular joint (jaw) disorders.[26] Shiatzu has been used with handicapped children. Seventy-four per cent improved in tests of co-ordination, communication, emotional, and physical wellbeing.[27] Recently, the use of acupressure at the nasal philtrum has been found to rapidly prevent epileptic fits, a clear indication of the kind of energetic action at a distance that is the operation of Qi.[28] Research has identified that inflammation and even injury of a nerve is a rare but possible adverse effect of inappropriate shiatzu,[29] so as with all manual medicine, a sensitive and trained practitioner should be sought.

Applied kinesiology

Applied kinesiology (AK) was created in 1965 through the efforts of Dr George Goodheart, a chiropractor. He discovered that the kinesiological tests used to determine relative muscle strength and tone over the range of movement of the joints could also give qualitative information about the functions of body organs—the liver, kidneys, small intestines, etc. Using knowledge of chiropractic, of the trigger or reflex points on the body, and of acupuncture meridians and their relationship to organs and muscle groups, he developed a consistent diagnosis and treatment system.[30] Its theoretical basis rests on the assumption that muscle weakness is the result of the functional state of the nervous system, expressed in the muscle-nerve connections (motor neurone facilitation). The organs express their function via nerves to specific muscle groups.

AK is used to detect incorrect joint function, spinal lesions, muscle weakness, organic dysfunction, psychological effects on the function of the body as a whole, and sometimes even nutritional needs, and allergies. These last two factors have however aroused considerable controversy within the health care professions.[31]

A simple muscle test, for example, involves the practitioner applying a downward pressure on the patient's extended right arm while the patient is sitting. If the patient's arm 'locks' in that position it indicates the general strength of the group of muscles in the shoulder; if the arm does not lock and feels 'spongy' then a weakness is indicated. Individual muscles can then be isolated by placing the arm into different positions and re-testing, so giving an accurate picture of the weakened muscles.

Different muscle groups can be tested to diagnose different kinds of organic dysfunction. The precise location of muscle weakness also aids in the traditional chiropractic or osteopathic diagnosis. Treatment of the weakened muscle is secondary to treatment of any underlying problem revealed by AK. However, working on the appropriate reflexes and meridians with finger-pressure strengthens the weak muscles and restores structural balance. AK is now used in American dental practice and in international sports medicine, as well as in chiropractic and osteopathic practices in Europe, the USA, Australia, and New Zealand. The research on AK so far is inconclusive.[32] Muscle strength testing does seem to reveal changing internal mind-body conditions.[33] However a study which tested kinesiological diagnosis of nutritional deficiencies with laboratory tests of actual deficiencies found no correlation.[34]

Spinal touch treatment

The recognition of the effects of stress on the body is at the core of spinal touch treatment. The constant bombardment of pressures, problems, illness, and inadequate nutrition (not forgetting gravity), puts our bodies under constant stress. Stress is a positive factor in growth and development. However, when pushed beyond natural elastic limits, stress becomes strain. Muscles left in a condition of strain for a prolonged period of time will cause body distortion. This can reduce vitality because of an over-accumulation of fatigue poisons such as lactic acid.

Treatment begins with a complete plumb-line analysis of the patient to determine how far his posture has deviated from the norm, the most crucial point of reference being the lumbosacral joint—the centre of gravity of the body, and the point to which all stresses in the body are directed. The differences are noted, and the patient then relaxes in a prone (face-down) position on the treatment table and the practitioner begins treatment (lasting between 10 and 15 minutes) using a very light touch on a number of contact points on the gluteal muscles, along the spine, neck, and shoulders, base of skull, and abdomen. Touching these key areas redirects the body's energy, causing the muscles to relax and gently pulling the spine into its more natural position.[34] Several treatments are required to relax the tissues to the point where the body maintains the correct postural balance, although relief of symptoms and the restoration of proper functioning may take place after the first treatment.

Aromatherapy

Aromatherapy is the therapeutic use of essential oils extracted from plants.[35] The oils are not actually oils, more correctly aromatic volatile essences containing largely terpenes. They are concentrated from a large variety of plants, mostly by distillation. They are highly concentrated; sometimes more than a kilo of plant material is needed to make one gram of the essential oil. The oils are derived from medicinal and aromatic plants, and have certain advantages and disadvantages compared with herbal teas. They are strong and easy to use—one or two drops may have equivalent aromatic constituents to a cup of herb tea. They are absorbed through the skin and they work rapidly. There is evidence that within 20 minutes from external application the oils have pharmacological effects within the body.[36] On the other hand they can be quite toxic, and also they do not have all the herbal constituents in the original plant—only the aromatic, volatile ones. Therefore they tend to have a more limited range of actions on the body than the whole herbs, tending towards antibacterial and antifungal effects, antispasmodic, carminative, circulatory stimulation, and decongestant, and aiding mood and general well-being.[35]

In general, aromatherapy is used with massage and the oils applied externally only. They are always diluted in vegetable oils such as almond oil, often at a dilution of 2 per cent. When so applied, their effect on internal functions is mild. But they have a more potent effect on mood, emotion, and well-being, and they affect the skin and peripheral circulation. For example, neroli oil calms and relieves anxiety, it has an antispasmodic and anti-inflammatory effect. Lavender oil is one of the oils that is sometimes used neat, in first aid as an external antiseptic and healing oil used for burns, bites, and wounds. It also helps in insomnia, migraine, and menstrual problems. Juniper oil helps in urinary problems including stones, and for rheumatic joints. Eucalyptus oil, one of the main constituents of Oriental balms, is useful for respiratory problems, including bronchitis, catarrh, and influenza. With more training aromatherapists can use oils internally too, although there is currently debate within the profession on the wisdom of this since some oils can be quite toxic.

Aromatherapy is one of the fastest growing therapies in the UK and Europe because it is appealing and sensory, and so life-giving. In addition it is relatively easy to learn especially in the restricted form in which the oils are limited to external use. Research is in its infancy but some interesting new studies have recently been carried out, especially on the psychophysical effects of aromatherapy massage. In one recent study with patients in Intensive Care after cardiac surgery, a 20 minute foot massage with neroli oil (used for relief of anxiety and relaxation of involuntary muscles) clearly reduced anxiety and stress. However, in common with other studies, it was hard to find significant physiological changes arising from the treatment. The use of essential oil increased calmness, relaxation, and patient comfort compared with massage without it.[36] A similar finding has been reported for cancer patients.[7] A six-month pilot study at the John Radcliffe Hospital in Oxford with 585 mothers in labour used various essential oils: lavender to reduce anxiety and pain, peppermint to relieve nausea and vomiting, clary sage to increase contractions. The programme was a great success, and mothers reported a high degree of satisfaction and relief.[37] Six-hundred and thirty-five women participated in another randomized double-blind trial of lavender oil versus inert oil in the bath after childbirth. Perineal discomfort was mildly, but not significantly relieved with lavender compared with placebo.[38]

Essential oils have a powerful and penetrating scent and aroma which itself can have potent psychological effects, in addition to any direct pharmacological actions of the oil components on the tissues: 'Smells are surer than sounds or sights to make your heartstrings crack.' is a quote from Rudyard Kipling summarizing the findings of a psychological review of the effects of the scent of aromatic oils on the mind.[39] We have only to consider the powerful biological and largely unconscious role of pheromones to appreciate the possible changes in mood that might be induced by different scents.[40] One study with mice demonstrated that the scent of the oils calmed them when agitated, and could be detected in their blood.[41]

References

1. Kohnlechner, K. (1979). *Handbuch derNaturheilkunde* (2 volumes). Wilhelm Heyne Verlag, Munich.
2. Downing, George (1972). *The massage book*. Random House, New York. Hofer, Jack (1976). *Total massage*. Grosset and Dunlap, New York. Cohen, N. (1987). Massage is the message. *Nursing Times*, **83**, 19–20.
3. Stone, R. (1978). *Health building*. Parameter Press, Orange County, California.
4. Downing, George (1974). *Massage and meditation*. Random House, New York. McKechnie, A.A., Wilson, F., Watson, N., and Scott, D. (1983). Anxiety states: a preliminary report on the value of connective tissue massage. *Journal of Psychosomatic Research*, **27**, 125–9.
5. McMahon, R. and Pearson, A. (eds.) (1991). *Nursing as therapy*. Chapman and Hall, London. Rankin-Box, D. (1993). Innovation in practice: complementary therapies in nursing. *Complementary Therapies in Medicine*, 1, 30–3.
6. Fraser. J. and Kerr, J. B. (1993). Physiological effects of back massage on elderly institutionalised patients. *Journal of Advanced Nursing*, **18**, 238–45.
7. The Centre for Cancer and Palliative Care Studies (1994). An evaluation of the use of massage and self-massage with the addition of essential oils on the wellbeing of cancer patients. Unpublished report. The Institute of Cancer Research, The Royal Marsden NHS Trust, London.
8. Ferrel-Tory, A. T. and Glick, O. J. (1993). The use of therapeutic massage as a nusing intervention to modify anxiety and the perception of pain. *Cancer Nursing*, **16**, 93–101.
9. Hill, C. F. (1993). Is massage beneficial to critically ill patients in intensive care units? A critical review. *Intensive and Critical Care Nursing*, **9**, 116–21.
10. Scafidi, F. A., Field, T. *et al.* (1993). Factors that predict which preterm infants benefit most from massage therapy. *Journal of Developmental and Behavioural Paediatrics*, **14**, 3–8. Kuhn, C. M., Schanberg, S. M. *et al* (1991). Tactile-kinetic stimulation effects on adrenocortical function on pre-term infants. *Journal of Paediatrics*, **119**, 434–40.
11. Groer, M., Mozingo, J. *et al.* (1994). Measures of salivary secretory immunoglobulin A and state anxiety after a nursing back rub. *Applied Nursing Research*, **7**, 2–6. Field, T. and Morrow, C. (1992). Massage reduces anxiety in child and adolescent psychiatric patients. *Journal of American Academy of Child and Adolescent Psychiatry*, **31**, 1–8.
12. Goats, G. C. (1994). Massage—the scientific basis of an ancient art: Part 2. Physiological and therapeutic effects. *British Journal of Sports Medicine*, **28**, 153–7. Hovind, H. and Nielson, S. L. (1974). Effect of massage on blood flow in skeletal muscle. *Scandinavian Journal of Rehabilitation Medicine*, **6**, 74–7. Ernst, E., Matrai,

A., Magyarosy, I., Liebermeister, R. G. A., and Eck, M. (1987). Massages cause changes in blood fluidity. *Physiotherapy*, **73**, 43–5.

13. Goats, G. C. and Keir, K. (1991). Connective tissue massage. *British Journal of Sports Medicine*, **25**, 131–3. Hansen, T. I. and Kristensen, J. H. (1973). Effect of massage, shortwave diathermy and ultrasound upon[133] Xe disappearance rate from muscle and subcutaneous tissue in human calf. *Scandinavian Journal of Rehabilitation Medicine*, **5**, 179–82.

14. Pflug, J. J. (1975). Intermittent compression in the management of swollen legs in general practice. *Practitioner*, **215**, 69–76.

15. Harris, B. and Lewis, R. (1994). Pain management: a hands on approach—part 2. *International Journal of Alternative and Complementary Medicine*, **12**, 17. Kaada, B. and Torsteinbo, O. (1989). Increase of plasma B-endorphins in connective tissue massage. *General Pharmacology*, **20**, 487–9.

16. Bayly, D. (1982). *Reflexology today*. Thorsons, Harper Collins, London.

17. Grinberg, A. (1989). *Holistic reflexology*. Thorsons, Harper Collins, London.

18. Sahai, S. (1993). Reflexology—its place in modern healthcare. *Professional Nurse*, **8**, 722–5. Booth, B. (1994). Reflexology. *Nursing Times*, **90**, 38–40.

19. Oleson, T. and Flocco, W. (1993). Randomized controlled study of premenstrual symptoms treated with ear, hand, and foot reflexology. *Obstetrics and Gynecology*, **82**, 906–11.

20. Kesselring, A. (1993). Foot reflex zone massage. *Schweizer Medizinische Wochenschrift*, Supplement 62, 88–92.

21. Rolf, I. (1977). *Rolfing—The integration of human structures*. Dennis Landmann, Santa Monica, California.

22. Cottingham, J. T. *et al.* (1988). Shifts in pelvic inclination angle and parasympathetic tone produced by rolfing soft tissue massage. *Physiological Therapy*, **68**, 1364–70.

23. Blate, M. (1982). *The natural healers acupressure handbook: G-J fingertip technique*. Routledge and Kegan Paul, London.

24. Namikoshi, Tokujiro (1977). *Shiatzu therapy, theory and practice*. Wehmann Brothers, New Jersey. Ohashi, Watani (1990). *Do-it-yourself shiatsu: how to perform the ancient Japanese art of acupuncture without needles*. Unwin, London.

25. Harris, B. and Lewis, R. (1995). Acupressure and Traditional Chinese Massage. *International Journal of Alternative and Complementary Medicine*, **13**, 8. Kurland, H. D. (1976). Treatment of headache pain with autoacupressure. *Diseases of the Nervous System (USA)*, **37**, 127–9.

26. Matsumura, W. M. (1993). Use of acupressure techniques and concepts for nonsurgical management of TMJ disorders. *Journal of General Orthodontics*, **4**, 5–16.

27. St. John, J. (1987). Acupressure therapy in a school environment for handicapped children. *American Journal of Acupuncture*, **15**, 227–32.

28. Pothmann, R. and Schmitz, G. (1985). Acupressure in the acute treatment of cerebral convulsions. *Alternative Medicine*, **1**, 63–7.

29. Herskovitz, S. *et al.* (1992). Shiatsu massage-induced injury of the median recurrent motor branch. *Muscle Nerve*, **15**, 1215.

30. Birdwhistell, R. L. (1970). *Kinesics and context: essays on body motion communication*. University of Pennsylvania Press, Philadelphia.

31. Klinkoski, B. and Leboeuf, C. (1990). A review of research papers published by the International College of Applied Kinesiology from 1981–1987. *Journal of Manipulative and Physiological Therapeutics*, **13**, 190–4.

32. Webb, D. E. and Fagan, J. (1993). The impact of dream interpretation using psychological kinesiology on the frequency of recurring dreams. *Psychotherapeutics and Psychosomatics.*, **59**, 203–8.

33. Kenney, J. J., Clemens, R., and Forsythe, K. D. (1988). Applied kinesiology unreliable for assessing nutrient status. *Journal of American Dietetic Association*, **88**, 698–704.
34. Thie, J. and Marks, M. (1973). *Touch for health*. De Vorss Press, Santa Monica, California.
35. Tisserand, R. B. (1994). *The art of aromatherapy*. C. W. Daniel, Saffron Waldon, Essex.
36. Stevenson, C. J. (1994). The psychophysiological effects of aromatherapy massage following cardiac surgery. *Complementary Therapies in Medicine*, **2**, 27–35.
37. Burns, E. and Blamey, C. (1994). Soothing scents in childbirth. *International Journal of Aromatherapy*, **6**, 24–8. Burns, E. and Blamey, C. (1994). Complementary medicine. Using aromatherapy in childbirth. *Nursing Times*, **90**, 54–60.
38. Dale, A. and Cornwell, S. (1994). The role of lavender oil in relieving perineal discomfort following childbirth: a blind randomized clinical trial. *Journal of Advanced Nursing*, **19**, 89–96.
39. King, J. R. (1994). The scientific status of aromatherapy. *Perspectives in Biology and Medicine*, **37**, 409–15.
40. van Toller, S. and Dodd, G. H. (eds.) (1992). *Fragrance, the psychology and biology of perfume*. Elsevier Science, London.
41. Buchbauer, G., Jurovetz, L. *et al.* (1993). Fragrance compounds and essential oils with sedatory effects upon inhalation. *Journal of Pharmaceutical Science*, **82**, 600–4.

17
Mind-body therapies

The mind in disease

Apart from obvious mental diseases, medicine has more or less ignored the mind as a cause of sickness ever since therapeutics ousted magic. However, in the last 20 years research on the subject has forced the medical establishment to adjust its attitudes.[1] It was Hans Selye who first showed that animals under experimental stress developed some of those diseases so common today: indigestion and gastric ulcer, heart problems, and disturbance of the immune defensive systems of the body. He incorporated classical 'fight or flight' physiology in a new model which suggested how psychological disease caused physical disease.[2]

Much of human physiology is designed to maintain a balanced, calm, clement, and constant inner environment. As soon as threat or change is perceived by our senses and interpreted by our minds, physiology adopts a defensive posture to maintain this balance that results from the continual and delicate compensation by the most sensitive of scales.[3] The physiology of the mobilization of body defences is now very well understood. It involves the sympathetic nervous system and adrenaline and steroid hormones of the adrenal glands under the hormonal and nervous direction of the lower brain, the hypothalamus, and pituitary glands. The cascade of defence reactions is profound, arousing the mind, altering muscle action, blood circulation, heart action, metabolism, breath, and digestion. The emotions can be visualized as ancient internal mechanisms for marshalling these forces.

These body responses are however a two-edged sword. For when challenges or over-arousal persist, described as a state of stress, continued defensive readiness produces a profound deterioration in health. For example, there is clear evidence that stress or anxiety, arising for example from bereavement, inability to cope, or depression can undermine the immune system, and thus lower resistance to almost any disease. This is under intensive investigation at the present time, being described as the new field of psychoneuroimmunology.[4]

There is also a good deal of research which demonstrates that the stress hormones of people who do not 'switch off' properly get used to a round-the-clock mobilization, leading directly to tiredness, 'burn-out', irritability, insomnia, and then on to serious psychosomatic disease.[1,5] Anxiety, tension, over-stimulation, clock-watching, restlessness, ambition, guilt, fear, and so on are all psychological postures which cause persistent stress reactions.

The diseases that result occur frequently. This does not only mean those diseases which have always been known to be psychosomatic (that is directly related to stress and mental processes), such as indigestion, gastric ulcer, migraine, high blood pressure, disturbances of heart function, asthma, and obesity, but also many very serious and widespread diseases which have previously been thought of as having exclusively an external 'accidental' origin, such as cancer, atherosclerosis, rheumatic conditions, and chronic infections. This is not to say that diet and environment do not contribute, but that personality, stress, and mental attributes also have an influence. The psychogenic contribution to cardiovascular disease, for example, is now thoroughly accepted by the medical world.[6] It is also accepted that the mind has an effect on the origin and development as well as the regression of cancer,[7] and considerable evidence is now emerging as to how this happens. Depression and anxiety and other kinds of psychological stress causes disturbances in the hypothalamic/pituitary control of the endocrine system, particularly the corticosteroids. This in turn reduces or exhausts the thymus and the circulating lymphocytes which normally weed out nascent tumour cells.[8]

There have been other findings relating to the mind's connection with health. The placebo response, that is healing occurring solely as a result of belief in the treatment, is now better understood and utilized in treatment.[9] Research has linked it to changes in brain neuropeptides. It is these same substances which are associated with acupuncture effects, the relief of pain, and the control of stress in the body.[10]

It is not surprising that some authorities consider these brain substances to be a third nervous system bridging mind and body, with powerful controls over states of energy, health, and constitution.[11] Nevertheless, this is only a beginning. Most complementary practitioners, and anyone who holds a more subtle expansive view of man, can only state that all disease has a psychological as well as physical, environmental, social, and sometimes even spiritual dimension. This is the assumption underlying all traditional medical systems.

The mind in treatment

There are a considerable number of different psychotherapeutic or psychosomatic methods now available within complementary medicine for preventing and treating disease. These include meditation (especially visualization), relaxation, bioenergetics, prayer and faith, stress management regimes, yoga, concentrative breathing exercises, counselling, autogenic therapy, and biofeedback. They all have certain features in common. First, they may begin with therapy but they all move on to growth, self-awareness, and personal development. To a greater or lesser extent these are therapies for the healthy as well as the sick. Secondly, they all attempt to elicit self-healing capacities. In each case they do so by giving them room to work, usually by removing, dissipating, or neutralizing attachments, negative emotions, anxieties, and destructive thought processes that lead to negative physiological reactions and negative behaviour patterns such as compulsions. Thirdly, these methods are largely non-specific, that is they do not apply specifically to a certain set of symptoms discovered by a therapist as a result of diagnosis. Fourthly, the therapist is normally an instructor or even priest, and the patient a trainee. The trainee must work on himself, largely by himself. The prognosis or outcome is as much his responsibility as anyone else's.[1,12]

There are few precautions or side-effects with these methods, providing they are competently taught and executed. Perhaps the only real danger is that a person with a serious organic condition may not receive appropriate complementary or conventional treatment if he chooses a psychological therapy in the absence of a proper diagnosis. Therefore, anyone who is ill, or suspects disease, ought to have a diagnosis by a doctor or complementary practitioner, and make arrangements for his condition to be monitored. Then psychological methods can be used as an adjunctive, or where appropriate, sole treatment. Other problems might arise where the trainee dabbles and muddles different methods, where failure leads to psychological problems, where the method dredges up material from deep within the mind which neither the trainee nor an inexperienced trainer can handle, and so on. These risks are endemic to any psychotherapeutic undertaking.

The many body-oriented psychotherapies as well as yoga therapy, T'ai-chi, bioenergetics (Reichian psychotherapy), and so on, are, for reasons mentioned in the Preface (p. ix), outside the scope of this book. However the Bibliography lists interesting further reading and the books by Matson, Rowan, Assagioli, and Dychtwald are particularly recommended. The body-orientated psychotherapies are also described in the American holistic medicine books listed in the general section of the Bibliography. Relaxation, autogenic therapy, and biofeedback are discussed below since they are systems which are fully available and taught in a therapeutic setting in the UK. Hypnotherapy has close connections to autogenic therapy, which is a type of hypnotic meditation. Hypnotic induction also utilizes standard relaxation techniques. However, this is described in fuller detail in Chapter 15.

Much can be achieved with counselling, which is gaining acceptance as a helpful addition to medical treatment for diseases such as cancer. Psychotherapeutic counselling is outside the scope of this book. However its significant impact both on long-term survival of cancer patients and on their quality of life has been repeatedly proven.[13] Counselling has also been demonstrated to be effective in other conditions conventionally thought to be purely physical, such as irritable bowel disease.[14] Therefore it should be taken into account in the mind-body treatment of all disease. Sometimes even complementary medicine can become technique-oriented, assuming that methods such as relaxation will be sufficient, when actually they need to be combined with emotional discharge, feelings of empowerment and control over a patient's environment, reassurance and support, and so on.

Relaxation techniques

Relaxation is surprisingly difficult to achieve for people who are not naturally relaxed. Lying down is easy but a very great deal of tension will still remain in the body unless the mind too can be stilled. People relax in front of the television but the postures they take, and the tiredness they feel afterwards, demonstrates the opposite; that their physiology continues its state of sympathetic activation and arousal. True relaxation implies a profound shift in many physiological systems, a release of muscle tension and holding patterns, the mind barely ticking over, a deep surrendering of the body to its supports, and a slow and regular breath.

Relaxation methods are progressive. First, a setting is arranged so as to induce calm and contentment. Harsh surroundings, such as fluorescent lights, are to be avoided. The setting should establish cues that tend to remind a trainee of previous occasions of deep relaxation. After preparatory introduction and information, the trainee is sometimes taken through limbering, loosening, and stretching exercises to encourage subsequent rest.

The trainee is usually helped towards a comfortable posture, often lying corpse-like on the floor with hands outwards. Instructions are gradually introduced to relax parts of the body in turn, releasing tensions, sinking down and contacting and trusting the earth below, and eventually ending with the instructions to the mind to 'let go'.

There may follow sessions of guided imagery, colours, or reflections on pleasurable and absorbing memories.[15] There may be music, or there may be occasional reminders to concentrate on breathing sensations. The breath is often used as a bridge to reach an individual's calm, confident centre, unavailable through his web of discursive thoughts.[16] Relaxation programmes may also be combined with sessions in which people learn to control stressful influences. Useful rule-of-thumb techniques are taught, for example, to shift to abdominal breathing when situations get tense.

It is obvious that there is a great deal of overlap between relaxation, meditation in its beginning stages, yoga relaxation, and so on.[17] In fact, in terms of physiology, deep relaxation produces the same alteration in skin resistance, brain waves, breath patterns, and other measures of arousal, as transcendental meditation.[18] The quietening down of the sympathetic nervous system is striking and similar in all of these techniques.[19] A classical survey of the world medical and scientific literature on meditation and other self-control strategies came to the conclusion that various kinds of meditation, relaxation methods, yoga and biofeedback were equivalent from the point of view of health benefits.[20]

This does not mean that meditation is 'no more than' these other self-regulation methods, for obviously it goes very much further, indeed it is the logical conclusion of all these methods. However, the differences relate to the selftransforming experiences undergone by the meditator, not the reduction of stress and removal of psychogenic diseases.

Studies on the results of progressive relaxation have concentrated on certain psychosomatic conditions. For example, controlled studies of relaxation showed that it can significantly decrease asthma, especially of the large airway.[21] Irritable Bowel Syndrome has also been found to respond well to relaxation. At least two-thirds of patients who had long-standing illness showed a lasting improvement.[22] Relaxation has been sucessfully tested many times in the prevention of chemotherapy-induced nausea, and in general in improving mood, vitality, and resistance to toxic drugs in cancer patients.[23] Several studies have looked at chronic pain, especially headache, and found long-term improvements in at least 50 per cent of cases, especially in the frequency rather than severity of headache.[24]

For example, Dr Chandra Patel has reported several controlled studies in which patients who are at risk of developing heart problems were taught relaxation, with the result that many of their predisposing signs, such as high blood pressure, were reduced. The improvements in cardiovascular health persisted over several years compared with a control group. This has been recently confirmed in high quality clinical studies.[25] Through the additional use of visualization as a therapy, which is the intense concentration on specific images, a further range of health benefits, particularly the regression of cancer, may be possible in some people, given aptitude and will.[26]

As with meditation, relaxation will give an opportunity for thoughts and materials which have been suppressed by cerebral censorship to well up. There is therefore a possibility of increased anxiety, restlessness, and withdrawal in some sensitive or disturbed people. This could hardly be described as a side-effect, and it is often preferable to denial, but it is important to be aware of it, and perhaps utilize it as the basis for further psychotherapeutic work. In addition, relaxation techniques may be inappropriate where they are used as avoidance, or where a person is of a disposition that requires arousal and alertness rather than the opposite.

Biofeedback

The learning of all human abilities requires feedback. When a child learns to speak there is a constant two-way flow of attempts and corrections which are gradually refined down to a communicable tongue. This feedback is an unconscious strategy; however, there are many cases where feedback programmes are designed to supplement or replace those naturally available to man, for example in teaching a deaf person to speak or in teaching the re-use of limbs in the disabled. Biofeedback is the use of programmes of this kind, not to replace but to extend control into areas not normally manipulable by the will. That is, to control so-called 'involuntary' mental and physical processes.

The origins of biofeedback are found in the psychological experiments demonstrating basic conditioning or learning procedures that have occupied a good deal of experimental psychology for many years. Conditioning is a learning procedure by which some aspect of normal voluntary behaviour is elicited by rewards, a classic being ice-cream for good behaviour. However, researchers such as Kemmel and Miller demonstrated that responses that are normally automatic, or involuntary, such as heart rate, blood pressure, peristalsis of the intestines, blood flow in vessels, or skin temperature, could also be learnt by animals in the laboratory by rewarding them appropriately.[27]

It was not long before people hooked themselves up to the plethora of medical machinery used by doctors and researchers to monitor automatic physiological processes: the electroencephalograph (EEG) to measure brain waves, the electromyograph (EMG) to measure muscular activity, blood pressure and heart rate recorders, the electrical skin resistance metre (ESR), and so on. Not only could people learn to control their responses fairly quickly, but clear health benefits ensued. When muscle tension was reduced, the whole body became relaxed; headaches, stress, and anxiety were reduced too; when finger temperature was increased people lost their tensions, relieved their migraines, improved their circulation, and could sleep better at night.

In fact, in order to learn a specific ability, biofeedback trainees must enter a state of relaxed awareness. Physiological changes, such as a reduction in skin resistance and a redistribution of blood supply to the periphery of the body ensue, and all these are superimposed on the original ability. It follows that biofeedback is as good as other procedures in relieving stress-related conditions,[17] such as anxiety and insomnia. High blood pressure and tachycardia have shown to respond very well to biofeedback of blood pressure metering or muscle tension using an electromyograph,[28] and so do tension headaches.[29] However, in addition there are certain areas where it excels, for it can bring internal processes under more specific control than is possible by other relaxation methods. For example, learning to raise finger temperature or lower forehead temperature has shown excellent results in the treatment of migraine.[30] A Birmingham clinic found that some 80 per cent of migraine patients improved with this method. The same method is one of the best available for the treatment of Raynaud's disease, trench foot, and some other problems arising from inadequate circulation in the small blood vessels of the limbs. The temperature in the fingers has been clearly shown to rise, although this does not seem to be due to decreased activation of the sympathetic nervous system: the mechanism is still unknown.[31] It has been used very successfully in increasing blood pressure in those confined to wheelchairs, in re-training incontinent people,[32] and in restoring function to specific damaged muscles. An interesting example was published recently of the successful use of biofeedback along with autogenic training (see below) in controlling involuntary muscular spasms (myoclonus) after brain damage.[33] It raised the point that biofeedback can be a very useful adjunct to relaxation and autogenic training (see below), for biofeedback allows the patient to clearly visualize his increased control over body processes. In fact, most biofeedback today is usually combined with relaxation and other mind-body methods.

In practice a trainee must learn the signal language of the equipment he is using, while in a normal aroused state. He then endeavours to alter the metre, tone, or light by any means at his disposal in a state of relaxation. Gradually, he learns to alter the readings of the instrument above his own, now familiar, baseline. Eventually he becomes used to the state of mind which he has empirically found to be successful, and can then dispense with the feedback. The last stage is perhaps the most difficult. For many biofeedback practitioners have found that their subjects learn quickly and can re-create the desired state easily when hooked up to the machinery in a therapeutic setting. However, when the subject goes home the ability is gradually lost.[29] Daily life, of course, tends to distract from entry into states where automatic functions are controllable. There are several possible strategies that avoid this. Training should be extended, should include sessions with the machine switched off, should alter the response upwards and downwards, and should use responses relating directly to the condition, that is resistance of the air passages for an asthma patient rather than a more unconnected response such as heart rate.[34] The fall-off has limited the use of biofeedback alone in controlling high blood pressure. Success is possible only where biofeedback is combined with other methods.[28,35]

Biofeedback is in the unique position of being a science-based therapeutic procedure, with some 2500 papers to its credit, at the same time as an exciting self-development tool. The same rational behavioural procedure as is utilized to prevent headaches, when used with equipment to monitor brain waves, can become a stepping stone to explore altered states of consciousness.[36] In the UK, biofeedback is taught more as a self-monitoring procedure than a self-training one. That is, in contrast to the American school, trainees are instructed to regard the biofeedback tools as a check on progress in reaching desired psychophysical states. This helps to avoid dependence on the instrumentation.

Autogenic therapy

Johannes Schultz was a German psychiatrist and neurologist, working in Berlin in the 1930s. He was perhaps one of the first to develop practical self-help strategies incorporating scientific discoveries on the physiology of arousal and relaxation. This arose out of his use of hypnosis, for he observed how those entering the hypnotic state became relaxed and passively aware. He reasoned that if people could be taught to enter this state at will, the recuperative and health benefits of hypnosis would become generally available. He constructed an exact system which is something like a mixture of progressive relaxation, self-hypnosis, and meditative affirmations. The essence of the technique is passive (that is relaxed and unconcerned) attention to various parts of the body. There are several stages to the method.

The first stage is autogenic training itself. The practitioner or instructor, after taking a personal and medical history, will instruct the trainee in an appropriate relaxed posture, and the technique of passive awareness of parts of the body. Then he gives the trainee an exercise. The first one involves passively attending to the right arm while holding the thought that 'my right arm is heavy'. The heaviness is then extended to the other limbs. The second exercise suggests warmth in the extremities, the third calms the heartbeat, the fourth calms and regularizes the breath, the fifth warms the solar plexus, and the sixth cools the forehead. The trainee goes through the training gradually, keeping a record, with the instructor checking and guiding along the way.

Neither the trainee nor the trainer will direct the technique towards the cure of a specific illness, for it is felt that the innate *vix medicatrix naturae* is sufficiently powerful to achieve a cure once it is unleashed by a receptive state. Schultz records many cures in thousands of well-documented case studies, particularly from peptic ulcer, indigestion, circulatory problems, heart arrhythmias and angina, obsessive behaviours, sexual problems, diabetic pathologies, asthma, migraine, and anxiety.[37] The conditions treated are similar to those treatable by biofeedback, relaxation, and hypnosis, with which autogenic therapy has much in common. It also, naturally, has a strong preventive role. There are, as yet, far fewer research studies on autogenic therapy than on hypnosis or biofeedback, partly because success takes a considerable time, and because the trainee integrates the practice into his daily life from which it is hard to extricate it for research purposes. However, a recent comprehensive review and meta-analysis summarizes several controlled clinical studies on asthma, on hypertension, anxiety, eczema, and Raynaud's disease.[38] In all cases, clear but not dramatic positive results were found compared with no treatment or 'placebo' such as psychotherapy/discussion. In general, AT was effective to the same degree as relaxation training and hypnosis, but in severe problems, such as Raynaud's disease, biofeedback had the best outcome. For example in a study of 56 patients with tension headache, both AT and self-hypnotic techniques were equally effective in reducing pain and stress. The effects lasted over several months, especially for those patients 'who attributed pain reduction obtained during therapy to their own efforts'.[39] In another eight-month study with asthma patients, AT was found to be much more effective than simple psychotherapy in restoring respiratory function as measured by a battery of physiological tests.[40] Both AT and hypnosis dramatically reduced anxiety and panic attacks in short-term hospital out-patient treatment. The effect was noticeable after three months, but the degree of relief at that time depended on the frequency of doing the exercises at home.[41]

Like the other mind-body therapies, autogenic training is also the springboard for further work into growth, self-fulfilment, and extending capabilities. The next stage after autogenic training is autogenic modification, which amplifies the training and directs it to develop specific areas. For example, 'my lower abdomen is warm' will be used to stimulate the colon, 'my sinuses are cool and my chest is warm' will be used in the case of asthma sufferers. There are also behaviour control and development formulae, which can be used by athletes or performers to remove fears and blocks and develop their powers. Another stage beyond this is autogenic neutralization which focuses on psychological postures and problems in the same state of passive acceptance. The next stage is autogenic meditation which makes use of visualizations, contemplation of ideas, and contact with deeper levels of a person's being. These more advanced procedures are available to trainees with a good grounding in the basic autogenic training.

The Bates method of eyesight training

William Bates was a highly respected eye doctor in New York. During the course of his long career, in which he examined some 30000 eyes, he came to the conclusion that defects in vision are not irreversible, as is the current medical view. The accommodation of the eye to distance is controlled by muscles which pull the lens. Bates reasoned that many of the defects in vision were due to tensions and poor function in these muscles. In addition, there was a psychological aspect to the quality of vision. For example, he saw that children who were under stress, such as when their parents went away, had problems in proper seeing and focusing, but then their sight improved if the stress was removed, as when their parents returned. He developed a system of re-training of vision which obeys the same general principles as those described in other sections of this chapter. That is, the use of the mind and relaxation techniques gradually to relax and re-align muscles and alter customary habits.

One of his great successes was the restoration of full sight to a virtually blind Aldous Huxley who then wrote:

'I have been treated by men of the highest eminence in their profession; but never once did they so much as faintly hint that there may be a mental side to vision, or that there may be wrong ways, unnatural and abnormal modes of visual functioning as well as natural and normal ones . . . My own case is in no way unique. Thousands of other sufferers from defects of vision have benefited by following the simple rules of that Art of Seeing which we owe to Bates and his followers.'[42]

There are now many teachers of Bates's methods all over the world. Their fundamental statement is that the eyes are not mechanical lifeless tools. They are not slaves which we rely on completely without giving them any attention. Instead they are living, adaptable, functions, that can change and respond to the way we use them, just like any other mind-body function. The method has several components. A basic relaxation method known as palming involves shutting all light out with the hands, followed by a deep progressive relaxation of the body. In the dark, the mind's eye is sharpened and perceptions are focused. For example, an object is imagined to be moving from the observer without losing its clarity. Another exercise involves swinging rhythmically from side to side, with the eyes focused in the distance but moving, relaxedly, with the head. The sun is also used, as a centre of light which is contemplated with eyes shut in order to regenerate and renew the tissues. An eye chart records progress, and is used in exercises of relaxed seeing, without staring and without strain. Above all, the exercises teach us awareness of the eyes within the whole process of perception; to sense the world more fully, and sense the eyes more fully.

Some Bates practitioners explore the psychological dimensions of the defective vision in the same way as those working with posture explore and release locked-up early experiences that led to the locked-in tensions. Short- and long-sightedness as well as astigmatism and squint can all be treated in this way. However, as it is an instructional technique, the treatment depends on the patient's will and persistence.

References

1. Monro, R., Trevelyan, J. E., and West, R. (1987). *Mind-body therapies: a select bibliography of books in English.* Mansell, London. Pelletier, K. (1977). *Mind as healer, mind as slayer: A holistic approach to preventing stress disorders.* Delacorte, New York. Pelletier, K. (1994). *Sound mind, sound body.* Simon & Schuster, New York. Lehrer, P. M. and Woolfolk, R. L. (eds.) (1993). *Principles and practice of stress management.* Guilford, New York.
2. Selye, Hans (1976). *The stress of life.* McGraw-Hill, New York.
3. Cannon, W. B. (1939). *The wisdom of the body.* Norton, New York.
4. Solomon, G. F. (1985). The emerging field of psychoneuroimmunology. *Advances*, **2**, 6–19. Cousins, N. (1989). *Head first: the biology of hope.* Dutton, New York. Editorial (1987). Depression, stress and immunity. *Lancet*, **2**, 1467–8. This field is covered in several journals including *Psychoneuroimmunology* and *Advances*.
5. Cassileth, B. R. and Drossman, D. A. (1993). Psychosocial factors in gastrointestinal disease. *Psychotherapy Psychosomatics*, **59**, 131–43. Ramirez, A. *et al.* (1989). Stress and relapse of breast cancer. *British Medical Journal*, **298**, 291–3. Schedlowski, M., Jacobs, R., Alker, J., Pröhl, F., Stratmann, G., Richter, S. *et al.* (1993). Psychophysiological, neuroendocrine and cellular immune reactions under physiological stress. *Neuropsychobiology*, **28**, 87–90.
6. Pelosi, A. J. and Appleby, L. (1992). Psychological influences on cancer and ischaemic heart disease. *British Medical Journal*, **304**, 295–8. Friedman, M. and Rosenman, R. (1974). *Type A behaviour and your heart.* Fawcett, New York. Mattiasson, I. and Lindgärde, F. (1993). The effect of psychosocial stress and risk factors for ischaemic heart disease on the plasma fibrinogen concentration. *Journal of Internal Medicine*, **234**, 45–51.
7. Guex, P. (1993). *An introduction to psycho-oncology.* Routledge, London. Ramirez, A. J. *et al.* (1989). Stress and relapse of breast cancer. *British Medical Journal*, **298**, 291–3. Stoll, B.A. (ed.) (1979). *Mind and cancer prognosis.* Wiley, Chichester.
8. Conway, A. (1988). Cancer and the mind: a conditioned sensitization model. *Holistic Medicine*, **3**, 85–90. Sabbioni, M. E. E. (1993). Psychoneuroimmunological issues in psychooncology. *Cancer Investigation*, **11**, 440–50. Snyder, B. K., Roghmann, K. J. and Sigal, L. H. (1993). Stress and psychosocial factors: effect on primary cellular immune response. *Journal of Behavioural Medicine*, **16**, 143–61. Riley, V. (1981). Psychoneuroendocrine influences on immunocompetence and neoplasia. *Science*, **212**, 1100–9.
9. Oh, V. M. S. (1994). The placebo effect: can we use it better? *British Medical Journal*, **309**, 69–70. Raskova, H. and Elis, J. (1978). The role of the placebo in therapeutics. *Impact of Science on Society*, **28**, 57.
10. Gracely, R. H. Dubner, R., Wolskee, P. J., and Deeter, W. R. (1983). Placebo and naloxone can alter post-surgical pain by separate mechanisms. *Nature*, **306**, 264–5.
11. de Wied, D. and Jolles, J. (1976). Hormonal influences on motivational learning and memory processes. In: *Hormones, behaviour and psychopathology.* Raven Press, New York.

12. NICABM. (1993). *Pathways to health: a vital reference to mind/body medicine*. National Institute for Clinical Application of Behavioural Medicine, Mansfield Centre, Conneticut. Goleman, D. and Gurin, J. (eds.) (1993). *Mind/body medicine: how to use your mind for better health*. Consumer Reports Books. New York. Garfield, S. and Bergin, A. E. (1986). *Psychotherapy and behaviour change*. Wiley, Chichester.

13. Fawzy, F. L., Fawzy, M. O. *et al.*, (1993). Malignant melanoma: effects of an early structured psychiatric intervention, coping, and affective state on recurrence and survival 6 years later. *Archives of General Psychiatry*, 50, 681–9. Spiegel, D., Bloom, J. R., Kraemer, H. C., and Gottheil, E. (1989). Effect of psychosocial treatment on survival of patients with metastatic breast cancer. *The Lancet*, 2, 888–91.

14. Guthrie, E., Creed, F., Dawson, D., and Tomenson, B. (1993). A randomized controlled trial of psychotherapy in patients with refractory irritable bowel syndrome. *British Journal of Psychiatry*, 163, 315–21.

15. Morse, D. R., Martin, J. S., Furst, M. L., and Dubin, L. L., (1977). A physiological and subjective evaluation of meditation, hypnosis and relaxation. *Psychosomatic Medicine*, 39, 304–24.

16. Geba, Bruno (1974). *Breathe away your tension: an introduction to Gestalt body awareness therapy*. Random House, New York.

17. Benson, H. (1976). *The relaxation response*. Morrow, New York. Silver, B. V. and Blanchard, E. B. (1978). Biofeedback and relaxation training in the treatment of psychophysiological disorders; or are the machines really necessary? *Journal of Behavioural Medicine*, 1, 217–19.

18. Thomas, D. and Abbas, K. A. (1978). Comparison of transcendental meditation and progressive relaxation in reducing anxiety. *British Medical Journal*, 4, 1749.

19. Hoffman, J. W., Benson, H., Arns, P. A., Stainbrook, G. L., Landsberg, L., Young, J. B., and Gill, A. (1982). Reduced sympathetic nervous system. Responsibility associated with the relaxation response. *Science*, 215, 190–2.

20. Shapiro, D. M. (1982). Overview: Clinical and physiological comparison of meditation with other self-control strategies. *American Journal of Psychiatry*, 139, 267–74.

21. Erskine, M. J. and Schonell, M. (1981). Relaxation therapy in asthma: critical review. *Psychosomatic Medicine*, 43, 365–72. Lehrer, P. and Hochron, S. (1986). Relaxation decrease in large airway but not small airway asthma. *Journal of Psychosomatic Research*, 30, 13–25.

22. Shaw, G. and Srivastava, E. D. (1991). Stress management for IBS: a controlled trial. *Digestion*, 50, 36–42. Lynch, P. M. and Zanble, E. (1987). Stress management training for IBS: a preliminary investigation. *Clinical Biofeedback and Health*, 10, 123–34.

23. Burish, T. G. and Lyles, J. N. (1981). Effectiveness of relaxation training in reducing adverse reactions to cancer chemotherapy. *Journal of Behavioural Medicine*, 4, 65–78. Mastenbrock, I. and McGovern, L. (1991). The effectiveness of relaxation techniques in controlling chemotherapy induced nausea. *Australian Occupational Therapy Journal*, 38, 137–42. Bridge, L. R., Benson, P., Pietroni, P. C., and Priest, R. G. (1988). Relaxation and imagery in the treatment of breast cancer. *British Medical Journal*, 297, 1169–72.

24. Turner, J. A. and Chapman, C. P. (1981). Psychological intervention in chronic pain: A critical review. I. Relaxation and biofeedback. *Pain*, 12, 1–21. Blanchard, E. B., Applebaum, K. A. *et al.* (1987). 5-year prospective follow-up on treatment of chronic headache with biofeedback and/or relaxation. *Headache*, 27, 580–3. Duckro, P. N. and Cantwell-Simons, E. (1989). A review of studies evaluating biofeedback and relaxation training in the management of pediatric headache. *Headache*, 29, 428–33.

25. Benson, H., Rosner, B. A., Marzetts, B. A., and Klemchuk, H. (1974). Decreased blood pressure in pharmacologically treated hypertensive patients who regularly elicited

the relaxation response. *Lancet*, 1, 289–91. Patel, C., Marmot, M. G., Terry, D. J., Carruthers, M., Hunt, B., and Patel, M. (1985). Trial of relaxation in reducing coronary risk. A 4-year follow-up. *British Medical Journal*, 290, 1103–6. Johnston, D. W., Gold, A. *et al.* (1993). Effect of stress management on blood pressure in mild primary hypertension. *British Medical Journal*, 306, 963–6.

26. Meares, A. (1981). Regression of recurrence of carcinoma of the breast at mastectomy site associated with intensive meditation. *Australian Family Physician*, 10, 218–19. Achterberg, J. (1985). *Imagery in healing: shamanism and modern medicine.* Shambhala, Boston.

27. Miller, N. E. (1969). Learning of visceral and glandular responses. *Science*, 163, 434–5.

28. Fahmion, S.L. (1991). Hypertension and biofeedback. *Primary Care*, 18, 663–82. McGrady, A., Williams, S., Woerner, M., Bernal, G. A., and Higgins, J. T. (1986). Predictors of success in hypertensives treated with biofeedback-assisted relaxation. *Biofeedback and Self-Regulation*, 11, 95–103.

29. Coh, A. *et al.* (1992). Long term efficacy of combined relaxation biofeedback treatments for chronic headache. *Pain*, 51, 49–56. Burke, E. J. and Andraisik, F. (1989). Home versus clinic-based biofeedback treatment for pediatric migraine: results of treatment through one-year follow-up. *Headache*, July, 434–40.

30. Orne, M. T. (1979). The efficacy of biofeedback therapy. *Annual Review of Medicine*, 30, 489–503.

31. Freedman, R. R. *et al.* (1993). Plasma catecholamine levels during temperature biofeedback training in normal subjects. *Biofeedback Self-Regulation*, 18, 107–14.

32. Tries, J. and Eisman, E. (1993). The use of biofeedback in the treatment of urinary incontinence. *Physiological Therapy Practitioner*, 2, 49–56.

33. Duckett, S. and Kramer, T. (1994). Managing myoclonus secondary to anoxic encephalopathy through EMG biofeedback. *Brain Injury*, 8, 185–8.

34. Colgan, M. (1981). Medical uses of biofeedback: principles and case studies. *New Zealand Medical Journal*, 93, 49–51.

35. Patel, C., Marmet, M. G., and Terry, D. J. (1981). Controlled trial of biofeedback-aided behavioural methods in reducing mild hypertension. *British Medical Journal*, 282, 2005–8.

36. Cade, C. M. and Coxhead, N. (1987). *The awakened mind—biofeedback and the development of higher states of awareness.* Element, Shaftesbury, Dorset.

37. Luthe, W. (1976). *Creative mobilisation technique.* Grune and Stratton, New York.

38. Linden, W. (1994). Autogenic training: a narrative and quantitative review of clinical outcome. *Biofeedback and Self-Regulation*, 19, 227–64.

39. Spindhoven, P., Linssen, A. C. G., van Dyck, R., and Zitman, F. G. (1992). Autogenic training and self-hypnosis in the control of tension headache. *General Hospital Psychiatry*, 14, 408–15.

40. Henry, M., de Rivera, J. L. G., Gonzalez-Martin, I. J., and Abreu, J. (1993). Improvement of respiratory function in chronic asthmatic patients with autogenic therapy. *Journal of Psychosomatic Research*, 37, 265–70.

41. Stetter, F. *et al* (1994). Ambulatory short-term therapy of anxiety patients with autogenic training and hypnosis. Results of treatment and three month follow-up. *Psychotherapy, Psychosomatics and Medical Psychology*, 44, 226–34.

42. Huxley, A. (1974). *The art of seeing.* Montanu Books, Seattle.

18

Naturopathy and nutrition therapy

Background

Naturopathy, to quote the manifesto of the British Naturopathic and Osteopathic Association, is 'a system of treating human ailments which recognises that healing depends upon the vital curative force within the human organism'. This fundamental tenet underlies all natural therapies and certainly naturopathy. In practice it may range widely for, according to the American Naturopathic Association, it is 'a therapeutic system embracing a complete physianthropy employing nature's agencies, forces, processes, and products'.

It is customary for many systems of medical care to claim Hippocrates as their founder. Naturopathy can, perhaps, justify this claim more than most. When Hippocrates laid down guidelines for the maintenance of health in terms of the correct balance of rest and exercise, adequate nourishment and emotional stability, he was advocating those principles of bodily hygiene which are the foundations of naturopathy. These principles, preserved by Avicenna in Medieval Arabic medicine and then lost, only came to be appreciated again in the past 150 years or so by a pioneering few.[1] A revival in vitalism began in nineteenth-century Europe when they discovered and developed the use of simple measures such as water applications, plain food, and herbs as ways of promoting the healing mechanisms of the body. The discoveries were generally empirical, rather than deliberately created under clinical conditions in the way that osteopathy or homeopathy were.

In the small village of Grafenberg, in the Silesian mountains, a farmer, Vincent Priessnitz, advocated fresh air, applications of cool water, and wholesome fare consisting of black bread, vegetables, and fresh milk from cows fed on the mountain pastures. Others learned from Priessnitz or discovered for themselves the value of nature's agents. Khune, a weaver, became famous for his dietary treatments, another farmer, Johannes Schroth, evolved a strict dietary regime combined with hydrotherapy for the treatment of rheumatic disorders which, in spite of its stringency, was, and still is, greatly esteemed by many sufferers from this complaint. However, it was to Father Sebastian Kneipp of Bad Worishösen in

Bavaria that the tremendous popularity of hydrotherapy was due. Spas utilizing the methods he advocated were established throughout Europe.

Sometimes a chance observation led to the discovery of a system of treatment or diagnosis. Thus it was that a Prussian priest, Edmund von Peczely, founded the art of iris diagnosis, widely used by naturopaths to assess the vitality and the constitutional weaknesses of their patients. Von Peczely had a pet owl and, one day, when handling it, he accidentally broke its leg. He noticed that a blemish appeared in its eye which gradually changed in texture as the leg healed and this led him to pursue his observations; this became the foundation of modern iridology.

Fundamental concepts

As a system of health care which grew out of practical experience, naturopathy's philosophical concepts were not really laid down until an American doctor, Henry Lindlahr, wrote his *Philosophy of natural therapeutics* in the early part of this century. According to Lindlahr, 'health is the normal and harmonious' vibration of the elements and forces composing the human entity on the physical, mental and moral planes of being in conformity with the constructive principle in nature'.[1] Disease is generally the result of the disobedience of nature's laws leading to an inharmonious vibration of those same elements and forces.

To the sceptic these definitions may seem to be gross over-simplifications; indeed they are, but they crystallize the thought that lies behind naturopathic practice. If the body possesses the capacity to heal cuts or mend broken bones then it must ultimately be capable of resolving other disorders. The concept of homeostasis, the self-regulating mechanism of the body, is generally accepted, and the immune process is under intense study in modern medicine. However, in concentrating attention on the minute biochemical details of disease, medicine has narrowed its view of the origin of disease and the requirements for recovery. Whereas the allopathic view might suggest that recovery is aided by removal of inflamed or degenerative tissue, destruction of bacteria, or intervention in a specific metabolic pathway, the naturopath would take steps to promote the body's ability to restore its own equilibrium.

Lindlahr wrote of the body's response to inimical forces by crisis which, if prolonged, would lead to exhaustion and devitalization of its resources. This is exemplified by the tendency for acute superficial disorders, if suppressed by drugs or unsatisfactorily resolved, to become chronic and lead to pathological change and degeneration. However, it was Professor Hans Selye, of Montreal, who first postulated in some detail the concept of a general adaptation syndrome. This is the adaptive process by which we have survived as a species.[2]

According to Selye, the body's response to any stress, be it emotional or physical, initiates a three-phase sequence. Initially in the *alarm stage* there is pain (due, for example, to injury), shock (from bad news), or inflammation (due to friction). Then, as the body adjusts to the crisis, there is a *stage of resistance* in which we adapt to, or withstand the 'invasion' (stiffen to protect a joint, or suppress the hurt feeling, etc.). If the traumas or emotional stresses are prolonged the body or the group of cells under siege can no longer adapt. It then enters a *stage of exhaustion* and collapse or degeneration occurs.[3]

Naturopaths attach great importance to this adaptive capacity of the body and recognize that symptoms, such as inflammation or fever or pain, are signs of the defences at work and not to be suppressed. Furthermore, the process of recovery from chronic ailments may necessitate a return to the stage of resistance—known in natural therapy as the *healing crisis*.

Therapeutic procedures are directed to the restoration of normality in all aspects of the human function but first it is necessary to determine at what level in the adaptive functions the breakdown has occurred.

Diagnosis

The patient who visits a naturopath for advice about a particular disorder may be surprised to be questioned about seemingly irrelevant aspects of his body function or lifestyle. Examination of the eyes or measurement of the blood pressure may not be expected by a person seeking advice about a gastric ulcer. For the naturopath, diagnosis is only partly the collection of data to arrive at a defined disorder. It is also an assessment of the total functional capacity of the individual. Naturopaths aim to diagnose the patient rather than the disease, although in practice they must do both.

Symptoms are relevant as indicators of breakdown in adaptive mechanisms. Whilst palliative measures may be necessary it is the underlying disorder of bodily processes which must be corrected if the patient is to recover satisfactorily. Thus, when confronted with a skin rash, the naturopath is not particularly concerned with categorizing it among the host of medically defined dermatoses for he recognizes that it is most probably a manifestation of a deeper imbalance. That could be a disturbance in the metabolism of nutrients, or a blood dyscrasia (and the naturopath would check for these by the normal diagnostic procedure such as urine and blood analysis), but more often it may be a phase in the eliminative response to an underlying functional disturbance of organs such as the lungs or liver. It is this deeper cause of the rash which has to be sought.

Naturopathic assessment is also aimed at assessing the patient's vital reserve—his ability to respond to treatment. This information will be gleaned by standard methods of medical investigation which may, however, be interpreted cautiously. Levels of blood sugar or of certain vitamins or minerals which are considered within the 'normal range' may not always be acceptable to the naturopath, because under stress, these levels may be pushed way up or down. If this happens repeatedly, chronic, sometimes irreversible, changes take place. The most common example of this is what one naturopath Martin L. Budd, has called a twentieth-century epidemic—hypoglycaemia.[4] This condition, otherwise known as low blood sugar, may occur in phases induced by repeated intake of refined carbohydrates (sugar, white flour), starchy snacks, and caffeine (in coffee, tea, or canned beverages). These are absorbed so rapidly that the pancreas becomes over-sensitive and produces too much insulin. The excess insulin reduces blood sugar below normal, which when repeated often, may eventually give rise to chronic disorders such as migraine, allergies, hyperactivity, depression, obesity, or alcholism. The hypoglycaemic pattern is fairly obvious from clinical signs and symptoms but it may be confirmed by a six-hour glucose tolerance test, which measures changes in the blood sugar level at regular intervals after administration of 50 g of glucose by mouth. Treatment is the stabilization of blood sugar levels by diet.

The nutritional status as well as general vital reserve may be gauged by observation of skin tone, complexion, and the state of mucous membranes of the mouth and tongue. The nails can, for example, exhibit white spots, or leukonychia, which may suggest a deficiency of the trace element zinc. Some naturopaths use hair analysis as a means of assessing the levels of both the essential minerals and also the toxic metals such as aluminium, cadmium, and lead, which may cause insidious damage. Interpretation of hair analysis is still experimental; however it seems that the body's need for certain nutrients is not always reflected in the levels revealed by the more acceptable methods of assessment.

Iris diagnosis is among the most valuable diagnostic tools of the naturopath. It has not, thus far, been possible to establish definite anatomical evidence for a connection between the eye and other parts of the body but it is possible that fine nervous connections do exist via the optic chiasma. The legacy of von Peczely's owl has become a sophisticated system of diagnosis which is now used the world over. The system was developed in Europe during the nineteenth century and there are now some German Heilpraktikers who rely almost exclusively on this method of diagnosis. Some practitioners take photographs of the iris as a permanent record whilst many others rely on direct observation with suitable illumination and magnification. It has, however, been impossible to confirm the truth of iridology by objective research.[5]

Iris diagnosis is based on the principle that the general tone and level of inflammatory activity in various body tissues is reflected in the iris of the eye. Each system, such as stomach, intestines, autonomic nervous system, lymphatics, or skin, is represented in circular zones with radial divisions indicating the state of individual organs and mental faculties. Observation of the iris reveals the overall vital reserve of the patient and the areas of inherent weakness. Interpretation of the signs in the iris is made in functional terms, for example underactivity of skin, rather than a specific diagnosis such as eczema.

The treatment

The information accumulated by questioning, observation, and examination now has to be co-ordinated to form an overall impression of the patient and his requirements. The therapeutic regime will depend on a number of factors other than those immediately obvious from the examination, for example hereditary tendencies, constitution (both of which play a significant part in naturopathic assessment), past history, and previous treatments, especially use of drugs.[6]

From this information a decision can be reached as to whether therapy must be primarily anabolic (building up) or catabolic (breaking down). If the patient is devitalized, nutritionally deficient, and suffering from a chronic ailment he may need to be moved out of an over-stimulating catabolic phase requiring instead anabolic and tonic measures: a wholefood diet, rest and relaxation, and gentle manipulative procedures, with a constructive mental outlook. Nutritional measures will often be used to add the elements required by the patient, either by altering diet, or more usually by prescribing supplements of those substances to be taken orally or, in some instances (e.g. vitamin B^{12}), administered intramuscularly. For example, many micronutrients and trace elements have been shown to be important in treating conditions such as hypoglycaemia.[7]

In other cases, toxic accumulations must first be cleared by catabolic purificatory methods. Indeed, these eliminative methods in naturopathy used to rule supreme, especially in the early days of naturopathic hydros. Controlled catabolic activity is a necessary process in the management of chronic disorders to promote the functions of skin, lungs, or bowels. This may be done by dietary restriction or fasting, by hydrotherapy, both internal and external, and more stimulating exercise and manipulative procedures.

There are schools of naturopathy that still rely entirely on eliminative methods, with considerable success. The pure hygienic methods, pioneered by Shelton, will not admit of any external supplements or aids.[8] Spas and hydros offer a number of purificatory treatments, such as hot and cold spring and mineral baths, mud packs for skin conditions, bubbling aerated water, steam baths, and so on.[9]

It is sometimes necessary to promote a fever as a means of enabling the body to burn up toxic waste. This may be achieved by means of heat treatment and hydrotherapy, or the use of herbal substances. The stage at which these stimulating forms of treatment are introduced will depend upon the vitality of the patient—in those with sufficient vital reserve such treatments would be introduced at an early stage. These procedures may occasionally promote a crisis, and unless the naturopath can keep his patient under close observation, as, for example, in a residential clinic, he would be less inclined to impose prolonged eliminative procedures.

Fasting and other restricted diets

Under proper supervision the fast may be regarded as a most constructive, health-restoring procedure and should not be confused with starvation. The fact that it has been an important part of religious rituals in many parts of the world bears out its intellect-sharpening as well as physical benefits. Fasting constitutes a physiological rest which enables the body to divert its energy to the process of removing metabolic waste and restoring homeostasis. It can be highly effective even in chronic conditions such as rheumatoid arthritis.[10] Some authorities suggest that the element of metabolic shock in fasting induces an immune response. Fasting need not be total. A mono-diet is one in which a food or group of foods is eaten almost exclusively for a period of time. The most famous of these is the grape cure first advocated by Dr Johanna Budwig but graphically described by Basil Shackleton, who lived only on grapes (in South Africa where they are abundant) for almost 50 days and wrote '. . . after the twenty-third day an abscess came away from my one and only kidney and I was completely cured after all medical treatment had failed and made my condition worse'.[11]

The single most consistent factor in naturopathic practice has been the advocacy of a wholefood high fibre diet, preferably of foods which have been organically grown and are free from chemical additives.[6,7,12] For decades naturopaths have pointed out the harmful effects of chemicals and pesticide residues in food and, after encountering much opposition, are now finding more widespread acceptance and corroboration in medical research.[13]

The dynamics of structure

The need for an adequate transport system to and from each cellular unit is implicit in the requirement of good nutrition and adequate elimination. Freedom of circulation for the blood and lymph is, therefore, of paramount importance and the naturopath is very concerned with the removal of any obstacles to these in the form of joint restrictions and muscular spasm. Some naturopaths are also trained as osteopaths and can therefore bring to certain disorders, such as joint problems, the added dimension of the 'total lesion concept'. This means viewing restrictions of mobility and alignment not just from a mechanical standpoint but considering nutritional integrity, tissue tone, muscle balance, and even the influence of the emotions on the patient's postural habits.

The body-mind amalgam

The holistic view of health cannot ignore the powerful influence of thought, conscious or subconscious, on physical well-being. Naturopaths place varying degrees of emphasis on the role of the emotions in causing physical illness. A number of practitioners devote considerable time to counselling and other psychological approaches to physical illness. The fact that naturopaths give a great deal of time to their patients means that the social and psychological aspects of their ailments can be considered in some depth. Some also teach relaxation methods. In general, where 'outrageous fortune' burdens the patient with stresses, such as marital disagreements or unreasonable work pressures, the naturopath will emphasize the need for sound nutrition to improve the person's ability to withstand the 'slings and arrows'.

The long-term effects of under-nutrition, or the constant abuse of digestive organs by over-refined or over-concentrated foods create a sensitivity to a wider and wider range of substances. Lack of vitamins or sensitivity to such common foods as eggs or milk have been found to precipitate quite severe mind-body disorders. Exclusion of the offending foods or supplementation achieves improvement although naturopathy attaches more importance to attaining the stability of the internal milieu.[14]

Nutrition therapy

Nutrition therapy, or nutritional medicine, is a daughter specialization of naturopathy. It has grown so fast that the child is as big as, and in America towers over, its parent. It is the science of treating disease and promoting health by the use of specific nutritional factors, together with the elimination of toxic and allergenic materials from the diet.[7] It differs from naturopathy in several respects. First, it is more specialized: practitioners do not pay so much attention to hygienic, physical, or hydrotherapeutic aspects of traditional naturopathy. Secondly, it is more scientific. Practitioners draw their inspiration more from the 1000 nutritionally oriented scientific publications published in the world literature every year, than from the tenets of Hippocrates, Priessnitz, and Lindlahr. Thirdly it is more prescriptional: minerals, vitamins, essential fatty acids, amino acids, and other supplements are taken in therapeutic doses for a medicinal effect. Many naturopaths regard this as too interventionist for comfort, deviating from the basic naturopathic principles of self-cure.[6,15]

The basic principles of nutritional medicine are well defined in the summary issued by the British Society for Nutritional Medicine:

1. Man's diet, even in industrialised societies, may very often have only a borderline or indeed low content of certain essential nutrients. A 'normal' diet is not necessarily a healthy or optimum one.

2. Requirements for essential nutrients vary from individual to individual depending on genetic, physiological, lifestyle and other influences. What is adequate for one person may not be for another.

3. Illness is inevitably linked with an abnormal biochemistry and an alteration in the metabolism of nutrients and their by-products.

4. Specific nutrients such as vitamins, minerals, essential fatty acids and amino acids, as well as dietary manipulation in general, provide a potent means of influencing body biochemistry and thus disease processes.

5. By correcting fundamental biochemical abnormalities by nutritional means one can prevent certain diseases or alter the course of disease processes for the better.

In the last few years nutritional medicine has rapidly increased in popularity among both conventional and complementary health professionals. Doctors gain a set of options in addition to drugs to help manage some of the more intractable problems which reappear in their surgeries. For example, magnesium supplements, along with dietary changes, have been found useful as part of a combined treatment of high blood pressure and arrhythmias.[16] Antioxidants are now recommended in coronary care.[17] Evening primrose oil containing gamma-linolenic acid (GLA) is used for premenstrual, menopausal, rheumatic, allergic, and other conditions,[18] zinc and vitamin C for healing,[19] B vitamins in certain psychosomatic conditions,[20] and so on. Some clinical nutritionists who may or may not be medically qualified, use dietary factors as a health care system in its own right. Diagnosis would be essentially naturopathic, but would add hair mineral analysis, and a complete analysis of the diet and toxic constituents (including drugs) which the patient consumes. Treatment is given as a personally designed daily cocktail of vitamin, mineral, and other supplements.[6,7]

Nutritional therapists also pay attention to the possibility of food allergies, or more commonly, food sensitivities. Diseases such as infant gastrointestinal conditions, eczema, asthma, hyperactivity and sleep disturbance in children, migraine, colitis, obesity, malaise, headache and various so-called psychosomatic symptoms, yeast (*Candida*) infections, and autoimmune related conditions have all been associated with food allergies or sensitivities in a proportion of patients.[21] There is increasing medical research evidence to support this, for example studies at the Institute of Child Health have found that roughly two-thirds of children with hyperactivity and insomnia are cured by the removal of allergenic additives, particularly colourants and preservatives, from their diet.[22] Food allergies are diagnosed, classically, by a fast after which foods are restored one by one and the reactions carefully assessed. However, this method is difficult for patients to manage, and newer, less conventional methods are now employed, including testing of the reaction of the white blood cells of the patient, sublingual tests, applied kinesiology, and certain electrical equipment (see electroacupuncture p.138). These practices await solid clinical research backing. In particular, it is not known to what extent patients treated by the elimination of additives and contaminants to the diet are responding because of elimination of allergic reactions, or the addition of necessary dietary factors along with the elimination of toxins and 'empty calories'. In addition, according to a large new study covering 7500 UK households, there is a strong psychological component in supposed food allergies and sensitivities that needs to be taken into account.[23]

Research

Because of its complex, multidisciplinary approach, naturopathy as a complete therapy has rarely been subject to controlled research. Yet some of its main tenets, such as the harmful effects of dietary animal fats and lack of fibre, have been 'discovered' by conventional medical experts, and then tested in academic establishments. This research has produced a very large body of evidence to support much of naturopathic theory, referred to in references 6 and 7 with some further examples below.

A stimulus towards acceptance of naturopathic tenets has been observation of the health and longevity of primitive tribal communities, or religious groups practising abstinence, particularly the Pennsylvania Amish.[24] At first this lent support to the view that the rich animal fat diet of the civilized world produced the degenerative disease load in its wake. However, subsequent analysis showed that some healthy tribes, such as the Masai and the Eskimos, eat a lot of meat. This drew attention of researchers to salt, milk and milk products, refined foods, a lack of certain polyunsaturated fatty acids and trace elements, combined with inadequate exercise and relaxation.[25]

Recently, more profound understanding of the primitive diet has emerged from a lengthy study of the nutritional status of early man.[26] Not only was his diet ten times richer in vitamin C than the recommended daily allowance today, but the ratio of polyunsaturated to saturated fats was three times that of today's diet. The meat of wild animals has eight times less fat than that of farm animals and contains the important protective fatty acid eicosapentanoic acid (EPA) which is in fish oil, but absent from today's meat. Together with a great deal of pharmacological and clinical work, the above evidence shifts the emphasis away from the question of dietary fat as such, towards consideration of content and quality.[27] EPA itself has been implicated in the prevention of cardiovascular, arthritic, and malignant conditions.[27] The recent Lyon heart study, with heart patients, has confirmed the health benefits of a simple natural diet, in this case the country diet of Crete—olive oil, salads, bread, and white cheese and herbs such as purslane. Heart attacks and death rates were reduced by three-quarters compared with the controls.[28]

There has been a tremendous amount of research on the effects of vitamins and micronutrients on health and recovery from disease. The reader is referred to a number of books on the subject that review the evidence.[6,7,29] To cite one or two examples more or less at random, recent studies reported in the major medical journals include the finding of a protective effect of selenium and vitamins A and E against cancer,[30] and their support for a healthy cell-mediated immunity.[31] Vitamin E has also been shown in some very large recent studies to protect against cardiovascular risk, presumably by preventing lipid peroxidation and platelet stickiness.[32] It is useful in the treatment of peripheral vascular disease and neurological conditions.[33] Other studies on specific dietary constituents have pinpointed the toxic effects of small amounts of metals in the diet, particularly lead,[34] and have questioned the wisdom of fluoridation which may affect immunity and bone function in the long term.[35]

The use of specific nutritional factors in treatment of diseases, though an improvement on potentially toxic drugs, still misses the point of naturopathy, which is to help the body to restore its own health and basic vitality. There is some recent impressive evidence on the positive therapeutic effects of a complete naturopathic intervention. In particular, the paper by Dean Ornish and collaborators demonstrated that naturopathic treatment can achieve what was always assumed to be impossible by conventional medicine, that is to significantly reverse even severe atherosclerotic blockage of the arteries.[36] Fasting and dietary treatment on a health farm has been shown to reduce all the symptoms of rheumatoid arthritis, an effect which was clearly noticeable even a year later.[10,37] Twelve per cent of the UK population no longer eat meat, and 4.5 per cent have become vegetarians. The evidence for the improvements in health available from a vegetarian or vegan diet have now been amply confirmed by researchers. A very large scale study demonstrated a 40 per cent reduction in mortality over 12 years in vegetarians compared with meat eaters.[38] Vegetarians have thinner blood and lower blood pressure, which may help to prevent cardiovascular diseases.[39] Diet is very helpful in the treatment of premenstrual syndrome (PMS), and vegetarian women have a hormone pattern after the menopause that would tend to reduce the incidence of postmenopausal symptoms.[40]

As far as non-dietary aspects of naturopathy are concerned, research is limited. The effectiveness of hydrotherapy is rarely explored outside Germany.[41] There is some work on the positive health benefits of negative ions in the atmosphere, which may account for some of the value of fresh air, especially by the sea or in the mountains.[42] There is also a great deal of new evidence on the value of colonic hydrotherapy, one of the mainstays of naturopathic detoxification.[43] Research has also confirmed the importance of probiosis, that is the maintenance of a healthy gastrointestinal flora, without which overgrowth of pathogenic organisms can lead to poor vitality and perhaps allergies and autoimmune diseases.[44] Biorhythms and natural cycles, particularly of the endocrine system, have been investigated to a limited extent.[45]

Uses and risks

Naturopathy is first and foremost a preventive system. The naturopath sees an important part of his work as that of education in the fundamentals of health—mechanical, biochemical, and mental/emotional—and does not, therefore, attach great importance to the classification of disease. Nevertheless, there are certain categories of illness which naturopathy treats most effectively.

For example, respiratory disorders such as colds, coughs, tonsilitis, and sinusitis may be regarded as self-limiting but recovery is aided by naturopathic measures. Skin diseases are often closely related to lung disorders and are often successfully treated by naturopathy although inevitably there are cases in both categories which prove resistant to therapy. Sometimes this may be because the vital response of the patient has been considerably modified by previous therapy with drugs. Disorders of the gastrointestinal system can frequently be present without any evident cause in medical terms. These disorders may be associated with an inappropriate lifestyle and improve with a review of the patient's dietary habits and work on stress and mind-body health. Diseases of the heart and circulation may have a functional basis which responds well to naturopathic treatment aimed at restoring adaptability. In some cases naturopathic treatment can be the only genuine way to reverse long-standing chronic cardiovascular disease, in particular atherosclerosis.

The normalizing procedures of naturopathy are, however, best utilized in treating functional disorders before they become degenerative. If they advance to irreversible degenerative pathology, for example in osteoarthrosis or valvular heart disease, naturopathy can develop existing resources to aid the body's compensations for its physical shortcomings. The reduction of catarrh in the patient with chronic bronchitis, or emphysema, coupled with breathing exercises and osteopathic mobilization of the chest and back will at least improve the patient's capacity and reduce the occurrence of infections. Naturopathy cannot claim to have any special answer to disorders such as cancer or severe neurological disorders but it has a definite contribution to make in terms of raising general resistance and improving nutrition and outlook.

Children are particularly amenable to naturopathic treatment. They have a much greater vital response and can, therefore, be subjected to more stimulating forms of treatment, such as hydrotherapy. Naturopaths commonly treat children with acute or chronic respiratory disorders, allergies, and urinary disturbances such as nocturnal frequency. The naturopath also has an important role to play in the care of the elderly by the application of constructive nutritional measures and the use of neuromuscular techniques for the alleviation of musculoskeletal disorders.

The naturopath aims to make his patient self-sufficient with regard to health but the attainment of that level of function may take weeks or months, and sometimes complete self-sufficiency may not be possible at all. The chronic arthritic, for example, may find periodic treatment necessary, perhaps every month or two for an indefinite period. There are no risks with properly qualified naturopathic practitioners, although in some cases fasts and purificatory procedures might make a patient feel temporarily worse and should be closely monitored by a practitioner.

References

1. Lindlahr, V. H. (1975). *Philosophy of natural therapeutics*. Maidstone osteopathic clinic, Maidstone, Kent. Lindlahr, V. H. (1990). *Natural therapeutics* (2 vols). C.W. Daniel, Saffron Walden. Lafaille, R. and Hiemstra, H. (1990). The regimen of Salerno, a contemporary analysis of a medieval healthy lifestyle program. *Health Promotion International*, 5, 57–74.
2. Cannon, W. B. (1939). *The wisdom of the body*. Norton, New York.
3. Selye, Hans (1976). *The stress of life*. McGraw-Hill, New York.
4. Lesser, M. (1985). *Nutrition and vitamin therapy—the dietary treatment of mental and emotional ill-health*. Thorsons, Harper Collins, London.
5. Kriege, T. (1969). *The fundamental basis of iridiagnosis*. Fowler, London. Knipschild, P. (1988). Looking for gall bladder disease in the patient's iris. *British Medical Journal*, 297, 1578–81.
6. Murray, M. and Pizzorno, J. (1990). *Encyclopaedia of natural medicine*. Macdonald Optima, London.
7. Werbach, M. (1993). *Nutritional influences on illness*, Third Line Press, Tarzana, California. Holford, P. (1983). *The whole health guide to elemental health*. Thorsons, Harper Collins, London.

8. Shelton, H.M. (1969). *The hygienic system*. Health Research, Mokelumne Hill, California.

9. Roberts, P. (1981). Hydrotherapy: its history, theory and practice. *Occupational Health*, **33**, 235–44.

10. Kjeldsen-Kragh, J., Haughen, M., Borchgrevink, C. F., Laerum, E., Eek, M., Mowinkel, P. *et al.* (1991). Controlled trial of fasting and one-year vegetarian diet in rheumatoid arthritis. *Lancet*, **338**, 899–902.

11. Brandt, J. (1971). *The grape cure*. Benedict Lust, Simi Valley, California.

12. Davies, S. and Stewart, A. (1987). *Nutritional medicine*. Pan, London. Robbins, J. (1991). *Diet for a new America*. Stillpoint, Walpole, Hew Hampshire.

13. The National Cancer Institute in the USA acknowledges that the consumption of fruits and vegetables reduces the risk of certain cancers: Palmer, S. and Bakshi, K. (1983). Diet, nutrition and cancer, interim dietary guidelines. *Journal of the National Cancer Institute*, **70**, 1151–70. The UK's Committee on Medical Aspects of Food Policy now recommends a 50 per cent increase in fruits and vegetables and complex carbohydrates, and a switch to monounsaturated fats: Lipley, N. (1994). New diet guidelines. *General Practitioner*, **18** November, 14. WHO Study Group (1990). *Diet, nutrition and the prevention of chronic diseases*. World Health Organization, Geneva.

14. Wurtman, R. J. (1983). Behavioural effects of nutrients. *Lancet*, **1**, 1145–8. Schoenthaler, S. J., Moody, J. M., and Pankow, L. D. (1991). Applied nutrition and behaviour. *Journal of Applied Nutrition*, **43**, 31–9. Benton, D. and Roberts, G. (1988). Effect of vitamin and mineral supplements on intelligence of a sample of schoolchildren. *Lancet*, **1**, 140–3.

15. Chaitow, L. (1984). Will the real naturopathy stand up? *Journal of Alternative Medicine*, **2**, 20.

16. Woods, K.L. *et al.* (1994). The second Leicester intravenous magnesium trial [LIMIT-2]. *Lancet*, **343**, 816–19. Stamier, R., Stamier, J., Grimm, R., Gosch, F. C., Elmer, P., Dyer, A., Berman, R., Fishman, J., Van Neel, N., Civinelli, J., and MacDonald, A. (1987). Nutritional therapy for high blood pressure. Final report of a four-year randomized controlled trial. *Journal of the American Medical Association*, **257**, 1484–91.

17. Arens, U. (1994). Antioxidants: can they prevent coronary heart disease? *British Journal of Cardiology*, **1**, 126–7. Voelker, R. (1994). Recommendations for antioxidants; how much evidence is enough? *Journal of the American Medical Association*, **271**, 1148–9. Mason, R. S. (1993). Vitamin E and cardiovascular disease. *Complementary Therapies in Medicine*, **1**, 19–23.

18. Kleijnen, J. (1994). Evening primrose oil. *British Medical Journal*, **309**, 824–5. Gamma-Linolenic Acid Multicenter Trial Group (1993). Treatment of diabetic neuropathy with gamma-linolenic acid. *Diabetes Care*, **16**, 8–15. Leventhal, L. J., Boyce, E. G., and Zurier, R. B. (1993). Treatment of rheumatoid arthritis with gammalinolenic acid. *Annals of Internal Medicine*, **119**, 867–73.

19. Goode, H. F. *et al.* (1992). Vitamin C depletion and pressure sores in elderly patients with femoral neck fracture. *British Medical Journal*, **305**, 925–6. Pasantes, M., Morales, H., Wright, C.E., and Gaull, G.E. (1986). Protective effect of taurine, zinc and tocopherol on retinol-induced damage to human lymphoblastoid cells. *Journal of Nutrition*, **114**, 2256–61.

20. Crook, W. G. (1987). Nutrition, food allergies and environmental toxins. *Journal of Learning Disabilities*, **20**, 260–1. Ghadirian, A. M., Anath, J., and Engelsman, F. (1980). Folic acid deficiency and depression. *Psychosomatics*, **21**, 926–9. Harrel, R. *et al.* (1981). Can nutritional supplements help mentally retarded children? An exploratory study. *Proceedings of the National Academy of Science*, **78**, 574–8.

21. Lewith, G., Kenyon, J., and Dowson, D. (1992). *Allergy and intolerance: a complete guide to environmental medicine.* Green Print, London.
22. Egger, J., Wilson, J., Carter, C. M., Turner, M. W., and Soothill, J. F. (1983). Is migraine a food allergy? *Lancet*, 2, 865–9. Egger, J., Stolla, A. *et al.* (1992). Controlled trial of hyposensitisation in children with food-induced hyperkinetic syndrome. *Lancet*, 339, 1150–3.
23. Young, E. *et al.* (1994). A population study of food intolerance. *Lancet*, 343, 127–9.
24. Dubos, René (1968). *So human and animal.* Scribners, New York.
25. Temple, N. J. and Burkitt, D. P. (1994). *Western diseases.* Humana Press, New Jersey.
26. Eaton, B. and Kooner, M. (1985). Paleolithic nutrition. *New England Journal of Medicine*, 312, 283–9.
27. Harker, L. A. *et al.* (1993). Interruption of vascular thrombus formation and vascular lesion formation by dietary n-3 fatty acids in fish oil in non-human primates. *Circulation*, 87, 1017–29. Woodcock, B. E., Smith, E., Lambert, W. H., James, W. M., Galloway, J. H., Greaves, M., and Preston, F. E. (1984). Beneficial effect of fish oil on blood viscosity in peripheral vascular disease. *British Medical Journal*, 288, 592–4. Bittiner, S. B., Tucker, W. F. *et al.* (1988). A double blind controlled trial of fish oil in psoriasis. *Lancet*, 1, 378–80.
28. McKeigue, P. (1994). Diets for secondary prevention of coronary heart disease. Can linoleic acid substitute for oily fish? *Lancet*, 343, 1445. de Lageril, M. *et al.* (1994). Mediterranean alpha-linoleic rich diet in secondary prevention of coronary heart disease. *Lancet*, 343, 1454–9.
29. Null, G. (1984). *The complete guide to health and nutrition.* Arlington, London. Bland, J. (ed.) (1986). *Yearbook of nutritional medicine.* Keats Publishing, New Canaan, Connecticut.
30. Colditz, G., Branch, L. G. L., Lipnick, R. J., Willett, W. C., Rosner, B., Posner, B. M., and Hennekens, C. H. (1985). Increased green and yellow vegetable intake and lowered cancer deaths in an elderly population. *American Journal of Clinical Nutrition*, 41, 32–6. Lupulescu, A. (1994). The role of vitamins A, beta-carotene, E and C in cancer cell biology. *International Journal of Vitamin and Nutrition Research*, 64, 3–14. Garewal, H. (1994). Chemoprevention of oral cancer: beta carotene and vitamin E in leukoplakia. *European Journal of Cancer Prevention*, 3, 101–7. Block, G. (1991). Epidemiological evidence regarding Vitamin C and cancer. *American Journal of Clinical Nutrition*, 54, 1301S–14S.
31. Penn, N. D., Purkins, L. *et al.* (1991). Effect of diet supplement with vitamins A, C and E on cell-mediated immune function in elderly long-stay patients: a randomised controlled trial. *Age and Ageing*, 20, 169–74. Bates, C. (1993). Commentary. *Lancet*, 341, 28.
32. Stampfer, M. J. *et al.* (1993). Vitamin E consumption and the risk of coronary disease in women. *New England Journal of Medicine*, 328, 1444–9. Horwitt, M. K. (1991). Data supporting supplementation of humans with vitamin E. *Journal of Nutrition*, 121, 424–9.
33. Piesse, J. (1984). Vitamin E and peripheral vascular disease. *International Journal of Clinical and Nutritional Reviews*, 4, 178–82. Egan, M. F. *et al.* (1992). Treatment of tardive dyskinesia with vitamin E. *American Journal of Psychiatry*, 149, 773–7. Seddon, J. M. *et al.* (1994). Dietary carotenoids, vitamins A, C and E and advanced age-related macular degeneration. *Journal of the American Medical Association*, 272, 1413–20.
34. Brodie, R. (1995). Mercury toxicity in dental amalgams. *Journal of Alternative and Complementary Medicine*, 13, 29–31.
35. Gibson, S. L. M. (1992). Effects of fluoride on the immune system. *Complementary*

Medicine Research, **6**, 111–14. Bayley, T. A., Harrison, J. E., Murray, T. M. *et al.* (1990). Fluoride-induced fractures: relation to osteogenic effect. *Journal of Bone Mineral Research*, **5**, (Supplement 1) s217–22.

36. Ornish, D., Brown, S. E., Scherwitz, L. W., Billings, J. H., Armstrong, W. T., Ports, T. A. *et al.* (1990). Can lifestyle changes reverse coronary heart disease? *Lancet*, **336**, 129–33.

37. Darlington, L. G., and Ramsey, N. W. (1993). Review of dietary therapy for rheumatoid arthritis. *British Journal of Rheumatology*, **32**, 507–14.

38. Thorogood, M., Mann, J., Appleby, P., and McPherson, K. (1994). Risk of death from cancer and ischaemic heart disease in meat and non-meat eaters. *British Medical Journal*, **308**, 1667–71.

39. Ernst, E. and Franz, A. (1995). Blood fluidity score during vegetarian and hypocaloric diets—a pilot study. *Complementary Therapies in Medicine*, **3**, 70–1. Editorial (1984). *Lancet*, **1**, 671–3.

40. Armstrong, B. K., Brown, J. B., Clarke, H. T., Crooke, D. K., Hahnel, R., Masarei, J. R., and Ratajczak, T. (1981). Diet and postreproductive hormones: a study of vegetarian and non-vegetarian postmenopausal women. *Journal of the National Cancer Institute*, **67**, 761–7. Stewart, A. C., Tooley, S., and Stewart, M. (1991). The effect of a nutritional programme on premenstrual syndrome: a retrospective analysis. *Complementary Medical Research*, **5**, 8–11.

41. Golland, A. (1981). Basic hydrotherapy. *Physiotherapy*, **67**, 258–62. O'Hare, J., Heywood, A., Summerheyes, C., Lunn, G., Evans, J. M., Walters, G., Corrall, R. J. M., and Dieppe, P. A. (1985). Observations on the effects of immersion in bath spa water. *British Medical Journal*, **291**, 1747.

42. Finnegan, M. J., Pickering, C. A., Gill, F. S., and Ashton, I. (1987). Effect of negative ion generators in a sick building. *British Medical Journal*, **294**, 1195–6.

43. Kelvinson, R. C. (1995). Colonic hydrotherapy: a review of the available literature. *Complementary Therapies in Medicine*, **3**, 88–92.

44. Fuller, R. (ed.) (1992). *Probiotics: the scientific basis*. Chapman and Hall, London. Bernet, M. F. *et al.* (1994). Lactobacillus LA1 binds to cultured human intestinal cell lines and inhibits cell attachment and cell invasion by enterovirulent bacteria. *Gut*, **35**, 483–9. Gorbach, S. L. (1990). Lactic acid bacteria and human health. *Annals of Medicine*, **22**, 37–41. Polson, R. J. (1992). Pseudomembranous colitis associated with antibiotics. *Prescribers Journal*, **32**, 137–40.

45. O'Neil, B. and Phillips, R. (1975). *Biorhythms: how to live with your life cycles*. Signet, New York.

19
Osteopathy

Background and fundamental concepts

Andrew Taylor Still was born in Virginia. His father was a Methodist minister who farmed and cared for the sick, as well as preached. This background influenced Still's devout behaviour and fierce opposition to alcohol. He was also an excellent mechanic. Shattered by the loss of three of his children in an epidemic of meningitis, Still was mystified by the impotence of the doctors, although he praised their attention and skill.[1] He turned his mind to the problem of health and disease, and developed an interesting but simplistic theory.

God, he reasoned, had created man in his own likeness and therefore the design of the human body was perfect. How then could man become ill? Because, as with the machines Still understood so well, man's structure got out of adjustment; if readjusted it would function normally. Still extended his loathing of alcohol to drugs. He could not believe the God he worshipped could have designed man without including in the package all necessary equipment and chemicals. He believed the body was its own medicine chest.

Still's theories were not based on observation but on personal and religious conviction, yet contemporary accounts of his successful treatment of many ailments show that he was soon putting them to the test. He announced his theory of osteopathy in 1874 when he was 46, and tried hard to gain acceptance by the medical profession of his methods of treating disease. The doctors would not listen and the local Methodist minister denounced him as being in league with the devil, forcing him to move to another town: Kirksville in Missouri. Here, in 1892, he founded the first school of osteopathy.

Within a few years John Martin Littlejohn enrolled as a student. Littlejohn had studied physiology for three years at Glasgow University as part of a study of forensic medicine for which he was awarded the William Hunter Gold Medal in 1892. It has been said that Littlejohn 'took A.T. Still's osteopathy and . . . dipped it well and truly in a bath of physiology and what is more, kept it there'.[2]

It was Littlejohn who first expressed the idea of osteopathy in what we would recognize as holistic terms. He called it the science of adjustment. Man as an organism lived in an environment which had physical, social, occupational, dietetic, and many other aspects. Health was present when man was in balance with these influences and enjoyed a capacity to adjust to them within a range. Ill health occurred when there was a breakdown in this adjustment and the task of the osteopath was to adjust the patient back to normal. This of course implies knowledge of psychology and dietetics as well as anatomy, physiology, and manipulative skills. Littlejohn returned to England in 1913 and set up the British School of Osteopathy in 1917.

Still's concept of pathology was naïve. He describes an early experience with a small child with severe diarrhoea. The child's spine was hot and its abdomen cold so he simply tried to move the heat to the cold parts. He was amazed at the child's rapid recovery. He ultimately came to the conclusion that minor strains, slips, dislocations, and subluxations caused pressure on arteries which impeded blood flow. Reduction in arterial blood flow was the key: 'Unobstructed blood will never form a tumor', he wrote. His method of treatment was to examine a patient for evidence of these factors and to devise a large number of manual techniques to resolve these problems to his satisfaction. However, Still's students had great difficulty in learning from him. They thought his diagnosis clairvoyant and he performed techniques so quickly that they could not follow him. Frequently he would use a technique only once. It was many years before satisfactory methods of teaching manual skills were devised.

There has been a gradual evolution in the interpretation of spinal diagnosis. Still was concerned only with variations from the normal position of the vertebrae. By the 1930s vertebral diagnosis was interpreted in terms of the range of motion of one bone on another. Also, by the 1930s many of the explanations advanced for successful treatment had dismissed the concept of arterial pressure in favour of that of disturbance of reflex activity.

The term *osteopathic lesion* was used early in the twentieth century to describe vertebral diagnostic observations. It is useful in terms of identifying a segment at which the examining fingers perceive something to be wrong but has led critics erroneously to deride osteopaths for having their own concept of pathology. The Americans dropped the term in favour of the less specific *somatic dysfunction* which was subsequently adopted by the World Health Organization. In the early 1970s the British School of Osteopathy dropped the term in favour of a diagnostic system which sought more specifically to identify the tissue that was responsible for the malfunction or pain and thus led to selection of more specific techniques.

Today, osteopathy largely treats back pain, cases of which have reached epidemic proportions, and spinal problems generally.[3] Many osteopaths, however, still see their role as being wider than this and will undertake to assist in disturbances of function of the respiratory, gastrointestinal, genitourinary, and cardiovascular systems, although they are selective in the conditions they undertake to treat. Those skilled in cranial techniques also tend to treat head symptoms, including some types of sinus problem and giddiness, and problems in infants and children which are related to birth injuries. Additionally, some osteopaths train in a combination of osteopathy and naturopathy and so view osteopathy from the standpoint of natural medicine; this colours the way in which they approach the patient and his treatment.

A suitable definition of an osteopath is therefore a practitioner who is an expert in the examination, treatment, and interpretation of abnormalities of function of the musculoskeletal system.

Diagnosis

The osteopath will first take the patient's history which will give him the patient's view of the onset, duration, characteristics, and so on of current and other problems. The patient is then observed standing still and performing active movements. He is then observed sitting. Areas which exhibit potential problems are examined more minutely using palpation and passive movements. The osteopath will also carry out various accepted clinical procedures employing percussion hammer, stethoscope, ophthalmoscope, auriscope, etc. He may order or carry out X-rays and tests on blood and urine. At the end of this he is able to decide whether or not the patient needs further investigation, or referral and whether or not he is likely to respond to osteopathic treatment.

The osteopath now has an overall and detailed assessment of the patient's musculoskeletal system.[4] He may, for example, have detected the overall tension resulting from anxiety, or the solid, stiff feel of degenerative changes in the spine.[4] He will certainly have a detailed picture of spinal function, segment by segment, which he must be able to relate to the symptoms. Symptoms are traced back into the patient's life habits. A pain in the lower back, for example, may be related to such features as an inequality of leg length, an area of stiffness in the thorax, altered gait caused by new footwear, loss of the long arch of one or both feet, or pressure at work or at home. Thus the treatment prescription will be individual and will seek to restore the individual to a harmonious relationship with his or her environment in its broadest sense as well as secure a better level of physical function.

Treatment

The techniques open to osteopaths have been classified in many ways. One of the simplest is to divide them into direct and indirect techniques. The best known, especially in the United Kingdom, are the direct techniques.

Direct techniques

1. *Soft tissue techniques* suggest to the patient that he is being given a general massage but in fact only those tissues which need treatment are handled. Direction, amplitude, speed, and force are modified from moment to moment so that the practitioner almost appears to be enjoying a dialogue with the tissues under his hands. Soft tissue treatment may be a treatment in itself if the problem is confined

to the muscles, or may be a preliminary to another technique which requires prior relaxation of the muscles. One special technique is called neuromuscular technique (NMT). The osteopath searches the soft tissue with a probing thumb, looking for stress bands, or tense, fibrosed, or contracted locations.[5] The easing of the tensions can release physical knots, easing neighbouring joint problems. Tender 'trigger points' can also be massaged, which, like reflexology, can aid function of organs within the same reflex zone. It has to be remembered that owing to the inter-relationship of all tissues the osteopath may well treat a disc problem merely by using soft tissue techniques. The change in the soft tissues not only releases some pressure but creates a situation in which circulatory changes may occur, initiating healing.

2. *Articulatory techniques* involve the passive movement of joints. Techniques may be used to stretch or break down adhesions, stretch shortened ligaments, promote fluid movement, and exchange or treat muscles by stretching them. The osteopath is able to sense which tissue is restricting motion by the feel of the quality of the motion and the nature of its end-point. Again the essential feature is the impression of dialogue, one hand sensing the response in the tissues while the other provides the motive power and control. Springing is another form of articulation often used to provide shearing forces between joints which are not strictly speaking normal anatomical movements. It is often used on joints which normally have little active movement, for example sacro-iliac joints.[6]

3. *High velocity thrust techniques* are sudden movements, often followed by a crack or pop, which startle the patient although in skilled hands they are painless. These techniques can be applied to the spine or peripheral joints. Ironically they owe more to the traditional bonesetter than to the founder of osteopathy who did not use and indeed disparaged them. Occasionally the technique can be very successful in causing dramatic relief from spinal pain. However, it is often used uncritically by many osteopaths because the patients believe in it and expect it. It is not clear what the technique achieves in scientific terms although clinically there is often a dramatic reduction of muscle tension.

4. *Muscle energy techniques* evolved in the USA in the last 20 years. The patient supplies the motive power for these. The skill in this type of technique lies in the osteopath's sense of a barrier to motion. The joint is moved until a barrier is sensed. At this point the patient attempts to move the joint away from the barrier while the osteopath resists. The amount of power, the timing, and the patient's effort are all variables with therapeutic significance. The technique is fairly new to the UK but has been found valuable in certain acute cases, with nervous patients, or where thrust techniques may be contraindicated, for example, with elderly patients.

Indirect techniques

1. *Release techniques* also rely on a sense of barrier but here the patient is passive. The osteopath moves a joint to the point of barrier and then applies a small

extra force which is maintained. Frequently the osteopath becomes aware that the position is being maintained although the force has lessened, and relocates the boundary in its new position. On other occasions he becomes aware of the barrier slowly retreating to a new position. The technique is repeated until complete release has occurred or until it is judged that further release will not occur. This technique can also be used on soft tissue and organs, where accessible, in the abdominal and pelvic cavities.

2. *Functional techniques* were developed by Hoover, Bowles, and Johnston in the USA over the last 40 years.[7] Here the joint is moved, with the patient's co-operation, through ranges of flexion, extension, sidebending, rotation, forward/backward, and sideways movements. The osteopath assesses where the joint prefers to be with reference to the ease of motion. Again the sense of ease and barrier to motion is paramount. A composite is found for all ranges where the joint is in its most favoured position. The patient's breath is held at the point of maximal ease. The tissues are felt to change and the joint is checked for improved function in motion. These are subtle techniques requiring a different range of skills and again are of great value in acute cases, although they can also be used effectively in chronic cases. Like all the indirect techniques they are difficult to explain. No force is involved but a subtle positioning. Inevitably not all osteopaths are attracted to these techniques.

3. *Cranial techniques.* Even more difficult to rationalize are the techniques which owe their origin to William Garner Sutherland.[8] Sutherland postulated that the sutures of the human skull permit a small but essential degree of motion. Manual encouragement of this motion assists the circulation of cerebrospinal fluid. This could relieve local symptoms, and have more far-reaching effects, such as on pituitary function.[9] However, it is still a controversial technique, partly because holding a patient's head without apparently performing any active function smacks of faith healing and is as far from thrust techniques as any manual skill can possibly be. However, research relating symptomatology of the newborn and learning disabilities in children with diagnosed disturbances of cranial function[10] lends support to the protagonists of cranial techniques and although only some osteopaths are skilled in the technique at present, it is here to stay.

In an ideal situation all of these techniques would be taught at undergraduate level. One school is attempting this at present but the more conservative schools rely on the longer-established direct techniques, leaving postgraduate departments to provide opportunities for extending skills in indirect techniques.

Research and development

Most research has been carried out in the USA, beginning in the early part of this century. While it is inadequate by today's standards this early research yields some useful information: animal experiments suggested that vertebral lesions could affect the function of other tissues, and this has been occasionally confirmed in recent years,[11] although the mechanisms involved are unclear. One concept that was put forward in the 1950s was that tension in the musculoskeletal system affected nerves: at an osteopathic lesion there was an underlying alteration in neurological function: namely a facilitation of motor neurones.[12] Further research demonstrated that, with spinal defects, not only was motor function affected but the autonomic nervous system was also disturbed, leading to altered function in viscera and circulation. For example, animal studies have shown that strains of the vertebra result in changes in the structure of organs on the same embryological segment,[13] and it is well known that nerves act as channels, not only for electrical impulses, but also for substances needed by organs. However, the jump from such theories to practical outcomes is large, and as with chiropractic, it has been hard to demonstrate that osteopathic treatment can affect functional diseases. For example, spinal manipulation treatment does appear to aid gynaecological problems. A controlled study of spinal manipulation in women with dysmenorrhoea found a reduction in pain and discomfort in the pelvic area; another study found that soft tissue techniques were able to reduce pelvic pain, and also all other symptoms of menopause such as flushes, sweats, insomnia, etc., compared with placebo (that is false) manipulation.[14] However in both these cases, the role of placebo was significant and not entirely understood or accounted for. While gynaecological problems could be affected by relief of tension and restriction in the pelvic area, and might therefore be helped by massage and manipulative techniques, it would be harder to justify the osteopathic treatment of other chronic conditions such as asthma or ischaemic heart disease, and studies show that osteopathic treatment might make patients feel a bit better subjectively, but did not affect the course of the disease.[15] Like chiropractors, osteopaths have also stepped back from claiming to treat functional disorders, concentrating instead on specialist proficiency in the area of musculoskeletal problems, and offering adjunctive help where deeper disease creates musculoskeletal symptomatology.

There has been considerable clinical research on manipulation, and its role in musculoskeletal problems is now proven.[16] For reference to this work, see Chapter 9. Little attempt has been made to compare different forms of manipulative treatment in controlled studies. Until this is done, one can only conclude that the positive evidence to date applies equally to osteopathy, chiropractic, and other forms of manipulation. Controlled studies specifically on osteopathic manipulation have been carried out, and generally show equivalent results to other methods.[17] In addition, some gentle soft tissue techniques, which are the special province of osteopathy as opposed to chiropractic and medical manipulation, have shown some interesting positive results in special cases, such as after stokes.[18] However, it is extremely difficult to carry out trials in this area, not only because of the power of placebo, and impossibility of double blinding, but also because different osteopaths have various concepts of a patient's problem, and thus treatment will vary.[19] Thus one osteopath sees his findings in terms of altered positional relationships, another in terms of mobility, another in terms of muscle tones, another in terms of involuntary function, and so on. That makes it difficult to obtain clear results, and negative as well as positive findings become suspect.[20]

There is general agreement that one needs large scale, well-conducted trials to obtain clear results, and these have been lacking in osteopathy. Research so far has however helped to identify those for whom osteopathy will have best effect. These are patients whose musculoskeletal problems are of longer duration and those who go to an osteopath soon after the problem has occurred.[3,17] The advantage to patients is most discernable between 1 and 2 weeks after treatment, and is reduced thereafter.

Treatment almost invariably involves undressing down to underclothes. Gowns which tie up at the back allowing for complete exposure of the spine may be provided. For a first visit a patient may be required to attend for anything from 30 to 60 minutes while a subsequent treatment session may be 10 to 40 minutes, depending upon the osteopath and the type of problem. Courses of treatment may be just one session or extend over many months. The trained osteopath will always discuss the prognosis and the likely length and cost of treatment. There is occasionally some discomfort after treatment for a day or two. More severe reactions occur only very rarely, and have been well documented. The risks are very low.[21] In such instances the patient should always return to the osteopath who treated him as severe reactions can usually be quickly modified. Osteopathy is suitable for any musculoskeletal or joint problems, including rheumatic problems, sports injuries, etc.[22] Osteopathy in America today is very different to that of the UK and Europe, which may cause some confusion. American osteopathy is a medical speciality rather than a natural alternative to modern medicine.[23]

References

1. Still, A. T. (1910). *Osteopathy—research and practice*. Privately published, A. T. Still, Missouri.
2. Hall, T. E. and Wernham, J. (1978). *The contribution of John Martin Littlejohn to osteopathy*. Maidstone Osteopathic Clinic, Maidstone, Kent.
3. Burton, A. K. (1981). Back pain in osteopathic practice. *Rheumatology and Rehabilitation*, 20, 239–46. Pringle, M. and Tyreman, S. (1993). Study of 500 patients attending an osteopathic practice. *British Journal of General Practice*, 43, 15–18.
4. Chaitow, L. (1995). Learning how to assess postural muscles. *Journal of Alternative and Complementary Medicine*, 13, 11–14. Chaitow, L. (1991). *Palpatory literacy*. Thorsons, Harper Collins, London.
5. Chaitow, L. (1991). *Soft tissue manipulation*. Healing Arts Press, Rochester, Vermont. McKechnie, A. A., Wilson, F., Watson, N., and Scott, D. (1983). Anxiety states: a preliminary report on the value of connective tissue massage. *Journal of Psychosomatic Research*, 27, 125–9.
6. Lewit, K. (1992). *Manipulative therapy in rehabilitation of the locomotor system*. Butterworth Heinemann, London.
7. Johnston, W. L. (1966). Manipulative skills. *Journal of the American Osteopathic Association*, 66, 389–407. Shekelle, P. G. (1994). Spinal manipulation. *Spine*, 19, 85–7.
8. Upledger, J. and Vredevoord, J. (1983). *Craniosacral therapy*. Eastland Press, Chicago. Holmes, P. (1991). Cranial osteopathy. *Nursing Times*, 87, 36–7.
9. White, W. (1985). The relation of the craniofacial bones to specific somatic dysfunction:

a clinical study of the effects of manipulation. *Journal of the American Osteopathic Association*, **85**, 603–4.

10. Upledger, J. E. (1978). The relationship of craniosacral examination findings in grade school children with developmental problems. *Journal of the American Osteopathic Association*, 77, 640–69. Page, J. (1994). Why teach massage therapists to treat the craniosacral system? *Journal of Alternative and Complementary Medicine*, 12, 18–19.

11. Nicholas, A. *et al.* (1987). A somatic component to myocardial infarction. *Journal of the Americal Osteopathic Association*, 87, 123–9.

12. Denslow, J. S., Korr, I. M., and Krems, A. D. (1947). Quantitative studies of chronic facilitation in human motoneuron pools. *American Journal of Physiology*, 150, 229–38.

13. Korr, I. M., Wright, H. M., and Chace, J. A. (1964). Cutaneous patterns of sympathetic activity in clinical abnormalities of the musculoskeletal system. *Acta Neurovegetativa*, 25, 589–606. Korr, I. M. (1980). *The neurobiologic mechanisms in manipulative therapy*. Plenum, New York.

14. Kokjohn, K., Schmid, D. M., Triano, J. J., and Brennan, P. C. (1992). The effect of spinal manipulation on pain and prostaglandin levels in women with primary dysmenorrhea. *Journal of Manipulative and Physiological Therapeutics*, 15, 279–85. Cleary, C. and Fox, J. P. (1994). Menopausal symptoms: an osteopathic investigation. *Complementary Therapies in Medicine*, 2, 181–6.

15. Allen, T. W. and D'Alonzo, G. E. (1993). Investigating the role of osteopathic manipulation in the treatment of asthma. *Journal of the American Osteopathic Association*, 93, 654–9.

16. Koes, B. W., Assendelft, W. J. J., van der Heijden, G. J. M. G., Bouter, L. M., and Knipschild, P. G. (1991). Spinal manipulation and mobilisation for back and neck pain: a blinded review. *British Medical Journal*, 303, 1298–303.

17. Macdonald, R. S. and Bell, C. M. J. (1990). An open controlled assessment of osteopathic manipulation in nonspecific low-back pain. *Spine*, 15, 364–70. Cummings, M. (1986). Evaluation of changes associated with osteopathic treatment of the lumbosacral region: a pilot study. *Complementary Medicine*, 3, 10–12. Burton, A. K. (1986). Osteopathy in back trouble. *British Medical Journal*, 293, 1482.

18. Magnusson, M. *et al.* (1994). Sensory stimulation promotes normalization of postural control after stroke. *Stroke*, 25, 1176–80.

19. Fitzgerald, G. *et al.* (1994). Issues in determining treatment effectiveness of manual therapy. *Physical Therapy*, 74, 227–33.

20. Gibson, T., Grahame, R., Harkness, J., Woo, P., Blagrave, P., and Hills, R. (1985). Controlled comparison of short-wave diathermy treatment with osteopathic treatment in non-specific low back pain. *Lancet*, 1, 1258–61.

21. Sinel, M. and Smith, D. (1993). Thalamic infarction secondary to cervical manipulation. *Archives of Physical Medicine and Rehabilitation*, 74, 543–6.

22. Moule, T. G. (1980). Sports injuries: how osteopathy can help. *Nursing*, 4, 163–5.

23. Meyer, C. T. and Price, A. (1993). Osteopathic medicine: call for reform. *Journal of the American Osteopathic Association*, 4, 473–85.

20

Radionics and psionic medicine

Background

Radionics has been defined as a method of diagnosis and treatment at a distance, through the medium of an instrument, using what is known as the radiesthetic faculty, which is a form of extrasensory perception.

Radionics as a healing art emerged from the pioneering work and discoveries of the distinguished American physician Dr Albert Abrams, who was born in San Francisco in 1863. Something of a prodigy, Abrams completed his medical studies at such an early age that his degree could not be issued. He later became Professor of Pathology and Director of the Cooper Medical College of Stanford University, California. He wrote several successful medical textbooks and eventually won for himself a national reputation as a specialist in diseases of the nervous system.

At the beginning of this century Abrams made a strange discovery. In the course of a routine examination of a middle-aged male patient, who had a small cancerous growth on his lip, Abrams discovered that during the process of percussing the abdomen of the patient, the resonance of the note given off changed when the man faced west, and this in a very specific area above the navel. Abrams' curiosity was aroused and he went on to check a whole series of patients with cancer, all of whom without exception gave the same reaction. He then decided to check patients with other identifiable diseases, and found, for example, that those with tuberculosis exhibited the same repeatable phenomena, this time below the navel. Considering this to be an electromagnetic phenomenon, Abrams devised a box containing resistors, and by using this he found that he could measure the disease reactions in ohms, thus distinguishing one disease from another. He found that carcinoma reacted at 50 ohms, syphilis at 20, tuberculosis at 15 and so forth. In Abrams' next experiment he placed a dried spot of blood from a patient in the box, and found that he could diagnose very accurately what was wrong with the patient who had donated the blood spot.

When Abrams announced this procedure and his theories about it, there was quite naturally a very hostile response from the orthodoxy of the day. It was only in 1924, the year of Abrams' death, that a concerted effort was made to test his methods. A medical committee under the chairmanship of Sir Thomas Horder ran a series of tests under controlled conditions. The results proved an overwhelming vindication of Abrams, to the astonishment of the distinguished medical men involved.[1] In the 1930s Ruth Drown, a chiropractor who practised in Hollywood, California, developed new approaches to radionics and new instrumentation. Her work was to attract many chiropractors and osteopaths into this field and was seen as a pioneering effort to establish a new form of medicine, one that employed subtle healing energies as opposed to drugs and surgical procedures.

Following the Second World War the engineer George de la Warr set up laboratories in Oxford, thus beginning a new phase of growth from which emerged new instruments based on the same principles as Drown's. There can be no doubt that the fertile minds of George de la Warr and his assistants fostered a whole new era of radionic development, the 1950s being one of the most intensive periods of organized research in the radionic field. The bulk, if not virtually all the work, was carried out at Oxford.

Fundamental concepts

Basic to radionic theory and practice is the concept that all life forms, including man, are submerged in and interpenetrated by a common field of energy. At the lowest level this field registers as the electromagnetic spectrum but there are many levels or planes of energy which cannot be measured by scientific instrumentation, and which lie beyond the electromagnetic field. Any distortion in the life-field of an individual eventually registers as physical or psychological pathology.

Early radionic practitioners diagnosed and treated in medical and clinical terms. Today most practitioners have adopted a model of the body directly drawn from theosophical and Eastern teachings, such concepts fitting in more easily with the energetic view of man. They see man as being comprised of a totality of spirit, soul, and form, the latter being made up of the physical body, the etheric body (more recently referred to by some scientists as the bioplasmic body), the emotional body, and the mental body. The four-fold form is that aspect of man wherein disease manifests itself, and it is to these bodies that the practitioner directs healing energies through specific instrumentation.[2]

This model of man lends itself readily to modern radionic practice, because practitioners since Drown have diagnosed and treated at a distance. Drown discovered that it was not necessary for a patient to be present for purposes of diagnosis or treatment, due to the fact that the human mind, through the energy field in which it was immersed, could connect with the patient no matter where he or she was. She posited that a beam of energy literally connected practitioner and patient, and that along this beam information could be derived relevant to the patient's health; similarly energy for treatment purposes could be 'broadcast' to the distant patient, the blood spot on the instrument acting as a link.

Ruth Drown created a whole series of rates or numbers representing the parts of the human body, and of man's known diseases. Each body-part rate and each disease rate is in effect the vibrational identification pattern of that particular object. While in practice the method worked, her theories can be seen to be a conglomeration of beliefs derived from radio waves and metaphysics. These beliefs have been promulgated over the years, and certainly none of them stand up to scientific examination. There is no evidence to support the concept that some form of physical radiation generated by the rates set up on the instrument goes out or is broadcast from the set to the patient at a distance. Despite the view of Abrams, it is likely that the instruments, although useful as a focus for the mind of the practitioner, do not in themselves have any intrinsic value beyond the fact that they can be used to objectify a process going on at etheric levels. Mind connects the practitioner to the patient, and initiates the treatment process. Radionics is in fact a form of spiritual healing. When a practitioner tunes in to the patient, he literally brings that patient 'to mind' and on that plane of consciousness distance does not exist.

At this level the very act of making a diagnosis has a therapeutic impact upon the patient. This healing effect brought about by the diagnostic process has often been made clear to practitioners, by patients who telephone to exclaim how well they are feeling—and this before treatment in the accepted sense of the word has begun. There are cases where pain had been intractable for weeks, but cleared at the time the diagnosis was made, without the patient having any conscious knowledge of the work being done. Of course no practitioner should ever make a radionic analysis on an individual without his express permission; to do so is psychically to invade that patient, perhaps against his will. The only exceptions are in those cases of terminal illness where the patient cannot make his wishes known, and for children, where signed permission is given by the parents.

Diagnostic and therapeutic practices

The primary aim of all radionic diagnosis and treatment at a distance is to identify fundamental causes of disease and to set energies in motion which will eliminate these causes at their very root. In order to do this the practitioner employs a radionic diagnostic instrument.

The instrument usually takes the form of a box covered by a panel. On the panel is a set of dials. There is normally a circular metal plate upon which the patient's 'witness' is placed (the 'witness' is either a blood spot or a small snippet of hair). This is said to provide the link between the practitioner, instrument, and the patient at a distance. One method of diagnosis takes a specific symptom, and subsequently places the rate or numerical value for that symptom on the appropriate dials of the instrument. The practitioner, having tuned his mind to the patient, asks a series of questions to determine which body systems are involved in the symptom. The responses to these mentally posed questions are externalized in two ways, depending upon which method the practitioner uses. If he uses a pendulum, for he is literally dowsing for disease, then the pendulum will swing, as a rule, from a simple oscillation to a clockwise movement to give a 'yes'.

If a stick pad is built into the instrument, consisting of a rubber diaphragm over a rectangular metal plate, then the practitioner's fingers will literally stick to the pad instead of sliding easily across it as he mentally asks questions, giving a 'yes' in this way. Having pinpointed the exact areas of the body, the practitioner then proceeds to find out precisely what the causative agent is that is creating the disease. For example, with headaches, a practitioner may find that there are residual toxins from measles located in the meninges of the brain. These toxins, similar to the homeopath's 'miasms', may have been left over from when the patient contracted the disease as a child or they may have come from a vaccination against the disease. In any event such toxins could not be identified by orthodox clinical means, and it is here especially that radionics in identifying these residual toxins, may have a role to play. Information is available to the properly trained sensitive mind that cannot be determined by, or derived from, ordinary procedures.

Some practitioners also analyse the states of the *chakras* to see if they are overactive, underactive, or normally active. *Chakras*, according to Eastern philosophy, are a series of major force centres which lie along the cerebral spinal axis. They can be regarded as the points at which energy flows into the human system and maintains the integrity of the physical form by way of the etheric body. As such they provide a deep level at which treatment can occur.

The analysis of the patient can be extended beyond the *chakras* to include the quality and characteristics of the energies of the transpersonal self, the mental, emotional, and etheric/physical bodies, and those of the personality as a whole. When all of the imbalances in the various bodies and their energy systems have been identified and measured for intensity, and the cause or causes similarly dealt with, then the practitioner is ready to determine what form of treatment is needed to remove the causes of disease within the patient.

Radionic treatment is determined by placing the patient witness on the detector plate of the instrument or upon a treatment chart, and asking a series of mentally posed questions. The main idea is to find the correct, and thus the most effective, form of treatment to remove those causes of disease which have been identified in the analysis. Some practitioners may then put a phial of an appropriate homeopathic remedy, such as *Morbillinum* or *Aconite*, on the plate next to the patient witness, with the intention of modifying the energy directed to the patient in such a way as to speed up his response and clear, for example, the measles virus, more quickly.[3]

Treatment with instruments employing geometric cards provides a more versatile approach. For example three cards may be used to set up a treatment. For the measles virus in the meninges, a card for *Morbillinum* is placed in the first slot, in the second a card for the crown *chakra*, and in the third a card representing the meninges. In this way a flow of energy is symbolized; the healing remedy is placed into and through the crown *chakra* which governs the brain and from there to the meninges. Many practitioners use colour as a therapeutic agent in their practices and this can be 'broadcast' in the same way that homeopathic remedies are. Often remedies such as the biochemic tissue salts, Bach flower remedies, homeopathic medicines, or vitamins and minerals where indicated, are recommended to the patient to be taken orally as an adjunct to his radionic treatment. If other forms of treatment, such as allopathic, manipulation, or acupuncture are indicated, then the practitioner advises the patient accordingly. Diet too is taken into account, particularly in those cases where allergies have been identified.[4]

Applications and contra-indications

Radionics can be employed in the treatment of any form of disease; there do not appear to be any contra-indications at all. By its very nature it can be used whilst other forms of therapy are being applied without in any way interfering with the healing processes they are designed to initiate. Like psychic healing, radionics has been found to be particularly effective in terminal illness, especially in reducing pain and engendering in the patient a realistic, calm, and relaxed attitude towards his illness and its subsequent outcome.

Like most therapies it enjoys an average rate of success. Having the advantage of being able to determine the presence of deeply hidden causes, it gets good long-term results with chronic cases that have not responded to other forms of therapy. Radionics has an application in dentistry[5] and is also employed in the field of agriculture, increasing crop yields and body weight of stock. Animals respond very well to radionic treatment and some practitioners treat animals only.

Research and development

Radionics practitioners have not attempted to apply rigorous scientific tests to their work which would be hard to do. There is no such data published. Published studies have instead focused on patterns emerging from practice, with the intention of improving radionic skills. For example it has been observed that some children have exactly the same set of over- and underactive chakras as the mother, if during pregnancy the mother was highly tensed and subject to a great deal of stress. Radionics, as a form of healing and dowsing, will obviously benefit from research demonstrating parapsychological phenomena in general. Some intriguing studies on dowsing, for example, have indicated that muscles might be able to respond sensitively to magnetic fields by virtue of crystals of magnetite buried in the tissues.[6] (See also Chapter 12.)

Obtaining treatment

As with any form of therapy it is always best to seek out a fully trained and qualified practitioner. The UK is the centre of radionics in the world today and information about practitioners is readily available from the relevant organizations. Having decided upon a practitioner the patient fills in a case history sheet giving his past medical history and present problem, and returns this to the practitioner together with signed permission for investigation and a small snippet of hair. When the analysis has been completed the practitioner sends a report of findings to the patient. At this point, if the practitioner and patient have not met or spoken to each other, it is not a bad idea to make such a contact. Often practitioners never see or speak to patients, especially those who live far away. In these cases the whole process of contact can be carried out through correspondence, which is satisfactory provided the channels of communication are kept alive by means of a monthly report from the patient and appropriate responses from the practitioner.

Psionic medicine

Psionic medicine is a composite diagnosis and treatment method involving basically similar concepts and practices to those of radionics. It was developed in the UK by Dr Gorge Laurence. He developed an energetic theory of the origin of disease that owes much to MacDonagh's unitary theory of disease, as well as to the teachings of Rudolf Steiner. He sees the source of many chronic diseases as miasms or vestiges of previous acute conditions, and treats homeopathically. Diagnosis and treatment are selected largely by pendulum. Psionic medicine is practised mostly by GPs, and therefore it is sometimes combined with conventional medicine.[7]

References

1. Horder, T. (1925). The electronic reactions of Abrams. *British Medical Journal*, 1, 179–85.
2. Wilcox, J. (1976). Radionics. *Nursing Times*, 72, 568–70.
3. Silver, S. (1978). The radionic phenomenon, treatment at a distance. *MIMS Magazine*, 2, 377.
4. Westlake, T. (1973). *The pattern of health: a search for a greater understanding of the life force in health and disease*. Shambhala, Colorado.
5. Upton, C. (1980). Psionic medicine in dentistry. *Probe*, 22, 9–11.
6. Williamson, T. (1987). A sense of direction for dowsers. *New Scientist*, **19 March 1987**, 40–3.
7. Reyner, J. H., Laurence, G., and Upton, C. (1980). *Psionic medicine*. Routledge and Kegan Paul, London.

Bibliography

Complementary and holistic medicine—general

Albery, N., Elliot, G., and Elliot, J. (1994). *The natural death handbook*.

British Medical Association (1993). *Complementary medicine: new approaches to good practice*. Oxford University Press, Oxford.

Budd, S. and Sharma, U. (1994). *The healing bond. The patient-practitioner relationship and therapeutic responsibility*. Routledge, London.

Chopra, D. (1990). *Quantum healing: exploring the frontiers of mind/body medicine*. Bantam, New York.

Dossey, L. (1982). *Space, time and medicine*. Routledge & Kegan Paul, London. (A seminal philosophy of medicine, bringing it up to date with the new discoveries in physics.)

Foulkes, J. (1991). *Complementary medicine careers handbook*. Hodder & Stoughton, London.

French, S. (1993). *Practical research – a guide for therapists*. Butterworth-Heinemann, Oxford.

Guirdham, A. (1957). *A theory of disease*. Neville Spearman, London. (A classical pioneering philosophical discourse)

Hastings, A.C. (eds.) (1981). *Health for the whole person*. Westview Press, Boulder, Colorado. (Highly recommended)

Hill, R. and Gould, A. (1996). *Complementary medicine: its practice in the health service*, submitted.

Inglis, B. (1978). *Natural medicine*. Collins, London. (Highly recommended)

Inglis, B. and West, R. (1983). *The alternative health guide*. Michael Joseph, London. (Good popular guide)

Johannessen, H., Launso, L., Olesen, S.G., and Staugard, F. (ed.) (1994). *Studies in alternative therapy I. Contributions from Nordic countries*. Odense University Press, Odense, Denmark.

Johannessen, H. et al. (eds.) (1995). *Studies in alternative therapy. II. Bodies and nature in alternative medicine*. Odense University Press, Odense, Denmark.

Keegan, L. (1994). *The nurse as healer*. Delmar, New York.

Kenyon, J. (1986). *21st Century medicine: a layman's guide to the medicine of the future*. Thorsons, Wellingborough.

Leibrich, J., Hickling, J. and Pitt, G. (1987). *In search of well-being. Exploratory research into complementary therapies*. Health Services Research and Development Unit, Department of Health, Wellington, New Zealand.

Lewith, G.T. (ed.) (1985). *Alternative therapies. A guide to complementary medicine for the health professional*. Heinemann, London.

Lewith, G. and Aldridge, D. (1991). *Complementary medicine in the European community*. C.W. Daniel, Saffron Walden, Essex.

Lewith, G. and Aldridge, D. (ed.) (1993). *Clinical research methodology for complementary therapies*. Hodder & Stoughton, London.

Lowenberg, J.S. (1989). *Caring and responsibility: crossroads of holistic practice and traditional medicine*. University of Pennsylvania Press, Philadelphia.

Lewith, G., Kenyon, J., and Lewis, P. (1996). *Complementary medicine: an integrated approach*. Oxford University Press, Oxford.

Mintel (1993). *Alternative medicines: Mintel market intelligence report*. Mintel, 18 Long Lane, London EC1A 9HE.

Nesse, R. M. and Williams, G.C. (1994). *Why we get sick. The new science of Darwinian medicine*. Times Books, New York.

Olsen, C. (1992). *The encyclopaedia of alternative medicine*. Piatkus, London.

Oscar, J. and Goldberg, P. (1993). *A different kind of healing. Doctors speak candidly of their successes with alternative medicine*. Putnam, New York.

Pelletier, K.R. (1979). *Holistic medicine; from stress to optimum health*. Delta, N.Y.

Pietroni, P. (1990). *The greening of medicine*. Gollancz, London.

Rankin-Box, D. (1995). *The nurses' handbook of complementary therapies*. Churchill Livingstone, Edinburgh.

Reason, P. and Rowan, J. (ed.) (1981). *Human inquiry: a sourcebook of new paradigm research*. Wiley, Chichester.

Richman, J. (1987). *Medicine and health*. Longman, London.

Salmon, J.W. (ed.) (1985). *Alternative medicines: popular and policy perspectives*. Tavistock, London and New York. (First sociological text)

Saks, M. (1992). *Alternative medicine in Britain*. Oxford University Press, Oxford.

Sharma, U. (1995). *Complementary medicine today: practitioners and patients*. Routledge, London.

Sobel, D. (1979). *Ways of health: holistic approaches in ancient and contemporary medicine*. Viking, New York.

Stanway, A. (1994). *Alternative medicine: guide to natural therapies*. Penguin, Harmondsworth, Middlesex.

Strohecher, J. (ed.) (1994). *Alternative medicine*. Future Medicine Publishing, Puyallyup, Washington.

Thomson, R. (1989). *Loving medicine; patients experiences of personal transformation through the holistic treatment of cancer*. Gateway, UK.

Trevelyan, J. and Booth, B. (1994). *Complementary medicine for nurses, midwives and health visitors*. Macmillan, London.

Vickers, A. (1993). *Complementary medicine and disability: alternatives for people with disabling conditions*. Chapman & Hall, London.

Watt, J. (ed.) (1988). *Talking health. Conventional and complementary approaches*. Royal Society of Medicine, London.

Weil, A. (1991). *Health and healing: understanding conventional and alternative medicine*. Houghton Mifflin, Boston, Massachusetts.

Weil, A. (1995). *Spontaneous healing*. Alfred Knopf, New York.

Weil, A. (1990). *Natural health, natural medicine*. Houghton Mifflin, Boston, Massachusetts.

Werbach, M.R. (1986). *Third line medicine*. Routledge, London.

Critiques of conventional medicine

Adams, P. and Mylander, M. (1993). *Gesundheit!* Healing Arts Press, Rochester, Vermont.

Banit, E., Courtenay, M., Edler, A., Hull, S., and Julian, P. (1993). *The doctor, the patient and the group*. Routledge, London.

Carlson, R.J. (1975). *The end of medicine*. Wiley—Interscience, New York. (Pioneering work)

Carter, J.P. (1993). *Racketeering in medicine. The suppression of alternatives*. Hampton Roads Press, Norfolk, Virginia.

Dossey, L. (1992). *Meaning and medicine*. Bantam, New York.

Dubos, Rene (1968). *Man, medicine and environment*. Praeger, New York.

Fulder, S. (1995). *How to survive medical treatment*. C.W. Daniel, Saffron Walden, Essex.

Gape, J., Kelleher, D., and Williams, G. (1994). *Challenging medicine*. Routledge, London.

Gould, D. (1985). *The Black and White Medicine Show*. Hamish Hamilton, London.

Howe, G.M. (1977). *Man, environment and disease in Britain*. Pelican Books, Harmondsworth, Middlesex. (Invaluable statistical and historical review)

Illich, I. (1977). *Medical nemesis: The expropriation of health*. Bantam, New York. (Highly recommended)

Inglis, B. (1981). *Diseases of civilisation*. Hodder & Stoughton, London.

Karpf, A. (1988). *Doctoring the media*. Routledge, London.

Lafaille, R. and Fulder, S. (eds.) (1933). *Towards a new science of health*. Routledge, London.

Lock, M. and Gordon, D. (eds.) (1988). *Biomedicine examined*. Kluwer, Dordrecht, The Netherlands.

McKeown, T. (1979). *The role of medicine: dream, mirage or nemesis*. Rock Carling Memorial Lecture, Blackwells, Oxford.

Needleman, J. (1992). *The way of the physician*. Viking Arkana, London.

Mellville, A. and Johnson, C. (1982). *Cured to death, the effect of prescription drugs*. Secker & Warburg, London.

Richards, D. (1982). *The topic of cancer. When the killing has to stop*. Pergamon Press, Oxford and New York. (A strong case, by a scientist, against radical treatment of cancer.)

Rose, G. (1992). *The strategy of preventive medicine*. Oxford Medical Publications, Oxford.

Seale, C. and Pattison, S. (1994). *Medical knowledge: doubt and certainty*. Open University Press, Milton Keynes. Bowling, A. (1991). *Measuring health. A review of quality of life measurement scale*. Open University Press, Milton Keynes.

Walton, J., Barondess, J.A., and Lock, S. (1994). *The Oxford medical companion*. Oxford Medical Publications, Oxford.

Weitz, M. (1980). *Health shock: how to avoid ineffective and hazardous medical treatment*. Prentice-Hall, Englewood Cliffs, NJ; David and Charles, London.

Weir, A. (ed.) (1992). *Medicine in society*. Cambridge University Press, Cambridge.

History

Berman, M. (1990). *Coming to our senses: body and spirit in the hidden history of the West*. Unwin, London.

Bynum, W.F. and Porter, R. (eds.) (1993). *Companion encyclopedia of the history of medicine*. Routledge, London.

French, R. and Weir, A. (1989). *The medical revolution of the seventeenth century*. Cambridge University Press, Cambridge.

Gauld, A. (1992). *A history of hypnotism.* Cambridge University Press, Cambridge.

Griggs, B. (1988). *Green pharmacy.* Healing Arts Press, Rochester, Vermont.

Grossinger, R. (1980). *Planet medicine.* Shambhala, Colorado.

Hoizey, D. and Hoizey, M-J. (eds.) (1993). *History of Chinese medicine.* Churchill Livingstone, Edinburgh.

Inglis, B. (1979). *A history of medicine.* Fontana/Collins, London.

Siraisi, N. (1990). *Medieval and early Renaissance medicine. An introduction to knowledge and practice.* University of Chicago Press, Chicago, Illinois.

Smolan, R., Moffitt, P., and Naythons, M. (1992). *The power to heal: ancient arts and modern medicine.* Simon & Schuster, New York.

Cultural and traditional medicine

Bannerman, R.H., Burton, J., and Wen-Chieh, C. (1983). *Traditional medicine and health care coverage.* WHO, Geneva.

CIBA Foundation (1977). *Health and disease in tribal societies.* CIBA Symposium No. 49. Elsevier, Excerpta Medica, Amsterdam.

Foster, G.M. (1984). *Medical anthropology.* Wiley, New York.

Hakim, C. (1988). *The traditional healers' handbook.* Healing Arts, Rochester, Vermont.

Harner, M. (1990). *The way of the shaman.* Harper & Row, New York.

Helman, C. G. (1994). *Culture, health and illness: an introduction for health professionals.* Butterworth—Heinemann, Oxford.

Helman, C. (1985). *Culture, health and illness.* Wright, Bristol.

Hillier, S.M. and Jewell, J.A. (1984). *Health care and traditional medicine in China.* Routledge & Kegan Paul, London.

Hunan (Province) Revolutionary Health Committee. *A barefoot doctor's manual.* Routledge & Kegan Paul, London.

Landy, D. (ed.) (1977). *Culture, disease and healing: Studies in medical anthropology.* Macmillan, New York.

Lebra, W.P. (1976). *Culture-bound syndromes, ethnopsychiatry and alternative therapies.* Hawai University Press, Honolulu.

Lesley, C. and Young, A. (1992). *Paths to Asian medical knowledge.* University of California Press, Los Angeles.

Lupton, P. (1994). *Medicine as culture.* Sage, London.

McGuire, M. (1988). *Ritual healing in suburban America.* Rutgers University Press, Rutgers, California.

Maclean, U. (1971). *Magical medicine; a Nigerian case-study.* Penguin, Harmondsworth, Middlesex.

Phillips, D.R. and Verhasselt, Y. (1994). *Health and development.* Routledge, London.

Radley, A. (1995). *World of illness: biographical and cultural perspectives on health and disease.* Routledge, London.

World Health Organization, (1988). *Traditional medicine.* World Health Organization, Geneva.

Self-care (see also Mind–body and Naturopathy)

Benjamin, H. (1983). *Everybody's guide to nature cure.* Thorsons, Wellingborough.

Brewer, S. (1995). *The complete book of men's health.* Thorsons, Harper Collins, London.

Bricklin, M. (1990). *The practical encyclopedia of natural healing*. Rodale Press, Emmaus, Pennsylvania.

British Medical Association (1994). *Medicine and drugs*. Dorling Kindersley. London.

Brook, D. (1984). *Naturebirth: you, your body and your baby*. Penguin, Harmondsworth, Middlesex.

Brostoff, J. and Gamlin, L. (1989). *The complete guide to food allergy and intolerance*. Bloomsbury, London.

Chaitow. L. (1990). *Osteopathic self-treatment*. Thorsons, Harper Collins, London.

Christie, J. (1992). *Food for vitality*. Bantam, New York.

Curtis, S. and Fraser, R. (1994). *Natural healing for women*. Pandora Press, London.

Drake, K. and Drake, J. (1984). *Natural birth control*. Thorsons, Harper Collins, London.

Dries, J. (1995). *The new book of food combining*. Element, Shaftesbury. Wellingborough.

Forbes, A. (1976). *Try being healthy*. Health Science Press, Holsworthy. (Highly recommended)

Fulder, S. (1983). *An end to ageing?* Thorsons, Harper Collins, London.

Fulder, S. (1994). *How to survive medical treatment. A holistic guide to avoiding the risks and side effects of conventional medicine*. Daniel, Saffron Walden, Essex.

Grant, B. (1992). *An A—Z of natural healthcare*. Optima, London.

Halvorsen, B. (1987). *The natural dentist*. Century Arrow, London.

Inglis, B. and West, R. (1983). *The alternative health guide*. Michael Joseph, London.

Kenton, L. (1993). *Nature's child*. Ebury, London.

Kenton, L. (1995). *The new joy of beauty. The complete guide to lasting energy and good looks*. Vermillion, London.

Kenyon, J. (1992). *Acupressure techniques: a self-help guide*. Thorsons, Harper Collins, London.

Lockie, A. (1994). *The family guide to homeopathy*. Hamish Hamilton, London.

Lockie, A. (1995). *The complete guide to homeopathy*. Dorling Kindersley, London.

McIntyre, A. (1992). *Herbs for common ailments*. Gaia, Stroud, Gloucestershire.

McIntyre, A. (1994). *The complete woman's herbal*. Gaia Books, Stroud, Gloucestershire.

Mayes, A. (1991). *The A—Z of nutritional health*. Thorsons, Harper Collins, London.

Monte, T. (ed.) (1993). *World medicine—the East West guide to healing your body*. Jeremy Tarcher, Los Angeles.

Null, G. (1984). *The complete guide to health and nutrition*. Arlington, London.

Odent, M. (1994). *Birth reborn*. Souvenir, London.

O'Neill, B. and Phillips, R. (1985). *Biorhythms: how to live with your life cycles*. Signet, New York.

Polunin, M. and Robbins, C. (1992). *The natural pharmacy*. Dorling Kindersley, London.

Reid, D. (1995). *The complete book of Chinese health and healing*. Shambala, Boston, Massachusetts.

Schneider, M. and Larkin, M. (1994) *The handbook of self-healing*. Viking Arkana, London.

Shealy, C.N. (1993). *The self-healing workbook*. Element, Shaftesbury.

Smyth, A. (1994). *Gentle medicine. Thorsons' concise encyclopaedia of natural health*. Thorsons, Harper Collins, London.

Speight, L. (1992). *Homeopathy, a home prescriber*. C.W. Daniel, Saffron Walden, Essex.

Tiran, D. and Mark, S. (1994). *Complementary therapies for pregnancy and childbirth*. Ballière, London.

Weller, S. (1994). *The yoga back book*. Thorsons, Harper Collins, London.

Acupuncture

Auteroche, B., Gervais, G., Auteroche, M., Navailh, P., and Toui-Kan, E. (1992). *Acupuncture and moxibustion: a guide to clinical practice*. Churchill Livingstone, Edinburgh.

Beinfield, B. and Korngold, H. (1991). *Between heaven and earth: a guide to Chinese medicine*. Ballantine, New York.

Bensky, D. (1993). *Chinese herbal medicine—formulas and strategies*. Eastland Press, Seattle.

Bensoussan, A. (1991). *The vital meridian. A modern exploration of acupuncture*. Churchill Livingstone, Edinburgh.

Campbell, A. (1987). *Acupuncture: the modern scientific approach*. Faber & Faber, London.

Clifford, T. (1993). *Tibetan Buddhist medicine and psychiatry*. Snow Lion Press, Ithaca, New York.

Dummer, T. (1995). *Tibetan medicine and other health-care systems*. Snow Lion Press, Ithaca, New York.

Eisenberg, D. (1985). *Encounters with Qi. Exploring Chinese medicine*. Penguin, Harmondsworth.

Farquhar, J. (1994). *Knowing practice: the clinical encounter in Chinese medicine*. Westview, Oxford; Boulder, Colorado.

Fibrace, P. and Hill, S. (1994). *A guide to acupuncture*. Constable, London.

Gach, M.R. (1992). *Acupressure: how to cure common ailments the natural way*. Piatkus Books, London.

Ji-Lin, L. (1995). *Diet therapy in traditional Chinese medicine*. Churchill Livingstone, Edinburgh.

Kaptchuck, T. (1990). *Chinese medicine: the web that has no weaver*. Rider, London.

Kenyon, J.N. (1985). *Modern techniques of acupuncture: practical guide to electroacupuncture*. Thorsons, Wellingborough.

Lewith, G.T. (1992). *Acupuncture: its place in Western medical science*. Thorsons, Harper Collins, London.

Lewith, G.T. and Lewith, N.R. (1994). *Modern Chinese acupuncture*. Green Print, London.

Macdonald, A. (1984). *Acupuncture from ancient art to modern medicine*.

Maciocia, G. (1989). *The foundations of Chinese medicine*. Churchill Livingstone, Edinburgh. Unwin, London.

Maciocia, G. (1994). *The practice of Chinese medicine: the treatment of disease with acupuncture and Chinese herbs*. Churchill Livingstone, Edinburgh.

Mann, F. (1982). *The treatment of disease by acupuncture*. Part 1: *Function of acupuncture points*. Part 2: *Treatment of disease* (4th edn.). Heinemann Medical Books, London.

Mann, F. (1992). *Acupuncture: cure of many diseases*. Butterworth–Heinemann, Oxford.

Mole, P. (1992). *Acupuncture: energy balancing for mind and body*. Element Books, Shaftesbury, UK.

Needham, J. and Gwei-Djen, L. (1980). *Celestial lancets: a history and rationale of acupuncture and moxa*. Cambridge University Press. (Highly recommended)

O'Connor, J. and Bensky, D. (eds.) (1981). *Acupuncture: A comprehensive text*. Shanghai College of Traditional Medicine. Eastland Press, Chicago. (The best complete work available)

Pokert, M. *The theoretical foundation of Chinese medicine: Systems of correspondence*. MIT Press, Cambridge, Massachusetts. (Theoretical text)

Shanghai College of Traditional Chinese Medicine. (1990). *Acupuncture—a comprehensive text.* Eastland Press, Seattle.

Veith, I. (transl.) (1966). *The Yellow Emperor's classic of internal medicine. (The Nei Ching).* University of California Press.

Woollerton, H. and MacLean, C.J. (1983). *Acupuncture energy in health and disease.* Thorsons, Wellingborough.

Worsley, J.R. (1990). *Is acupuncture for you?* Element, Shaftesbury.

Yu, C.S. and Fei, L. (1993). *A clinical guide to Chinese herbs and formulae.* Churchill Livingstone, Edinburgh.

Zhao-pu, W. (1992). *Acupressure therapy.* Churchill Livingstone, Edinburgh.

Alexander and Feldenkrais Techniques

Alexander, F.M. (1971). (ed. E. Maisel) *The resurrection of the body.* Dell, New York. (The classic book by the originator of the technique)

Alexander, F.M. (1992). *The use of the self.* Gollancz, London.

Barlow, W. (1990). *The Alexander principle.* Gollancz, London. (A comprehensive description of the technique)

Feldenkrais, M. (1992). *Awareness through movement: health exercises for personal growth.* Harper & Row, New York. (The main book by the originator of the Feldenkrais Technique)

Gelb, M. (1994). *Body learning.* Society of Teachers of the Alexander Technique. London.

Gray, J. (1990). *Your guide to the Alexander technique.* Gollancz, London.

Jones, F.P. (1976). *Body awareness in action: a study of the Alexander Technique.* Schocken, New York. (Excellent section on research)

Maisel, E. (1969). *The resurrection of the body.* University Books, New York.

Park, G. (1989). *The art of changing. A new approach to the Alexander technique.* Ashgrove, UK.

Stevens, C. (1993). *Alexander technique.* Optima, London.

Anthroposophical medicine

Bott, V. (1985). *Anthroposophical medicine.* Thorsons, Harper Collins, London.

Bott, V. (1986). *Anthroposophical guide to family medicine.* Thorsons, Harper Collins, London.

Buhler, W. (1979). *Living with your body.* Rudolf Steiner Press, London.

Hauschke, M. (1979). *Rhythmical massage.* Rudolf Steiner Press, London.

Lievegoed, B. (1982). *Phases—crisis and development in the individual.* Rudolf Steiner Press, London.

Steiner, R. (1948). *Spiritual science and medicine.* Rudolf Steiner Press, London.

Steiner, R. (1979a). *The philosophy of freedom.* Rudolf Steiner Press, London.

Steiner, R. (1979b). *Occult science—an outline.* Rudolf Steiner Press, London.

Ayurvedic medicine

Fawley, D. (1989). *Ayurvedic healing. A comprehensive guide.* Morson, Sandy, New Mexico.

Kapoor, (1990). *CRC Handbook of Ayrvedic medicinal plants*. CRC Press, Boca Raton, Florida.

Khan, M.S. (1985). *Islamic medicine*. Routledge, London.

Lad, V. and Frawley, D. (1989). *The yoga of herbs: an ayurvedic guide to herbal medicine*. Lotus Press, Santa Fe, New Mexico.

Lad, V. (1994). *Ayurveda, the science of life*. Lotus Press, Santa Fe, New Mexico.

Morrison, J.H. (1995). *The book of Ayurveda*. Simon & Schuster, New York.

Svoboda, R.E. (1992). *Ayurveda—life, health and longevity*. Penguin Arkana, London.

Chiropractic (see also Osteopathy)

Bergman, T.F., Peterson, D.H., and Lawrence, D.K.J. (1993). *Chiropractic technique: principles and procedures*. Churchill Livingstone, Edinburgh.

Brennan, M.J. (ed.) (1981). *The resource guide to chiropractic: a bibliography of chiropractic and related areas*. American Chiropractors' Association, Washington, DC.

Byfield, D. (1994). *Chiropractic manipulative skills: fundamentals of clinical practice*. Butterworth—Heinemann, Oxford.

Copland-Griffiths, M. (1991). *Dynamic chiropractic today*. Thorsons, Harper & Row, London.

Cyriax, J. (1971). *Treatment by manipulation, massage and injection*. Williams & Williams, Baltimore, Maryland.

Haldman, S. (1992). *Principles and practice of chiropractic*. Appleton & Lange, East Norwalk, Connecticut.

King's Fund Centre. (1993). *Report of a working party on chiropractic*. King's Fund Centre, London.

Kunert, W. (1963). *The vertebral column, autonomic nervous system and internal organs*. Enke, Stuttgart.

Leach R.A. (1994). *The chiropractic theories*. Williams & Wilkins, Baltimore.

Maitland, G.B. (1964). *Vertebral manipulation*. Butterworths, London. (A classical medical text on manipulation—*not* chiropractic)

Moore, S. (1993). *Chiropractic*. Charles E. Tuttle, Boston, Massachusetts.

National Institute of Neurological Communicable Disorders and Stroke (1975). *The research status of spinal manipulative therapy*. Department of Health, Education and Welfare: NIH, Washington DC.

Plaugher, G. (ed.) (1993). *Textbook of clinical chiropractic: a specific biomechanical approach*. Williams & Wilkins, Baltimore.

Report of the Commission of Inquiry (1979). *Chiropractic in New Zealand*. New Zealand Government Printer, Wellington.

Thomas, J.E. (1991). *Chiropractic manual of low back and leg pain*. Appleton & Lange, East Norwalk, Connecticut.

Valentine, T. and Valentine, C. (1985). *Applied kinesiology: muscle response in diagnosis, therapy, and preventive medicine*. Thorsons, Harper Collins, London.

Wardwell, W.I. (1992). *Chiropractic: history and evolution of a new profession*. Mosby, St Louis.

White, A.A. (1983). *Your aching back*. Bantam, New York.

Creative and sensory therapies

Alvin, J. (1985). *Music therapy*. Hutchinson, London.

Birren, F. (1950). *Colour psychology and colour therapy: a factual study of the influence of colour on human life*. McGraw-Hill, New York.

Bunt, L. (1994). *Music therapy, an art beyond words*. Routledge, London.

Clark, L.A. (1975). *Ancient art of colour therapy*. Devin-Adair, Old Greenwich, Connecticut.

Gilroy, A. and Lee, C. (eds.) (1994). *Art and music: therapy and research*. Routledge, London.

Gimbel, T. (1994). *The book of colour healing*. Gaia, UK.

Halpern, S. and Savary, S. (1985). *Sound health: music and sounds that make us whole*. Harper & Row, New York.

Jennings, S., Cattanach, A., Mitchell, S., Chesner, A., and Meldrum, B. (1993). *The handbook of dramatherapy*. Routledge, London.

Jones, P. (1995). *Drama as therapy: theatre as living*. Routledge, London.

McLellan, R. (1989). *The healing forces of music*. Element, Shaftesbury.

McNiff, S. (1994). *Art as medicine. Creating a therapy of the imagination*. Shambalah, Boston, Mass.

Michel, D. (1985). *Music therapy: an introduction*. Charles C. Thomas, Springfield, Illinois.

Newham, P. (1995), *The singing cure. An introduction to voice movement therapy*. Shambalah, Boston, Massachusetts.

Ott, J.N. (1984). *Health and light: The effects of natural and artifical light on man and other living things*. Devin-Adair, Old Greenwich, Connecticut.

Stebbing, L. (1975). *Music therapy—a new anthology*. Knowledge Books, Horsham.

Warren, B. (1993). *Using the creative arts in therapy*. Routledge, London.

Healing

Angelo, J. (1991). *Spiritual healing*. Element, Shaftesbury.

Benor, D. (1993). *Healing research, Volumes 1–4*. Helix Editions, Deddington, Oxfordshire.

Bishop, B. (1989). *A time to heal*. New English Library, London.

Brennan, B. (1987). *Hands of light. A guide through the human energy field*. Bantam, New York.

Brennan, B. (1993). *Light emerging. The journey of personal healing*. Bantam, New York.

Courtenay, A. (1991). *Healing now*. Dent, London.

Dossey, L. (1993). *Healing words. The power of prayer and the practice of medicine*. Harper, San Francisco.

Easthope, G. (1987). *Healers and alternative medicine: a sociological examination*. Gower, Aldershot.

Eliade, M. (1964). *Shamanism: archaic technique of ecstasy*. Princeton University Press. (Highly recommended)

Gennaro, L., Guzzon, F., and Marsigli, P. (1986). *Kirlian photography*. East West Publications, London.

Gerber, R. (1988). *Vibrational medicine*. Bear, New Mexico; Element Books, Shaftesbury.

Halifax, J. (1982). *Shaman, the wounded healer*. Thames & Hudson, London.

Krippner, S. and Villoldo, A. (1976). *Realms of healing*. Celestial Arts, Millbrae, California.

Le Shan, L. (1985). *From Newton to ESP*. Viking, New York.

MacManaway, B. (1983). *Healing*. Thorsons, Harper Collins, London.

Sargant, W.W. (1973). *The mind possessed: a physiology of possession, mysticism and faith healing.* Heinemann, London.

Shealy, C.N. (1988). *The creation of health. Merging traditional medicine with intuitive diagnosis.* Stillpoint, US.

Taylor, A. (1992). *Healing hands.* Macdonalds Optima, London.

Valentine, T. (1973). *Psychic surgery.* Pocket Books, New York.

Young, A. (1983). *Spiritual healing: miracle or mirage?* De Vorss Press, Marina del Ray, California.

Wolman, B.B. (1977). *Handbook of parapsychology.* Van Nostrand Rheinhold, New York.

Herbalism

Bellamy, D. and Pfister, A. (1992). *World medicine: plants, patients and people.* Blackwell Publishers, Oxford.

Bradley, P.R. (ed.) (1992). *British herbal compendium. Vol. 1: a handbook of scientific information on widely used plant drugs.* British Herbal Medicine Association, Bournemouth.

British Herbal Medicine Association. (1990). *British herbal pharmacopoeia.* BHMA, Bournemouth, UK.

Chadwick, D.J. and Marsh, J. (eds.) (1994). *Ethnobotany and the search for new drugs.* CIBA Foundation Symposium No. 185, Wiley, New York.

Chang, H.K. (1993). *The pharmacology of Chinese herbs.* CRC Press, Boca Raton, Florida.

Culpeper, N. (1987). *Culpeper's complete herbal and English physician.* Meyerbooks, Glenwood.

Datamonitor (1993). *Opportunities in European herbal and homeopathic remedies.* Datamonitor, 106 Baker Street, London WIM 1LA.

De Smet, P.A.G.M. (1992). *Adverse effects of herbal drugs.* Springer-Verlag, Berlin.

De Vries, J. (1985). *Traditional home and herbal remedies.* Mainstream, London.

Duke, J. (1988). *CRC handbook of medicinal herbs.* CRC Press, Boca Raton, Florida.

Duke, J. (1992). *Handbook of biologically active phytochemicals and their activities.* CRC Press, Boca Raton, Florida.

Foster, S. (1994). *Herbal rennaisance. Growing, using and understanding herbs in the modern world.* Gibbs Smith, Salt Lake City, Utah.

Fulder, S. (1993). *Ginger, the ultimate home remedy.* Souvenir Press, London.

Fulder, S. (1993). *The book of ginseng, and other Chinese herbs for vitality.* Healing Arts Press, Rochester, Vermont.

Fulder, S. and Blackwood, J. (1991). *Garlic: nature's original remedy.* Healing Arts Press, Rochester, Vermont.

Grieve, M. (1982). *A modern herbal.* Jonathan Cape, London; Peregrine, Harmondsworth, Middlesex.

Griggs, B. (1981). *Green pharmacy: a history of herbal medicine.* Jill Norman, London. (Highly recommended)

Hoffman, D. (1986). *Holistic herbal way to successful stress control.* Thorsons, Harper Collins, London.

Hoffman, D. (1991). *The new holistic herbal.* Element Books, Shaftesbury.

Hoffman, D. (1994). *The information sourcebook of herbal medicine.* Crossing Press, Freedom, California.

Holmes, P. (1993). *The energetics of Western herbs. Vols I and II: An herbal reference integrating Western and Oriental herbal medicine traditions.* Snow Lotus Press, P.O. Box 1824, Boulder, Colorado 80306. (The largest and most important study of *materia medica* in the Western world, and the only one that attempts to integrate the qualities and actions of Western and Oriental herbs in both Western and Oriental concepts).

Kenner, D. and Requena, Y. (1995). *Botanical medicine: a European professional perspective.* Churchill Livingstone, Edinburgh.

Kloss, J. (1984). *Back to Eden.* Woodbridge Press, Santa Barbara, California.

Launert, E. (1981). *Edible and medicinal plants of Britain and Northern Europe.* Hamlyn, London.

Lewis, W.H. and Elvin-Lewis, P.F. (1977). *Medical botany: plants affecting man's health.* Wiley, New York.

McIntyre, M. (1989). *Herbal medicine for everyone.* Penguin, London.

Mills, S. (1992). *Out of the earth; the essential handbook of herbal medicine.* Viking Penguin, London.

Mills, S. (1993). *The essential book of herbal medicine.* Arkana Penguin, Harmondsworth, Middlesex.

Ody, P. (1993). *The herb society's complete medicinal herbal: herbal healing for all.* Dorling Kindersley, London.

Rose, J. (1976). *Jeanne Rose's herbal body book.* Grosset & Dunlop, New York.

Royal Pharmaceutical Society of Great Britain, (1993). *Herbal medicines; guide for health care professionals.* RPS, London.

Steiner, R.P. (1986). *Folk medicine, the art and the science.* American Chemical Society, Washington DC.

Stuart, M. (ed.) (1979). *The encyclopaedia of herbs and herbalism.* Orbis, London.

Tierra, M. (1980). *The way of herbs.* Unity Press, Santa Cruz, California. (Highly recommended)

Tierra, M. (1988). *Planetary herbology.* Lotus Press, Wilmot, Santa Fe, New Mexico.

Tsarong, T.J. (1995). *Tibetan medicinal plants.* Snow Lion Press, Ithaca, New York.

Tyler, V. (1994). *Herbs of choice. The therapeutic use of phytomedicinals.* Pharmaceutical Products Press, Haworth Press, Binghamton, New York.

Vogel, V.J. (1982). *American Indian medicine.* University of Oklahoma Press, Norman.

Wagner, H. and Wolff, P. (1977). *New natural products and plant drugs with pharmacological, biological and therapeutic activity.* Springer-Verlag, Heidelberg.

Weiss, R.F. (1988). *Herbal medicine.* Beaconsfield Publishers, Beaconsfield, UK.

Wichtl, M. and Bisset, N.G. (translator/editor.) (1994). *Herbal drugs and phytopharmaceuticals.* CRC Press, Boca Raton, Florida.

Wren, R.C. (1988). *Potter's new cyclopaedia of botanical drugs and preparations.* C.W. Daniel, Saffron Walden, Essex.

Homeopathy

Babbington Smith, C. (1986). *Champion of homeopathy, the life of Margery Blackie.* John Murray, London.

Blackie, M.G. (1984). *The patient, not the cure: the challenge of homeopathy.* Unwin, London. (An acclaimed personal book by one of the leading UK homeopaths)

—(1986). *Classical homeopathy.* Beaconsfield Publishers, Beaconsfield.

Blackie, M. (1986). *Classical homeopathy.* Beaconsfield Press, Beaconsfield.

British Association of Homeopathic Manufacturers (1994). *British homeopathic pharmacopoeia.* BAHM, Ilkeston, Derby.

Curtis, S. (1994). *Homeopathic alternatives to immunization*. Winter Press.

Endler, P.C. and Schulte, J. (eds.) (1994). *Ultra high dilution physiology and physics*. Kluwer, Norwell, Mass.

Harvery, C. and Cochrane, A. (1994). *The encyclopaedia of flower remedies*.

Kent, J.T. (1993). *Repertory of the homeopathic materia medica (with a revised word index and textual corrections)*. Homeopathic Book Service, London.

Lockie, A. and Geddews, N. (1992). *Women's guide to homeopathy*. Hamish Hamilton, London; Penguin, Harmondsworth, Middlesex.

Pharmacopoeia Convention of American Institute of Homeopathy (1979). *The homeopathic pharmacopoeia of the United States*. American Institute of Homeopathy, Falls Church.

Roy, M. (1994). *The principles of homeopathic philosophy: a self-directed learning course*. Churchill Livingstone, Edinburgh.

Shepherd, D. (1990). *The magic of minimum dose*. C.W. Daniel, Saffron Walden, Essex.

Shepherd, D. (1991). *Homeopathy for the first aider*. C.W. Daniel, Saffron Walden, Essex.

Smith, T. (1986). *The principles, art and practice of homeopathy*. Insight Publications, Worthing, Sussex.

Twentyman, R. (1989). *The science and art of healing*. Floris, UK.

Vithoulkas, G. (1986). *The science of homeopathy*. Thorsons, Wellingborough and Grove, New York. (An intelligent guide to homeopathy)

Vithoulkas, G. (1981). *Homeopathy—medicine of the new man*. Arco Press, New York. (Perhaps the best short introduction available)

Vithoulkas, G. (1991). *A new model for health and disease*. North Atlantic Books, Berkeley, California.

Weeks, Nora (1979). *Medical discoveries of Edward Bach, physician*. Keats Publishers, New Canaan, Connecticut.

Whitmont, E. C. (1993). *The alchemy of healing; psyche and soma*. North Atlantic Books, Berkeley.

Whitmore, E. (1981). *Psyche and substance*. North Atlantic Books, Richmond, California. (Highly recommended to those interested in the metaphysics of homeopathy)

Hypnosis (see also Mind-body)

Ambrose, G. and Newbold, G. (1980). *A handbook of medical hypnosis*. Ballière Tindall, Eastbourne.

Austin V. (1994). *Self-hypnosis*. Thorsons, Harper Collins, London.

Barber, T.X., Spanos, N.P., and Chaves, J.F. (1986). *Hypnosis, imagination and human potentialities*. Pergamon Press, Oxford and New York.

Cheek, D. and Le Cron, L. (1986). *Clinical hypnotherapy*. Grune and Stratton, New York. (The presentation of the authors' results on hypnosis in surgery, with the unconscious, and with ideometer methods)

Graham, H. (1995). *Mental imagery in health care: an introduction to therapeutic practice*. Chapman & Hall, London.

Hartland, J. (1971). *Medical and dental hypnosis*. Ballière & Tindall, London. (The classic book for medical professionals)

Hilgard, E.R. and Hilgard, J.R. (1984). *Hypnosis in the relief of pain*. William Kaufmann, Los Altos, California.

Rogers, C. (1973). *Client centred therapy*. McGraw-Hill, New York.

Shone, R. (1985). *Autohypnosis: a step by step guide to self-hypnosis*. Thorsons, Wellingborough.

Shreeve, C. and Shreeve, D. (1984). *Healing power of hypnotism*. Thorsons, Wellingborough.

Temple, R. (1989). *Open to suggestion*. Aquarian, UK.

Udolf, K. (1986). *Handbook of hypnosis for professionals*. Van Nostrand Rheinhold, New York.

Waxman, D. (1981). *Hypnosis: A guide for patients and practitioners*. Allen & Unwin, London. (Recommended)

Manual therapies

Bahr, F. (1982). *The acupressure health book*. Unwin, London.

Bayly, D. (1982). *Reflexology today*. Thorsons, Harper Collins, London.

Benjamin, H. (1992). *Better sight without glasses or contact lenses*. Thorsons, Harper Collins, London.

Blate, M. (1982). *The natural healers acupressure handbook: G-J fingertip technique*. Routledge & Kegan Paul, London. (Recommended)

Cassar, M. P. (1995). *Massage made easy*. People's Medical Society, Allentown, Pennsylvania.

Davis, P. (1990). *Aromatherapy: an A—Z*. C.W. Daniel, Saffron Walden, Essex.

Dougans, I. and Ellis, S. (1991). *Reflexology—foot massage for total health*. Element, Shaftesbury.

Dougans, I. and Ellis, S. (1992). *The art of reflexology: new approach using the Chinese meridian theory*. Element Books, Shaftesbury.

Dowding, G. (1989). *The massage book*. Viking Arkana, London.

Downer, J. (1992). *Shiatsu*. Hodder & Stoughton, London.

Downing, G. (1972). *The massage book*. Random House, New York. (Perhaps the best all-round book on massage)

Downing, G. (1974). *Massage and meditation*. Random House, New York.

Gach, M.R. (1990). *Acuyoga. Self-help techniques to relieve tension*. Harper & Row, New York and San Francisco.

Gach, M. (1992). *Acupressure: how to cure common ailments the natural way*. Piatkus, London.

Hofer, J. (1976). *Total massage*. Grosset & Dunlap, New York.

Holdway, A. (1995). *Kinesiology; muscle testing and energy balancing for health and well-being*. Element, Shaftesbury.

Kaye, A. and Matchan, D.C. (1985). *Reflexology: techniques of foot massage for health and fitness*. Thorsons, Harper Collins, London.

Kunz, K. and Kunz, B. (1985). *The complete guide to foot reflexology*. Thorsons, Harper Collins, London.

Lacroix, N. (1991). *Massage for total relaxation*. Dorling Kindersley, London.

Lataurelle, M. and Courtney, A. (1992). *Introductory guide to kinesiology*. Thorsons, Harper Collins, London.

Mansfield, P. (1992). *The Bates method. [eyesight training]*. Optima, London.

Montagu, A. (1972). *Touching: the human significance of skin*. Harper & Row, New York.

Nightingale, M. (1988) *Holistic first aid*. Optima, London.

Ohashi, W. (1993) *Do it yourself shiatsu*. Unwin, London.

Price, S. and Price, L. (1995). *Aromatherapy for health professionals*. Churchill Livingstone, Edinburgh.

Ridolfi, R. (1993). *Shiatsu*. Macdonald, London.

Rolf, I. (1977). *Rolfing—the integration of human structures*. Dennis Landmann, Santa Monica, California.

Rowley, N. (1992). *Hands on: basic skills for complementary practitioners*. Hodder, London.

Ryman, D. (1991). *Aromatherapy: the encyclopedia of plants and oils and how they help you*. Piatkus, London.

Stone, R. (1978). *Health building*. Parameter Press, Orange County, California. (On polarity therapy)

Stormer, C. (1992). *Reflexology*. Hodder & Stoughton, London.

Thie, J. and Marks, M. (1979). *Touch for health*. De Vorss Press, Santa Monica, California.

Tisserand, R. (1994). *The art of aromatherapy*. C.W. Daniel, Saffron Walden, Essex.

Yamamoto, S. (1990). *The shiatsu handbook*. Japan Publications, Tokyo.

Young, J, (1994). *Acupressure for health*. Thorsons, Harper Collins, London.

Mind–body therapies

Achterberg, J. (1985). *Imagery in healing – shamanism and modern medicine*. Shambhala, Boston.

Achterberg, J., Simonton, C., and Simonton, S. (1976). *Stress, psychological factors, and cancer*. New Medicine Press, Forth Worth.

Ader, R., Felten, D.L., and Cohen, N. (eds.) (1991). *Psychoneuroimmunology* II. Academic Press, New York and London.

Assagioli, R., (1971). *Psychosynthesis*. Hobbs, Dorman, New York. (Classic book on Assagioli's visualization and meditative psychotherapies)

Barasch, M.I. (1993). *The healing path. A soul approach to illness*. Tarcher/Putnam. New York.

Benson, H. (1976). *The relaxation response*. Morrow, New York. (The classic book on the psychophysiological effects of relaxation)

Borysenkio, J. (1988). *Minding the body, mending the mind*. Bantam, New York.

Brown, B. (1984). *New mind, new body. Biofeedback: new direction for the mind*. Irvington, New York.

Cade, C.M. and Coxhead, N. (1987). *The awakened mind – biofeedback and the development of higher states of awareness*. Element Books, Shaftesbury, Dorset. (Leading UK biofeedback researchers)

Carroll, D. (1984). *Biofeedback in practice*. Longmans, Harlow.

Dychtwald, K. (1977). *Bodymind*. Random House, New York. (Excellent summary of theory, methods and results of body awareness techniques of all kinds)

Elbert, T. (ed.) (1984). *Self-regulation of the brain and behaviour*. Springer-Verlag, Berlin and New York.

Garfield, S., Bergin, A.E. (1986). *Psychotherapy and behaviour change*. John Wiley, Chichester.

Goleman, D. and Guin, J. (1993). *Mind–body medicine*. Consumer Reports Books, Yonkers, New York.

Gratchel, R.J. (1979). *Clinical application of biofeedback: appraisal and status*. Pergamon Press, Oxford and New York.

Guex, P. (1993). *An introduction to psycho-oncology*. Routledge, London.

Hewitt, J. (1993). *The complete yoga book*. Rider, London.

Hewitt, J. (1993). *The complete relaxation book*. Rider, London.

Husband, J. (1993). *Behaviour and immunity*. CRC Press, Boca Raton, Florida.

Huxley, Aldous L. (1974). *Art of seeing*. Montanu Books, Seattle. (Aldous Huxley's account of the return of his sight using the Bates method)

Institute of Noetic Sciences and Moore, M. (1993). *The heart of healing*. Turner Publishing, Atlantic City.

James, G., Dennis, J., and Bresler, D. (eds.) (1981). *Mind, body and health: towards an integral medicine*. National Institute of Mental Health, Rockville, Maryland. (Summaries by many top authorities and practitioners of holistic methods of health care)

Kermani, K. (1992). *Autogenic training: the effective way to conquer stress*. Thorsons, Harper Collins, London.

Krakowski, A.J. and Chase, P. (1983). *Psychosomatic medicine, theoretical, clinical and transcultural aspects*. Plenum, New York.

Laskow, L. (1992). *Healing with love*. Harper Collins, London.

Levine, S. (1987). *Healing into life and death*. Anchor, Doubleday, New York.

Lowen, A. (1978). *Bioenergetics*. Penguin, London.

Luthe, W. (1976). *Creative mobilisation technique*. Grune & Stratton, New York. (Manual of autogenic therapy)

Meares, A. (1983). *Relief without drugs*. Fontana, London.

Nagarathna, R., Nagendra, H.R., and Monro, R. (1991). *Yoga for common ailments*. Gala, Stroud, Gloucestershire.

Pelletier, K. (1994). *Sound mind, sound body*. Simon & Schuster, New York.

Pelletier, K. (1977). *Mind as healer, mind as slayer: a holistic approach to preventing stress disorders*. Delacorte, New York. (Highly recommended)

Rosa, C. (1976). *You and autogenic training*. Dutton, New York.

Seem, M. and Kaplan, J. (1989). *Bodymind energetics. Towards a dynamic model of health*. Healing Arts Press, Rochester, Vermont.

Selye, Hans (1976). *The stress of life*. McGraw-Hill, New York. (Personal account of bio-chemical and physiological discoveries by the man who 'discovered' the stress response)

Siegel, B. (1989). *Love, medicine and miracles*. Rider, London.

Siegel, B. (1990). *Peace, love and healing: bodymind communication and the path to self-healing*. Rider, London.

Simonton, O.C., Matthews-Simonton, S., and Creighton, J. (1978). *Getting well again*. Tarcher Books, Los Angeles. (The book covers the use of visualization and meditation in overcoming cancer)

Wills, P. (1994). *Visualisation*. Hygeia Press.

Naturopathy and nutrition therapy (see also Self-care)

Adams, R. and Murray, F. (1985). *Body, mind and B vitamins*. Larchmont, New York.

Bland, J. (ed.) (1986). *Yearbook of nutritional medicine*. Keats Publishing, New Canaan, Connecticut.

Chaitow, L. (1994). *Water therapy*. Thorsons, Harper Collins, London.

Cheraskin, E. and Ringsdorf, W. (1980). *Psychodietetics: food as the key to emotional health*. Stein & Day, New York.

Cheraskin, E. Ringsdorf, W., and Clark, J.W. (1977). *Diet and disease*. Keats Publishing, New Canaan, Connecticut. (Recommended)

Colgan, M. (1982). *Your personal vitamin profile*. Blond & Briggs, London.

Davies, S. and Stewart, A. (1987). *Nutritional medicine*. Pan, London.

Davis, A. (1983). *Let's get well*. Unwin, London.

De Vries, J. (1992). *Skin diseases. [herbal medicine and naturopathy].* Mainstream, Edinburgh.

Dubos, R. (1968). *So human an animal.* Scribners, New York.

Fuller, R. (ed.) (1992). *Probiotics: the scientific base.* Chapman & Hall, London.

Garrison, R. and Somer, E. (1985). *Nutrition desk reference.* Keats Publishing, New Canaan, Connecticut.

Gerson, M. (1977). *Cancer therapy: a result of 50 cases.* Totality Books, Delmar, California.

Goodman, S. (1991). *Vitamin C, the master nutrient.* Keats, New Canaan, Connecticut.

Gunn, T. (1992). *Mass immunisation—a point in question.* Cutting Edge, London.

Horrobin, D. (ed.) (1982). *Clinical uses of essential fatty acids.* Eden Press, Montreal.

Kohnlechner, K. (1979). *Handbuch der Naturheilkunde* (2 vols). Wilhelm Heyne Verlag, Munich. (The comprehensive reference book of Heilpraktiker).

Kushi, M., Esko, E., and van Canwenberghe, M. (eds.) (1983). *The macrobiotic approach to major illnesses.* East West Foundation, Boston, Massachusetts

Lewith, G., Kenyon, J., and Dowson, D. (1992). *Allergy and intolerance: a complete guide to environmental medicine.* Green Print, London.

Lindlahr, V.H. (1983). *Natural therapeutics* (2 vols). C.W. Daniel, Saffron Walden. (The classical work)

Mayes, A. (1985). *Dictionary of nutritional health.* Thorsons, Wellingborough.

Newman-Turner, R. (1984). *Naturopathy.* Thorsons, Wellingborough. (Recommended)

Null, G. (1984). *The complete guide to health and nutrition.* Arlington, London.

Orenstein, N. and Bingham, S. (1987). *Food allergies.* Putnam, New York.

Ornish, D. (1993). *Program for reversing heart disease.* Ballantine, New York.

Pauling, L. (1986). *How to live longer and feel better.* W.H. Freeman, New York.

Pfeiffer, C.C. (1975). *Mental and elemental nutrients: a physician's guide to nutrition and health care.* Keats Publishing, New Canaan, Connecticut.

Pitchford, P. (1993). *Healing with whole foods. (Oriental traditions and modern nutrition).* North Atlantic Books, Berkeley.

Pizzorno, J. and Murray, M. (1985). *A textbook of natural medicine.* John Bastyr College Publications, Seattle.

Randolph, T. and Moss, R. (1989). *An alternative approach to allergies.* Lippincott & Cromwell, New York.

Rowland, I.R. (1988). *Role of the gut flora in toxicity and cancer.* Academic Press, New York and London.

Royal College of Physicians. (1981). *Medical aspects of dietary fibre.* Pitman Medical, London.

Simone, C.B. (1992). *Cancer and nutrition.* Avery, Garden City Park, New York.

Smith, C. and Best, S. (1989). *Electromagnetic man: health and hazard in the electrical environment.* Dent, London.

Stone, I. (1979). *Healing factor: Vitamin C against disease.* Grosset and Dunlap, New York.

Vogel, H.C.A. (1994). *The nature doctor.* Mainstream, Edinburgh.

Werbach, M.R. (1992). *Nutritional influences on illness. A sourcebook of Clinical research.* Third Line Press, Tarzana, California.

Williams, R.J. (1977). *A physicians' handbook of nutritional science.* Pergamon, Oxford.

Williams, R.J. (1979). *Biochemical individuality.* Wiley, New York.

Williams, R. (1981). *Nutrition against disease.* Bantam, New York. (Highly recommended)

Osteopathy (see also Chiropractic)

Belshaw, C. (1987), *Osteopathy: is it for you?* Element Books, Shaftesbury.
Chaitow, L. (1982). *Osteopathy: Head-to-toe health through manipulation*. Thorsons, Wellingborough.
Chaitow, L. (1987). *Soft tissue manipulation*. Thorsons, Wellingborough.
Hoag, J.M., Cole, W.V., and Bradford, S.G. (1980). *Osteopathic medicine*. McGraw-Hill, New York.
King's Fund. (1991). *Report of a working party on osteopathy*. King's Fund, London.
Korr, I.M. (1978). *The neurobiologic mechanisms in manipulative therapy*. Plenum, New York.
McCatty, R. (1988). *Essentials of craniosacral osteopathy*. Ashgrove, Bath.
Masters, P. (1988). *Osteopathy for everyone*. Penguin, Harmondsworth, Middlesex.
Still, A.T. (1910). *Osteopathy—research and practice*. (Privately published, A.T. Still, Missouri)
Upledger, J. and Vredevoord, J. (1983). *Craniosacral therapy*. Eastland Press, Chicago.

Radionics and psionic medicine

Baerlin, E. and Dower, H.L.G. (1980). *Healing with radionics*. Thorsons, Wellingborough.
Burr, H.S. (1973). *The fields of life*. Ballantine, New York.
Reyner, J.H., Laurence, G., and Upton, C. (1980). *Psionic medicine*. Routledge & Kegan Paul, London. (Highly recommended)
Tansley, D.V. (1980). *Dimensions of radionics*. Health Science Press, Holsworthy.
Tansley, D.V. (1982). *Radionics: Science or magic?* Daniel, Saffron Walden, Essex.
Westlake, A.T. (1973). *The pattern of health: a search for a greater understanding of the life force in health and disease*. Shambhala, Colorado.

Directory of UK organizations in complementary medicine

Note: The number of organizations in the UK has expanded dramatically since the second edition of this handbook. At the same time, many organizations that were mentioned in the previous edition have closed down. The author and researchers have made their best efforts to include all the major and significant colleges, professional bodies and other organizations involved with complementary medicine in the UK. The authors have made contact with virtually all the organizations at the addresses given below, so that as of July 1995 we are reasonably confident of the accuracy of the directory.

Organizations may have been omitted because in the opinion of the author and researchers of the *Handbook of alternative and complementary medicine* they were small, local, or offering inadequate training (for example, corespondence courses). Or they may have been untraceable, or did not reply to our calls, or were unwilling to be included. We have made our best efforts to ensure the accuracy and comprehensiveness of this list, but cannot take responsibility for errors or omissions—that is, omitting organizations that should have been included, or including organizations that should rightly have been omitted. We were unwilling and unable to act as judge during the preparation of this directory. It should also be borne in mind that addresses and particularly telephone numbers change rapidly, and some time has elapsed since July 1995.[1]

ALEXANDER TECHNIQUE

TRAINING COLLEGES

Alexander ReEducation Centre (STAT)
10 Langdon Avenue,
Aylesbury,
Bucks HP21 9UX
Tel 01296 23833

The Alexander Technique Training
  Course, Oxford (STAT)
63 Chalfont Road,
Oxford OX2 6TJ
Tel 01865 58477

Brighton Alexander Training Centre
  (STAT)
57 Beaconsfield Villas,
Brighton
East Sussex BN1 6HB
Tel 01273 501612

Bristol AT Training School Association
  (STAT)
37 Bellevue Crescent,
Bristol BS8 4TF
Tel 0117 9298582

[1] The following list is protected by copyright. Please contact the Publishers for permission to reproduce, reprint, circulate, or distribute the whole or any part of it.

The Centre for Alexander Technique
(STAT)
46 Stevenage Road,
London SW6 6HA
Tel 0171 731 6348

Centre for Training (STAT)
142 Thorpedale Road,
London N4 3BS
0171 281 7639
Fax 0171 281 9400

The Constructive Teaching Centre Ltd
(STAT)
18 Lansdowne Road,
Holland Park,
London W11 3LL
Tel 0171 727 7222

Essex Alexander School (STAT)
65 Norfolk Road,
Ilford,
Essex IG3 8LJ
Tel 0181 220 1630

Fellside Alexander School
Sepulchre Lane, Low Fellside
Kendal LA9 4NJ
Tel 01539 733045

Headington Alexander Training School,
Oxford (STAT)
10 York Road, Headington,
Oxford OX3 8NW
Tel 01865 65511

North London Teachers' Training Course
(STAT)
10 Elmcroft Ave.
London NW11 0RR
Tel 0181 455 3938

North of England Teaching Centre for the
F M Alexander Technique (STAT)
Flat 3, Park House,
39 Hanover Square,
Leeds LS3 1BQ
Tel 0113 244 9713

The Oxford Alexander Technique Training
Centre (STAT)
63 Chalfont Road,
Oxford OX2 6TJ
Tel 01865 58477

School of Use (STAT)
Foxhole,
Dartington, Devon
Correspondence to:
46 Grange Road, Warberry Heights,
Ellacombe, Torquay,
Devon TQ1 1LF
Tel 01803 201419

Victoria Training Course for the
Alexander Technique (STAT)
50A Belgrave Road,
London SW1
Tel 0171 821 7916

West of Scotland AT Teachers' Training
course (STAT)
28 Queens Drive,
Queens Park, Glasgow,
Scotland G41
Tel 0141 423 3617

West Sussex Centre for the Alexander
Technique (STAT)
5 Coates Castle,
Nr Pulborough,
West Sussex RH20 1EU
Tel 01798 865503

PROFESSIONAL ORGANIZATIONS

The Society of Teachers of the Alexander
Technique
20 London House,
266 Fulham Road,
London SW10 9EL
Tel 0171 351 0828
Fax 0171 352 1556

Alexander Teaching Network
PO Box 53,
Kendal,
Cumbria
LA9 4UP

SUPPORT ORGANIZATIONS

The Alexander Trust
(Address as STAT)

The Feldenkrais Guild UK
PO Box 370,
London N10 3XA

ANTHROPOSOPHICAL MEDICINE

TRAINING COLLEGES

Hibernia School of Artistic Therapy
Hawkwood College,
Painswick Old Road
Stroud, Glos
Tel 01453 751685

Training in Curative Eurythmy
Eurythmy School,
Peridur Centre for the Arts,
Dunnings Road,
East Grinstead,
Sussex RH19 4NF
Tel 01342 312527
Fax 01342 323401

The Speech School,
Peridur Centre for the Arts,
Dunnings Road,
East Grinstead,
Sussex RH19 3NF
Tel 01342 24384

Tobias School of Art
Coombe Hill Road,
East Grinstead,
Sussex
Tel 01342 313655

PROFESSIONAL ORGANIZATIONS

Anthroposophical Medical Association
Park Attwood Therapeutic Centre,
Trimpley, Bewdley,
Worcs DY12 1RE
Tel 01299 861 444

Association of Eurythmy Therapists
Rudolf Steiner House,
35 Park Road,
London NW1 6XT
Tel 0171 723 4400

ASSOCIATED ORGANIZATIONS

Anthroposophical Society of Great Britain
Rudolf Steiner House,
35 Park Road,
London NW1 6XT
Tel 0171 723 4400

SUPPORT ORGANIZATIONS

The Medical Group of the Anthroposophical
Society in Great Britain
Park Attwood Therapeutic Centre,
Trimpley, Bewdley,
Worcs DY12 1RE

AROMATHERAPY

(Only professional organizations are noted.
These will supply lists of affiliated
schools.)

PROFESSIONAL ORGANIZATIONS

Aromatherapy Organisations Council
   (*represents 10 organizations*)
3 Latymer Close, Braybrooke,
Market Harborough,
Leics LE16 8LN
Tel 01858 434242

Association of Holistic Therapists
39 Prestbury Road,
Cheltenham,
Glos GL25 2PT
Tel 01242 512 601

Association of Medical Aromatherapists
Abergare, Rhu Point,
Helensburgh, G84 8NF
Tel 0141 332 4924

Association of Natural Medicine
27 Braintree Road,
Witham,
Essex CM8 2DD
Tel 01376 502762

Association of Physical and Natural
   Therapists
68A The Avenue,
Worcester Park,
Surrey KT4 7HJ
Tel 0181 335 3202

English Societé de l'Institute Pierre
   Franchomme, France
Belmont House,
Newport,
Essex CB11 3RF
Tel 01799 540622

Holistic Aromatherapy Foundation
83 Harestone Hill,
Caterham,
Surrey CR3 6DL
Tel 01883 343419

International Federation of Aromatherapists
Stamford House,
2–4 Chiswick High Road
London W4 1TH
Tel 0181 742 2605

International Society of Professional
    Aromatherapists
Hinckley and District Hospital,
The Annexe, Mount Road,
Leics LE10 1AG
Tel 01455 637987
Fax 01455 890956

Register of Qualified Aromatherapists
PO Box 6491,
London N8 9HF
Tel 0181 341 2958

Societé de l'Institute des Sciences
    Biomedicales, France
Belmont House,
Newport,
Essex CB11 3RF
Tel 01799 540622

CHIROPRACTIC

TRAINING COLLEGES

Anglo-European College of Chiropractic
13–15 Parkwood Road,
Boscombe, Bournemouth,
Dorset BH5 2DE
Tel 01202 436200
(associated with British Chiropractic
    Association)

McTimoney Chiropractic School Ltd
The Institute of Pure Chiropractic,
14 Park End Street,
Oxford OH1 1HH
Tel 01865 246786
(associated with McTimoney Chiropractic
    Association)

Oxford College of Chiropractic (formerly
    Witney School of Chiropractic)
The Old Post Office,
Stratton Audley,
Nr Bicester,
Oxon OX6 9BA
Tel 01869 277 111
(associated with British Association for
    Applied Chiropractic)

PROFESSIONAL ORGANIZATIONS

British Chiropractic Association
29 Whitley Street,
Reading RG2 0EG
Tel 01734 757 557
Fax 01734 757 257

British Association for Applied
    Chiropractic
The Old Post Office
Stratton Audley, Nr Bicester
Oxon OX6 9BA
Tel 01869 277 111

McTimoney Chiropractic Association
PO Box 126,
Oxford OX2 8RH
Tel 01865 246 687

Scottish Chiropractic Association
30 Roseburn Place,
Edinburgh EH12 5NX
Tel 0131 346 7500;
Fax 0131 346 7502
(associated with BCA)

SUPPORT ORGANIZATIONS

The Chiropractic Advancement Association
8, Centre 1
Lysander Way, Old Sarum
Salisbury,
Wilts SP4 6BU
Tel 01722 415 027

European Chiropractors' Union
c/o 9 Cross Deep Gardens,
Twickenham,
Middlesex TW1 4QZ
Tel 0181 891 2546

CREATIVE AND SENSORY THERAPIES

Music Therapy

TRAINING COLLEGES

Anglia Polytechnic University
Faculty of Humanities, Arts and
    Education,
Division of Music and Performing Arts
East Road,
Cambridge CB1 1PT
Tel 01223 63271 (ext 2045)

Guildhall School of Music and Drama
The Barbican,
London EC2Y 8DT
Tel 0171 628 2571

Nordoff-Robbins Music Therapy Centre
2 Lissenden Gardens,
London NW5 1PP
Tel 0171 267 4496

Roehampton Institute
Roehampton Lane
London SW15 5PU
Tel 0181 392 3000

University of Bristol
Department of Continuing Education,
Wills Memorial Building,
Queens Road,
Bristol BS8 1HR
Tel 01272 303 616

PROFESSIONAL ASSOCIATIONS

Association of Professional Music
    Therapists
Chestnut Cottage, 38 Pierce Lane,
Fulbourne,
Cambridge CB1 5DL
Tel 01223 880377

Art Therapy
Postgraduate Training Courses available
    at:

Edinburgh University Settlement
School of Art Therapy
Wilkie House, Guthrie Street,
Edinburgh EH11 1JG

Goldsmith's College
Art Therapy Unit
27 Albury Street, Deptford,
London SE8
Tel 0171 919 7171

Hertfordshire College of Art and Design
Manor Road,
Hatfield,
Herts AL10 9TL
Tel 01707 279 000

University of Sheffield
Floor 0, Dept of Psychiatry
Art Therapy Training Programme,
Royal Hallamshire Hospital,
Glossop Road,
Sheffield S10 2JF

PROFESSIONAL ORGANIZATIONS

British Association of Art Therapists
11A Richmond Road,
Brighton,
Sussex BN2 3RL
Fax 01273 685 852
Enquiries to 01734 265 407

Dramatherapy

TRAINING COLLEGES
Postgraduate courses available at:

Central School of Speech and Drama
Embassy Theatre, Eton Avenue,
London NW3 3HY
Tel 0171 722 8183/4/5/6

City College Manchester
Arden Centre,
Sale Road, Northenden,
Manchester M23 0DD
Tel 0161 957 1500

The Institute of Dramatherapy at
    Roehampton
Digby Stuart College,
Roehampton Lane,
London SW18
Tel 0181 392 3215/3063

South Devon College of Arts and
    Technology
Newton Road, Torquay,
Devon TQ2 5BY
Tel 01803 291212

University of Hertfordshire
College of Art and Design,
10 Manor Road, St Albans,
Herts AL10 9LT
Tel 01707 284000

University of Ripon and York St John
Department of Drama, Film and
Television
Lord Mayor's Walk
York YO3 7EX
Tel 01904 656771

PROFESSIONAL ORGANIZATIONS

British Association for Dramatherapists
5 Sunnydale Villas,
Durlston Road, Swanage,
Dorset BH19 2HY

ASSOCIATED ORGANIZATIONS

British Society for Music Therapy
25 Rosslyn Avenue,
East Barnet,
EN4 8DH
Tel 0181 368 8879

International Association for Colour
Therapy
PO Box 3688, Barnes
London SW13 0XA

SUPPORT ORGANIZATIONS

Hygeia College of Colour Therapy
Hygeia Studios, Colour-Light-Art Research
Ltd,
Brook House, Avening,
Tetbury GL8 8NS
Tel 01453 832 150

ETHNIC MEDICINE

PROFESSIONAL ASSOCIATIONS

International Society for Ayurveda
7 Ravenscroft Ave,
London NW11 0SA

Mohsinn Institute
446 East Park Road,
Leicester LE5 5HH
Tel 0116 2734 633

SUPPORT ORGANIZATIONS

Ayurvedic Living Ltd
PO Box 188,
Exeter EX4 5AB
Tel 01392 52874

HEALING
(Professional Associations only are listed)

PROFESSIONAL ORGANIZATIONS

Confederation of Healing Organisations
113 High Street,
Berkhamsted
Herts HP4 2DJ
Tel 01442 870660

Association for Therapeutic Healers
Flat 5, 54–56 Neal Street,
Covent Garden,
London WC2
Tel 0171 240 0176

British Alliance of Healing Associations
26 Highfield Avenue,
Herne Bay,
Kent CT6 6LM
Tel 01227 373804

College of Healing
Runnings Park
Croft Bank, West Malvern,
Worces WR14 4DU
Tel 01684 573 868

College of Psychic Studies
16 Queensbury Place,
London SW7 2EB
Tel 0171 589 3292/3

Fellowship of Erasmus
Moat House, Banyard's Green,
Laxfield, Woodbridge,
Suffolk IP13 8ER
Tel 01986 798 682

Healer Practitioner Association
1A Northcote Street,
Cardiff, CF2 3BH
Tel and Fax 01222 481 139
(not CHO)

Maitraya School of Healing
1 Hillside, Highgate Road,
London NW3
Tel 0171 482 3293

National Federation of Spiritual Healers
The Old Manor Farm Studio,
Church Street,
Sunbury-on-Thames,
Middlesex TW16 6RG
Tel 01932 783164

(run National Healer Referral Service,
   available to anyone over age of 18; calls
   cost 49p/a minute, Tel 0891 616 01801)

Spiritualist Association of Great Britain
33 Belgrave Square,
London SW1X 8QB
Tel 0171 235 3351

Spiritualists' National Union
Redwoods, Stansted Hall,
Stansted Mountfitchet,
Essex CM24 8OD
Tel 01279 816 363; Fax 01279 812 034
(Not CHO)

Sufi Healing Order of GB
91 Ashfield Street,
Whitechapel,
London E1 2HA
Tel 0171 377 5873

The White Eagle Lodge
NewLands, Rake,
Brewells Lane,
Hampshire GU33 7HY
Tel 01730 893300

World Federation of Healing
33 The Park, Kingswood,
Bristol,
Avon BS15 4BL
Tel 0117 9673 154

SUPPORT ORGANIZATIONS

Aetherius Society
757 Fulham Road,
London SW6 5UU
Tel 0171 736 4187

Christian Fellowship of Healing (Scotland)
6 Morningside Road,
Edinburgh,
EH10 4DD
Tel 0131 228 6553

Doctor Healer Network
Hay Cottage, 19 Fore Street,
Bishops Stainton
Devon TQ14 9QR

Greater World Christian Spiritualist
   Association
3 Conway Street, Fitzrovia,
London W1P 5HA
Tel 0171 436 7555

The Guild of Health
Edward Wilson House
26 Queen Anne Street,
London W1M 9LB
Tel 0171 580 2492

Methodist Church: Division of Social
   Responsibility: Family Healing and
   Personal
Concerns Committee,
Methodist Church,
1 Central Buildings,
Matthew Parker Street,
Westminster,
London SW1H 9NH
Tel 0171 222 8010

The Seekers' Trust
Centre for Prayer and Spiritual Healing
The Close, Addington,
West Malling,
Kent ME19 5BL
Tel 01732 843 589

HERBAL MEDICINE

TRAINING COLLEGES

Faculty of Herbal Medicine
General Council and Register of
   Consultant Herbalists
18 Sussex Square,
Brighton,
East Sussex BN2 5AA
Tel and Fax 01243 267 126

Middlesex University (BSc degree)
Faculty of Social Science and Education,
Queensway, Enfield,
Middlesex EN3 4SF
Tel 0181 362 5000
(associated with NIMH)

School of Herbal Medicine (Phytotherapy)
Bucksteep Manor, Bodle Street Green,
Hailsham,
East Sussex BN27 4RJ
Tel 01323 833812/4

PROFESSIONAL ASSOCIATIONS

The General Council and Register of
  Consultant Herbalists
18 Sussex Square,
Brighton,
East Sussex, BN2 5AA
Tel 01243 267 126

National Institute of Medical Herbalists
56 Longbrook Street,
Exeter EX4 6AH
Tel 01392 426 022

SUPPORT ORGANIZATIONS

British Herbal Medicine Association
1 Wickham Road,
Boscombe,
Bournemouth BH7 6JX
Tel 01202 433 691

The Herb Society
134 Buckingham Palace Road,
London SW1W 9SA
Tel 0171 823 5583

HOMEOPATHY

TRAINING COLLEGES

British School of Homeopathy
  at Avon and Gloucestershire College
  of Health
Stapleton, Bristol
Address for correspondence:
Pump Cottage,
Compton Durville, South Petherton,
Somerset TA13 5ER
Tel and Fax 01460 242 486
(SoH)

The College of Classical Homeopathy
Othergates Clinic,
45 Barrington Street,
Tiverton,
Devon EX16 6QP
Tel 01884 258 143
(SoH)

The College of Homeopathy
Regent's College,
Inner Circle, Regent's Park,
London NW1 4NS
Tel 0171 487 7416; Fax 0171 487 7675
(SoH)

The College of Practical Homeopathy
  (London)
Oakwood House,
42 Hackney Road,
London E2 7SY
Tel 0171 613 5468; Fax 0171 613 5469
(SoH)

The College of Practical Homeopathy
  (Midlands)
186 Wolverhampton Street,
Dudley DY1 3AD
Tel 01384 233 664
(SoH)

The Faculty of Homeopathy
Royal London Homeopathic Hospital,
Great Ormond Street,
London WC1N 3HR
Tel 0171 837 9469
(Doctors only)

The Hahneman College of Homeopathy
164 Ballards Road,
Dagenham
Essex RM10 9AB
0181 984 9240

The London College of Classical
  Homeopathy, at Morley College
61 Westminster Bridge Road,
London SE1 7HT
Tel 0171 928 6199
Fax 0171 633 0110
(SoH)

The London School of Classical
  Homeopathy
1–4 Suffolk Street,
London SW1Y 4HG
Tel and Fax 0181 959 2968
(SoH)

The Northern College of Homeopathic
Medicine
First Floor, Swinburne House,
Swinburne Street, Gateshead,
Tyne and Wear NE8 1AX
Tel 0191 490 0276

The North West College of Homeopathy
23 Wilbraham Road,
Fallowfield,
Manchester M14 6FB
Tel and Fax 0161 257 2445
(SoH)

Purton House School of Homeopathy
Purton House, Purton Lane,
Farnham Royal,
Bucks SL2 3LY
Tel 01753 646625
(SoH)

The School of Homeopathic Medicine
(Sheffield)
44 Longmeadow Road,
Alfreton,
Derbyshire DE5 7PD
Tel 01773 831 291
(SoH)

The School of Homeopathy
Yondercott House, Uffcolme,
Cullompton,
Devon EX15 3DR
Tel and Fax 01873 856 872
Address for correspondence:
8 Kiln Road,
Llanfoist, Abergavenny
Gwent NP7 9NS
(SoH)

The Scottish College of Homeopathy
11 Lyndoch Place,
Glasgow G3 6AB
Tel 0141 332 3917

The Soluna School of Homeopathy
North Street,
Cromford, Nr Matlock,
Derbyshire DE4 3RG
Tel 01629 826 190
(SoH)

The Yorkshire School of Homeopathy
Lansdown, 24 Rosebank,
Burley-in-Wharfdale, Ilkley,
West Yorks LS21 1AX
Tel 01943 863 213
Fax 01943 862 549
(SoH)

PROFESSIONAL ORGANIZATIONS

Faculty of Homeopathy
2 Powis Place,
Great Ormond Street,
London WC1N 3HR
Tel 0171 837 2495
Fax 0171 278 7900
(Medically qualified only)

Society of Homeopaths
2 Artizan Road,
Northampton NN1 4HU
Tel 01604 214 00
Fax 01604 226 22

UK Homeopathic Medical Association
243 The Broadway,
Southall,
Middlesex UB1 3AN
Tel 01474 560 336

SUPPORT ORGANIZATIONS

British Association of Homeopathic
Veterinary Surgeons
Chinham House,
Stanford-in-the-Vale,
near Faringdon,
Oxon SN7 8NQ
Tel 01367 710 324/710 475
Fax 01367 718 243

The British Homeopathic Association
27a Devonshire Street,
London WIN 1RJ
Tel 0171 935 2163

British Association of Homeopathic
Chiropodists
F-4, 16/17 New North Street,
London WC1N 3PJ
Tel 0171 831 2962

British Homeopathic Dental Association
2b Franklin Road,
Watford,
Herts WD1 1QD
Tel 01923 233 336

Dr Edward Bach Centre
Mount Vernon,
Sotwell, Wallingford,
Oxon OX10 0PD
Tel 01491 834 678

The Homeopathic Trust for Research and
    Education
Hahnemann House,
2 Powis Place,
Great Ormond Street,
London WC1N 3HT
Tel 0171 837 9469

International Podiatric Association of
    Homeopathic Medicine
134 Montrose Avenue,
Edgware,
Middlesex HA8 0DR
Tel 0181 959 5421

Society of Homeopaths Research Group
c/o Plough Cottage, Docking Road,
Sedgeford,
Norfolk PE36 5LR
Tel 01485 570377

Homeopathic hospitals

The Bristol Homeopathic Hospital
Cotham Hill,
Bristol BS6 6JU
Tel 01179 466 087; Fax 01179 238 759

The Glasgow Homeopathic Hospital
1000 Great Western Road,
Glasgow G12 0NR
Tel 0141 339 1824
Fax 0141 337 2276

Liverpool Clinic
The Mossley Hill Hospital, Park Avenue,
Liverpool, L18 8BU
Tel 0151 724 2355

Manchester Homeopathic Clinic
Brunswick Street,
Manchester M13 9ST
Tel 0161 273 2446

The Royal London Homeopathic Hospital
Great Ormond Street,
London WC1N 3HR
Tel 0171 837 8833;
Fax 0171 833 7269

Tunbridge Wells Homeopathic Hospital
Church Road,
Tunbridge Wells,
Kent TN1 1JU
Tel 01892 542 977; Fax 01892 542 244

Homeopathic Manufacturers

A. Nelson and Co. Ltd
Manufacturing Laboratories,
Broadheath House,
83 Parkside,
Wimbledon,
London SW19 5LP
Tel 0181 788 7888

Weleda (UK) Ltd
Heanor Road,
Ilkeston,
Derbyshire DE7 8DR
Tel 0115 9448 200

HYPNOTHERAPY

PROFESSIONAL ORGANIZATIONS

Association of Professional Therapists
55 The Spinney,
Sidcup,
Kent DA14 5NE
Tel 0181 308 0249

British Society of Medical and Dental
    Hypnosis
42 Links Road,
Ashtead,
Surrey KT21 2HJ
Tel 01372 273 522

also at: 17 Keppel View
Kimberworth, Rotherham,
Yorks
Tel 01709 554 558

British Society of Hypnotherapists
37 Orbain Road,
Fulham,
London SW6 7JZ
Tel 0171 385 1166

Central Register of Advanced
  Hypnotherapists
28 Finsbury Park Road,
London N4 2JY
Tel 0171 359 6991

National Association of Counsellors,
  Hypnotherapists and Psychotherapists
Aberystwyth,
Dyfed SY23 4EY
Tel and Fax 01974 241 376

National Council of Psychotherapists and
  Hypnotherapy Register
24 Rickmansworth Road
Watford WD1 7HD
Tel 01590 644 913

National Register of Hypnotherapists and
  Psychotherapists
12 Cross Street,
Nelson,
Lancs BB9 7EN
Tel 01282 699 378

SUPPORT ORGANIZATIONS

British Association for Autogenic Training
  and Therapy
Heath Cottage, Pitch Hill,
Ewhurst, Nr Cranleigh,
Surrey GU6 7NP

British Hypnosis Research
1 King Street,
Bakewell,
Derby DE45 1DZ
Tel 01629 814 491

MANUAL THERAPIES

(Professional organizations only are listed)

PROFESSIONAL ORGANIZATIONS

Reflexology

Association of Holistic Therapists
Rivendell Natural Therapies Clinic
Rivendell, Cwmbach Road,
Aberdare, Mid Glam
Tel 01685 875 237

Association of Physical and Natural
  Therapies
12 Cottage Road,
Stanford in the Vale,
Oxon SN7 8HX
Tel 01367 710 159

Association of Reflexologists
27 Old Gloucester Street,
London WC1N 3XX
Tel 01273 479 020

British Reflexology Association
Monks Orchard,
Whitbourne,
Worcs WR6 5RB
Tel 01886 821207

Foundation of Spiritual Healing and
  Guidance
Former Primary School,
Church Street, Seaford,
East Sussex BN25 1HH
Tel 01323 896 192

Holistic Association of Reflexologists
Holistic Healing Centre
92 Sheering Road,
Old Harlow,
Essex CM17 0JN
Tel 01279 429 060

International Federation of Reflexologists
76–78 Edridge Road,
Croydon,
Surrey CR0 1EF
Tel 0181 667 9458

International Institute of Reflexology
15 Hartfield Close,
Tunbridge,
Kent TN10 4JP
Tel 01732 350 629

Reflexologists' Society
7 Bristol Road,
Paulton,
Bristol BS18 5XX
Tel 01761 416 016

Scottish Institute of Reflexology
'Taymonth', Hill Crescent,
Wormit, Fife,
Scotland DD6 8PQ
Tel 01382 541 372

Massage

**British Massage Therapy Council
(umbrella body)**
Greenbank House
65a Adelphi Street,
Preston PR1 7BH
Tel 01772 881 063

Academy of Natural Health (BMTC)
7a Clapham Common Southside,
London SW4 7AA
Tel 0171 720 9506

**Bodywise Massage, Bodywise Health
Centre (BMTC)**
119 Roman Road,
London E2 0QN
Tel 0181 981 6938

Churchill Centre (BMTC)
22 Montagu Street,
London W1H 1TB
Tel 0171 402 9475

Essentials for Health (BMTC)
PO Box 2216
London E11 3TA
Tel 0181 556 8155

Lancashire Holistic College (BMTC)
Greenbank House,
65a Adelphi Street,
Preston PR1 7BH
Tel 01772 825 177

London College of Massage (BMTC)
5–6 Newman Place,
London W1P 3PF
Tel 0171 323 3574

Sequoia College (BMTC)
Units 1 & 2 Williams Court,
Cardiff CF1 5DQ
Tel 01222 238 599

Stress Matters (BMTC)
7 Ranelagh Road,
Harrow Green,
London E11 3JW
Tel 0181 519 5666

Clare Maxwell-Hudson (BMTC)
PO Box 457,
London NW2 4BR
Tel 0181 450 6494

**Sheffield School and Medical Association
(BMTC)**
289 Abbeydale Road,
Sheffield S7 1FJ
Tel 0114 258 6480

Guild of Professional Practising Therapists
42 Leominster Square,
London W2 4PU

**Independent Professional Therapists
International**
8 Oldsall Road,
Retford,
Notts DN22 7PL
Tel and Fax 01777 700 383

**Independent Register of Manipulative
Therapists Ltd**
32 Lodge Drive,
London N13 5JZ
Tel 0181 886 3120

**The London Counties Society of
Physiologists**
330 Lytham Road,
Blackpool FY4 1DW
Tel 01253 408443

SUPPORT ORGANIZATIONS

**Academy & Association of Systematic
Kinesiology**
39 Browns Road, Surbiton,
Surrey KT15 8ST
Tel 0181 399 3215
Fax 0181 390 1010

**BA in Therapeutic Massage/MA in
Therapeutic Bodywork**
(Validated by University of Westminster)
Marylebone Centre Trust
33 Queen Anne Street,
London
Tel 0171 255 3550

Bowen Technique
Bowtech England
38 Portway, Frome,
Somerset BA11 1QU
Tel 01373 461 837

Independent Therapists Examining
Council (ITEC)
James House, Oakelbrook Mill,
Newent,
Glos GL18 1HD
Tel 01531 821 875

The Metamorphic Association
67 Ritherden Road,
London SW17 8QE
Tel 0181 672 5951
The Rolfing Network

MIND-BODY THERAPIES

PROFESSIONAL ORGANIZATIONS

Association of Therapeutic Healers
c/o Neal's Yard Therapy Rooms
2 Neal's Yard,
London WC2

British Association for Autogenic Training
and Therapy
18 Holtsmere Close,
Garston, Watford,
Herts WD2 6NG

Energetics Association
72 Dumbarton Road,
Lancaster LA1 3BX
Tel 01524 67009

International Society of Polarity
Therapists
Shelaymah National Healing Centre
42 Braydon Road,
London N16 6QB
Tel 0181 800 2200

Polarity Therapy Association UK
Monomark House
27 Old Gloucester St,
London WC1N 3XX
Tel 01483 417 714
Tel 01203 670847

Polarity Therapy Educational Trust
Ashburton Hotel
79 East Street,
Ashburton,
Devon TQ13 7AL

Relaxation for Living
168–170 Oatlands Drive,
Weybridge
Surrey KT13 9ET
Tel 01932 831000

The Awakened Mind Ltd
9 Chatsworth Road
London NW2 4BJ
Tel 0181 451 0083

SUPPORT ORGANIZATIONS

British Wheel of Yoga
1 Hamilton Place,
Boston Road, Sleaford,
Lincs NG34 7ES
Tel 01529 306851

Institute for Neuro-physiological
Psychology
Warwick House, 4 Stanley Place,
Chester CH1 2LU
Tel 01244 311 414

International Stress Management
Association
Southbank University, LPSS
103 Borough Road,
London SE1 0AA
Tel 01702 584 025

The Relaxation Society
84 Herbert Gardens,
Willesden
London NW10 3BU
Tel 0181 969 6704

Yoga for Health Foundation
Ickwell Bury, Ickwell Green,
Northill, Biggleswade,
Bedfordshire,
Tel 01767 627 271

Yoga Biomedical Trust
PO Box 140,
Cambridge CB4 3SY
Tel 01223 67 301

NATUROPATHY AND NUTRITION THERAPY

TRAINING COLLEGES

British College of Naturopathy and
  Osteopathy
6 Netherhall Gardens,
London NW3 5RR
Tel 0171 435 6464
(GCRO)

Institute for Optimum Nutrition
13 Blades Court, Deodar Road,
London SW15 2NU
Tel 0181 877 9993

PROFESSIONAL ORGANIZATIONS
(some of whom also have their own colleges
that are not mentioned above)

General Council and Register of
  Naturopaths
Frazer House,
6 Netherhall Gardens,
London NW3 5RR
Tel 0171 435 8728

British Register of Naturopaths
328 Harrogate Road,
Leeds LS17 6PE
Tel 0113 2685 992

Incorporated Society of Registered
  Naturopaths
Kingston, The Coach House,
293 Gilmerton Road,
Edinburgh EH16 5UQ
Tel 0131 664 3435

Society for Promotion of Nutritional
  Therapy
PO Box 47, Heathfield,
East Sussex TN21 8ZX
Tel 01435 867 007

International Federation of Clinical
  Nutritionists
Research House, PO Box 131,
Fraser Road, Greenford,
Middlesex UB6 7DX
Tel 0181 810 5644

Council for Nutrition Education and
  Therapy
34 Wadham Road,
London SW15 2OR

Register of Nutritional Therapists
Hatton Green,
Warwick CV35 7LA
Tel 01926 484 596

SUPPORT ORGANIZATIONS

British Natural Hygiene Society
3 Harold Grove,
Frinton-on-Sea,
Essex CO13 9BD
Tel 01255 672 823

Community Health Foundation
188 Old Street,
London EC1V 9FR
Tel 0171 251 4076

Jewish Vegetarian Society
Bet Teva,
855 Finchley Road,
London NW11 8DX
Tel 0171 935 3924

McCarrison Society
23 Stanley Court,
Worcester Road,
Sutton,
Surrey

Society of Iridologists
998 Wimbourne Road,
Bournemouth BH9 2DE
Tel 01202 518 078

ORIENTAL MEDICINE

ACUPRESSURE
(There are other, smaller courses
elsewhere. Only the bigger colleges are
listed, mainly those offering over 500
hours of study over three years.)

TRAINING COLLEGES

Bristol School of Shiatsu
18 Lilymeade Avenue, Knowle,
Bristol BS4 2BX
Tel 0117 977 809

British School of Shiatsu
1st Floor, Block 2,
6 Erskine Road,
London
NW3 3AJ
Tel 0171 483 3776

Devon School of Shiatsu
The Coach House,
Buckyette Farm,
Littlehampton,
Devon TQ9 6ND
01803 762 593

European Shiatsu School
High Banks,
Lockeridge,
Nr Marlborough,
Wilts SN8 4EQ
Tel 01672 861 362

Healing/Shiatsu Education Centre
The Orchard, Lower Maescoed,
Pontrilas,
Herefordshire HR2 0HP
Tel 01873 87207

Ki Kai Shiatsu Centre
172a Arlington Road,
London NW1
0181 368 9050

Shen Tao Foundation
Middle Piccadilly Natural Healing Centre,
Holwell, Sherborne
Dorset
Tel 01963 23468

Shiatsu College
20a Lower Goat Lane,
Norwich,
Norfolk NR2 1EL
Tel 01603 632 555

PROFESSIONAL ORGANIZATIONS

The Shiatsu Society
5 Foxcote,
Wokingham
Berks RG11 3PG
Tel 01734 730836
Fax 01734 732752

ACUPUNCTURE

TRAINING COLLEGES

Academy of Chinese Acupuncture
52 Caldon Road,
London, E11 4EU
(PG courses for doctors and some others)

Academy of Traditional Chinese Medicine,
UK Ltd
12 Church Lane, Gosforth,
Newcastle-upon-Tyne NE3 1AR
Tel 0191 213 2464

British Academy of Western Acupuncture
c/o Carrick,
Tetchill, Ellesmere,
Shropshire SY12 9AI
Tel 01691 654 786
(Doctors, physiotherapists, and nurses
only)

British College of Acupuncture
8 Hunter Street,
London WC1N 1BN
Tel 0171 833 8164
(linked with BAcC)

Chung San Acupuncture School
15 Porchester Gardens,
London W2 4DB
Tel 0171 727 6778
(linked with BAcC)

College of Integrated Chinese Medicine
40 College Road,
Reading RG6 1QB
Tel 01734 263366
(linked with TAS – CFA)

College of Oriental Medicine International
Teaching Centre
The Lodge,
59 Whitham Road, Broomhill,
Sheffield S10 2SL
Tel 0114 267 1171
(linked with Association of Chinese
Acupuncture)

The College of Traditional Acupuncture
UK
Tao House, Queensway,
Leamington Spa,
Warwickshire, CV31 3LZ
Tel 01926 422121
(linked with Traditional Acupuncture
Society—CFA)

Fook Sang Acupuncture and Chinese
Herbal Practitioners' College
590 Wokingham Road,
Early, Reading,
Berks RG6 7HN
Tel 01734 665 454

The International College of Oriental
 Medicine
Green Hedges House,
Green Hedges Avenue,
East Grinstead,
Sussex RH19 1DZ
Tel 01342 313 106/7
(linked with International Register of
 Oriental Medicine—CFA)

London School of Acupuncture and
 Traditional Chinese Medicine
36 Featherstone Street,
London EC1Y 8QX
Tel 0171 490 0513
(linked with Register of Traditional
 Chinese Medicine—CFA)

Northern College of Acupuncture
124 Acomb Road,
York YO2 4EY
Tel 01904 785 120/784828
(linked with RTCM—CFA)

PROFESSIONAL ORGANIZATIONS

The British Acupuncture Council
 (*representing five professional bodies*)
Park House
206–208 Latimer Road,
London W10 6RE

Association of Auricular Therapy GB Ltd
106 Higher Lane,
Rainford, St Helens
Merseyside WA11 8AZ

Association of Chinese Acupuncture
Prospect House, 2 Grove Lane,
Retford,
Notts DN22 6NA
Tel/Fax 01777 704 411

British Medical Acupuncture Society
Newton House, Newton Lake,
Lower Whitley, Warrington,
Cheshire WA4 4JA
Tel 01925 730727
(Doctors only)

CHINESE HERBAL MEDICINE

East West College of Herbalism
Hartswood,
Marsh Green, Hartfield
East Sussex TN7 4ET
Tel 01342 822 312
Fax 01342 826 347

School of Chinese Herbal Medicine
Midsummer Cottage Clinic,
Nether Westcote,
Kingham
Oxon OX7 6SD
Tel 01993 830957

School of Kanpo Apprentice in Japanese
 Herbal Medicine
36 Bankhurst Road,
London SE6 4XN
Tel 0181 690 4840

The London Academy of Oriental Medicine
7 Newcourt Street,
London NW8 7AA
0171 722 5795

Tara College of Tibetan Medicine
45 East Trinity Road,
Edinburgh EH5 3DL
Tel 0131 552 1431
(associated with Association of Practitioners
 of Herbal Medicine)

PROFESSIONAL ORGANIZATIONS

Association of Practitioners of Tibetan
 Medicine
45 East Trinity Road,
Edinburgh EH5 3DL
Tel 0131 552 1431

Register of Chinese Herbal Medicine
PO Box 400,
Wembley,
Middlesex HA9 9NZ

Register of East West Certified Herbalists
Hartswood,
Marsh Green, Hartfield,
East Sussex TN7 4ET
Tel 01342 822 312; Fax 01342 826 347

SUPPORT ORGANIZATIONS

Samye Ling Tibetan Centre
Eskdalemuir
Nr Langholm,
Dumfrieshire DG13 0GL
Tel 01387 373 232

OSTEOPATHY

TRAINING COLLEGES

British College of Osteopathy and
  Naturopathy
6 Netherhall Gardens,
London N3 5RR
Tel 0171 435 6464
(GCRO)

The British School of Osteopathy
1–4 Suffolk Street,
London SW1Y 4HG
Tel 0171 930 9254
(GCRO)

College of Osteopaths
110 Thorkill Road,
Thames Ditton,
Surrey KT7 0UW

European School of Osteopathy
104 Tonbridge Road,
Maidstone,
Kent ME16 8SL
Tel 01622 671558
(GCRO)

The London College of Osteopathic
  Medicine
8–10 Boston Place,
London NW1 6ER
Tel 0171 262 5250
(associated with British Osteopathic
  Association—doctors only)

London School of Osteopathy
8 Lanark Square, Glengall Bridge,
London E14 9RE
Tel 0171 538 8344
(associated with Natural Therapeutic and
  Osteopathic Society)

College of Cranio-Sacral Therapy
9 St George's Mews,
Primrose Hill
London NW1 8XE
Tel 0171 483 0120
(associated with C-S TA)

Craniosacral Therapy Educational Trust
19 Carterknowle Road,
Sheffield S7 2DW
Tel 01742 586 290
(associated with C-S TA)

Karuna Institute
Natsworthy Manor
Widecombe in the Moor
Devon TQ13 7TR
Tel 01647 221 457
(associated with C-S TA)

PROFESSIONAL ORGANIZATIONS

General Council and Register of
  Osteopaths
56 London Street,
Reading,
Berks RG1 4SQ
Tel 01734 576585/566260

British Osteopathic Association
8–10 Boston Place,
London NW1 6ER
Tel 0171 262 5250
(Doctors only)

Cranio-Sacral Therapy Association of
  Great Britain
8 Warren Road,
Colliers Wood
London SW19 2HX
Tel 0181 543 4969

RADIONICS AND PSIONIC MEDICINE

SUPPORT ORGANIZATIONS

British Society of Dowsers
Sycamore Barn,
Hastingleigh, Ashford,
Kent TN25 5HW
Tel 01233 750253

Confederation of Radionic and
  Radiesthesic Organisations
The Maperton Trust,
Home Farm, Maperton,
Wincanton BA9 8EH
Tel 01963 32651,
Fax 01963 32626

De La Warr Society for Radionics
Raleigh Park Road,
Oxford OX2 9BB
Tel 01865 244 388

International Federation of Radionics
c/o Institute for Complementary Medicine
PO Box 194,
London SE16 1QZ
Tel 0171 237 5165

Radionics Association
Baerlein House,
Goose Green, Deddington,
Oxford OX5 4SZ
Tel 01869 338 852

A SELECTION OF GENERAL COMPLEMENTARY ORGANIZATIONS

Action against Allergy
24–6 High Street,
Hampton Hill,
Middlesex TW12 1PD
Tel 0181 943 4244

Affiliation of Crystal Healing Organisations
46 Lower Green Road,
Esher,
Surrey KT10 8HD
Tel 0181 398 7252

Alternative Health Information Bureau
12 Upper Station Road,
Radlett,
Herts WD7 8BX
Tel and Fax 01923 857 670

Association for New Approaches to Cancer
5 Larksfield,
Egham,
Surrey TW20 0RB
Tel 01784 433 610

The Bates Association (Eye Care)
c/o Peter Mansfield
Friars Court, Tarmount Lane
Shoreham by Sea,
Sussex BN43 6RQ
Tel 01273 452 623

Bristol Cancer Help Centre
Grove House,
Cornwallis Grove, Clifton,
Bristol BS8 4PG
Tel 01272 743216

British Complementary Medicine
   Association
39 Prestburg Road,
Cheltenham
Glos GL52 2PT
Tel 01242 226770
Fax 01242 226778

British Holistic Medical Association
Rowland Thomas House
Royal Shrewsbury Hospital (South)
Shrewsbury,
Salop SY3 8XF
Tel 01743 353 637/261 155

British Register of Complementary
   Medicine
Institute for Complementary Medicine
PO Box 194,
London SE16 1QZ
Tel 0171 237 5165

The Centre for the Study of Alternative
   Therapies
51 Bedford Place,
Southampton,
Hants SO1 2DG
Tel 01703 334 752

Complementary Medical Practitioners'
   Union
MSF
50 Southwark Street,
London SW18 2BR
Tel 0171 378 7255

Complementary Medicine Therapy and
   Research Centre
Health Services Research and Evaluation
   Unit
43 Albacore Crescent,
Lewisham,
London SE13 3EF

Council for Complementary and
   Alternative Medicine (CCAM)
Park House
206–208 Latimer Road,
London W10 6RE
Tel 0181 968 3862
Fax 0181 968 3469

Centre for Complementary Health Studies
Exeter University,
Streatham Court, Rennes Drive,
Exeter EX4 4PU
Tel 01392 33828

Green Library
9 Rickett Street,
London SW6 1RU
Tel 0171 385 0012

Guild of Complementary Practitioners
Alpha House
High Street, Crowthorne
Berks RG11 7AD
Tel 0131 44 761 715

Guild of Health
Edward Wilson House,
26 Queen Anne Street,
London W1M 9LB
Tel 0171 580 2492

Health Practitioners Association
187a Worlds End Lane,
Chelssfield,
Kent BR6 6AU

Institute of Allergy Therapy
Llangwyryfon,
Aberystwyth,
Dyfed SY23 4EY
Tel 01974 241 376; Fax 01974 7376

Institute for Complementary Medicine
15 Tavern Quay,
Plough Way, Surrey Quays,
London SE16 1QZ
Tel 0171 237 5175

Journal of Alternative and Complementary
  Medicine
(*see* Green Library)

Kirlian Institute
51 Rushton Road,
Kettering
Northants NN14 2RP

La Leche League
BM 3424,
London WC1N 3XX
Tel 0171 242 1278

Marylebone Centre Trust
33 Queen Anne Street,
London W1M 9FB
Tel 0171 255 3550

National Childbirth Trust
Alexandra House,
Oldham Terrace,
London W3 6NH
Tel 0181 992 8637

National Society for Research into Allergy
PO Box 45, Hinckley
Leics LE10 1JY
Tel and Fax 01455 851 546/291 294

Natural Health Foundation
159 George Street,
London W1H 5LB
Fax 0171 723 7256

Natural Health Network
2–4 Hardwicke Road,
Reigate,
Surrey
RH12 9HJ
Tel 01737 226 269

Natural Medicines Society
Market Chambers,
13a Market Place, Heanor,
Derby DE75 7AA
Tel 01773 710 002

Research Council for Complementary
  Medicine (RCCM)
60 Great Ormond Street,
London WC1N 3JF
Tel 0171 278 7412

Tyringham Naturopathic Clinic
Newport Pagnell,
Bucks MK16 9ER
Tel 01908 610450

The Vegan Society Ltd
7 Battle Road,
St Leonards on Sea
East Sussex TN37 7AA
Tel 01424 427 393 Fax 01424 717 064

Vegetarian Society
Parkdale, Dunham Road,
Altrincham,
Cheshire WA14 4QG
Tel 0161 928 0793

The UK Training College for
  Complementary Health Care Studies
St Charles Hospital,
Exmoor Street,
London W10 6DZ
Tel 0181 964 1206 Fax 0181 964 1207

Women's Nutritional Advisory Service
PO Box 268,
Lewes,
East Sussex BN7 2QN
Tel 01273 487 366

Index

Principal references are bold
Complentary Medicine has been abbreviate to CM

Abrams, Albert 266
absent healing 179, 181, 183
accreditation/standards 57–61
acupressure 130–1
  nausea treatment 137
  shiatzu 131, **225–6**, 302
  UK organizations 302
acupuncture **125–42**
  in Australia 107–8
  Codes of Practice 80–1
  ear acupuncture 138
  education/training issues 56, 58–60, 67
  electro-acupuncture 138
  equipment needed 51, 125, 130
  in Finland 104
  in France 99, 101–2
  health problems brought to 5, 38–9, 132–3
  historical aspects 12, 13, 125
  moxibustion 130
  needle hygiene 80–1, 130
  numbers seeking 32
  in Oxfordshire (UK) 36, 51
  professional bodies 56, 58–60, 67, 302–3
  research issues 9, 20–2, 25, 133–7
  SIA 101
  therapist numbers 36, 48
  therapist registration 73, 81
  UK organizations 302–3
  in the United States 97–8
  in Western Europe 99
  see also acupressure
additives (food) 251
advertising
  legal aspects 72
  standards 51, 77
Aesculapius 11
Africa 109–12
AIDS 36
  risks from acupuncture 81
Aldridge, David 172, 173
Alexander, F. Mathias 143
Alexander technique **143–5**
  for nurses 145–6

research issues 145
  therapist numbers 48
  training issues 57
  UK organizations 289–90
allergic conditions 36
  CM organizations 306
  food sensitivities 251
Alma-Ata conference (1977) 111
alternative medicine
  defined 3
  revival of 16–20
Alzheimer's disease 172
American Naturopathic Association 244
analgesia, *see* pain relief
Anglo-European College of Chiropractic 55, 168
anthroposophical medicine **147–56**
  art therapy 76, 152, **153**, 171–2, 173
  eurythmy 152
  training issues 56
  UK organizations 290–1
applied kinesiology 226–7, 300
aromatherapy **227–9**
  herbalism and 195
  training issues 61
  UK organizations 291–2
art therapy 76, 152, **153**, 171–2, 173
  UK organizations 290–1, 293
asthma
  acupuncture for 136–7, 139
  autogenic therapy for 239
  hypnotherapy for 216
  relaxation for 236
  statistics 14
auricular therapy 138, 303
Australia 107–9
  CM survey 37
autogenic therapy **238–40**
  training issues 57
  UK organizations 298, 300
Ayurvedic medicine 5, 115–18, **157–61**
  Siddha medicine 115–16, 158
  UK organizations 294
  Unani medicine 116, 158, 160

Bach flower remedies 208
  Dr Edward Bach Centre 297
back pain 36–7
  acupuncture for 134
  back pain statistics 168
  chiropractic for 165–6
  Cochrane Committee on 20, 166
  osteopathy for 259
Bad Worishoesen 100
barefoot doctors 114
Barlow, Wilfred 143–4
Bates Association 305
Bates eyesight training 240–1
Bates, William 240
Bayly, Doreen 222
Bedouin medicine 112
Belgium 99, 103
Benor, Daniel 180
Benviste, Professor 205
Bingham, Thomas 74
bioenergetics 234
  historical aspects 13
biofeedback 236–8
BMA (British Medical Association) 17
  on hypnosis 80
  Psychological Medicine Committee 80
  report on CM (1986) 18, 88–9
  report on CM (1993) 18–19, 47, 57, 62, 89
body therapy, *see* manual therapies
bonesetting 12, 13, 70, 162
Bordia, Professor 159
Braid, James 210
Bristol Cancer Help Centre 305
Bristol Homeopathic Hospital 79, 297
Bristol Natural Health Centre 52
British Acupuncture Accreditation Board
  56, 58, 65
British Acupuncture Association 67
British Acupuncture College 58
British Acupuncture Council 67, 303
British Chiropractors Association 163
British College of Acupuncture 58–9, 302
British College of Naturopathy and Osteopathy
  55, 301
British Complementary Medicine Association 48,
  66, 305
British Herbal Medicine Association 82, 86, 295
British Medical Association, *see* BMA
British Naturopathic and Osteopathic
  Association 244
British Psychological Society 80
British School of Osteopathy 55, 64, 259, 304
British Society for Nutritional Medicine 250
Budd, Martin L. 246
Budwig, Johanna 249
Bulgaria 106–7

Cade, Max 183
Camphill Villages 148

cancer
  Cancer Act (1933) 72
  psychogenic influences 233
  statistics 14–15
cancer treatment 15–16
  aromatherapy 228
  Association for New Approaches to Cancer
    305
  Bristol Centre 305
  complementary nursing care 94
  diet and cancer prevention 15
  hypnosis 216
  massage 221
  mistletoe (Iscador) 87, 151, 154–5
  patient satisfaction with CM 40, 41–2
  relaxation 236
  spiritual healing 183
cardiovascular problems 36
Cayce, Edgar 179
Centralised Information Service on CM
  (CISCOM) 22
Centre for Complementary Health Studies 306
Centre for the Integration of Orthodox and CM
  (USA) 98
Centre for the Study of Alternative Therapies
  306
chakras 269
Champneys (health resort) 53
Charles, Prince of Wales 18, 88
children 35
  acupuncture in 130, 139
  naturopathy in 254
Chinese medicine 112–15, 125–7
  eczema treatment 23, 137
  historical aspects 113, 186
  therapist numbers 48
  UK organizations 304
  see also acupuncture
chiropractic 162–70
  in Australia/NZ/South Africa 107–8
  education/training issues 54–5, 57, 62–3
  EEC rulings 104
  equipment needed 51, 165
  health problems brought to 38, 168
  historical aspects 13, 162–3
  insurance costs 73
  numbers seeking 32
  outmoded concepts 20
  research aspects 164, 165–8
  in Scandinavia 99, 104
  state registration 19, 20, 75
  therapist numbers 48
  UK organizations 292
  in the United States 97
  in Western Europe 99, 101, 103
chronic diseases 36–7
CISCOM (Centralised Information Service on
  CM) 22
clairvoyant diagnosis 9
clinical trials 23–6; *see also* research studies

Cochrane Committee on back pain 20, 166
College of Traditional Acupuncture 59, 303
colonic hydrotherapy 253
colour therapy 173–4
  UK organizations 293–4
comfrey root 83, 192
Complementary Medical Practitioners'
  Union 306
Complementary Medicine Therapy and
  Research Centre 306
Confederation of Healing Organizations
  (CHO) 48
confidentiality 72
consultation statistics 50–1
  with GPs 32–3, 49–51
conventional medicine
  diagnostic skills 8
  history of medicine 10–13
  modern crisis in 13–16
  patient satisfaction 39–43
  side-effects/risks 6
  see also doctors; GPs
Conway, Ashley 216
correspondence courses 56, 65
COST B4 project 22, 105
cost of CM 49
  reimbursement of fees 78
Council of Acupuncture 58
Council for Complementary and Alternative
  Medicine (CCAM) 58, 66, 81, 306
counselling 234
cranial osteopathy 259, 262
creative therapies 48, 171–3
  art therapy 76, 152, 153, 171–2, 173
  drama therapy 76, 172
  music therapy 172–3
  UK organizations 290–1, 292–4
Criminal Injuries Compensation
  Board 78
Cumberledge, Baroness 17, 85

Dangerous Drugs Act (1965) 82
Data Protection Act (1984) 72
de la Warr, George 267
De La Warr Society for Radionics 305
death certificates 78
Denmark 104
dermatitis (eczema) 23, 137
Dewey, John 144
diagnostic skills 7–9
diet
  Ayurvedic 158
  disease management and 15
  herbalism and 191
  monodiets 249
  nutrition therapy 12, **250–4**
  vegetarianism/veganism 253
dietetics, *see* nutrition therapy
Do-In 226

doctors
  registration of 71
  training in CM 18, 19, 63–4, 68, 100
  in Russia 106
  see also GPs
Dorrell, Stephen 89
double-blind trials 23–6
dowsing 9, 268–70, 305
drama therapy 76, 176
  UK organizations 293
Drown, Ruth 13, 267
drug therapy, *see* medicines
Dubois, Renˆ 14
Dundee, Professor 137

ear acupuncture 138
  Association of Auricular Therapy 303
Eastern Europe 106–7
eczema 23, 137
education/training issues **53–63**
  accreditation 57–61
  in Australia 108
  biomedical content 61–3
  competence/quackery 64–6
  for doctors 18, 19, 63–4, 68, 100
  EEC directives 76–7
  in India 116–17
  in West Germany 100
EEC, *see* European Union/EEC influence
eicosapentanoic acid (EPA) 252
elderly patients 35, 221, 254
electrical therapies 138
electro-acupuncture 138
Ellis, Tom 79
Enton Hall 53
equipment requirements 51
Eskimo medicine 112
Estebany, Oscar 177
European Herbal Practitioners Alliance 86
European School of Osteopathy 55
European Scientific Cooperation on
  Phytotherapy 86
European Union/EEC influence 104–6
  CM training issues 76–7
  herbal/homeopathic products 85–7
eurythmy 152, 291
evening primrose oil 251
Exeter University 57
eyesight training 240–1

Faculty of Homeopathy (UK) 64, 68, 117, 296
faith healing 177
  mechanisms 211–15
  in South Africa 112
Family Health Service Authorities 90–2
Far Eastern medicine
  Kanpo 132, 304
  shiatzu 131, **225–6**, 302

Tibetan 106, 131–2, 304
  see also Chinese medicine; Oriental medicine
fasting 248–9, 254
fees 49
  reimbursement of 78
Feldenkrais, Moshe 145
Feldenkrais technique 145
Finland 104
Fisher, Fleur 18
Fitzgerald, William 222
fluoridation of water 252
folk medicine, *see* traditional medicine
food additives 251
food sensitivities 251
France 101–2
  CM legal position 99
  use of homeopathy 32, 99
Furnham, Adrian 34, 41

Galen 11
garlic 1, 190
  for atherosclerosis 159
  garlic capsules 84
  research findings 193–4
General Chiropractic Council 75
General Council and Register of Osteopaths
  55, 67, 74
General Medical Council 17, 71, 87–8
General Osteopathic Council 67, 75
ginger 193, 194
Gingko biloba 194
Glasgow Homeopathic Hospital 79, 297
Goodheart, George 226
GPs
  CM in primary care 90–4
  consultation statistics 32–3, 50–1
  interest in CM 17–18, 90
  NHS reforms and 89–90
  numbers in UK 47
  training in CM 18, 19, 63–4
Grayshott Hall 53
group practices 51–2
Guild of Complementary Practitioners 66, 306
Guild of Health 306

Hahnemann College of Homeopathy 296
Hahnemann, Samuel 12, 199–200
hair analysis 251, 271
Hale Clinic 52
Hauschka, Margarethe 151
headache 37
  chiropractic for 167
  relaxation for 236
  shiatzu for 226
  see also migraine
healing therapies 176–85
  absent healing 179, 181, 183

faith healing 177, 211–15
  historical aspects 13
  laying on of hands 179, 181
  magnetic healing 178
  numbers seeking 32
  prayer 179
  in Russia 106
  social class and 36
  in South Africa 112
  spiritual healing 48, 176–85
  therapist numbers 47–8
  UK organizations 294–5, 299
  visualization method 179–80
Health and Safety at Work Act (1974) 72
Health Practitioners Association 306
health remedies *see* herbalism; medicines
health resorts 53
health spas 106, 245, 248
heart disease 14
Heilpraktikers 48, 99, 100
Herbal Practitioners Association 67
Herbal Remedies Order (1977) 82
herbalism 4, 5, **186–98**
  in Australia 108
  in Bulgaria 106
  education/training issues 55, 57, 60
  equipment needed 51
  in France 99, 102
  historical aspects 12, 186–8
  in India 158–60
  licensing of herbal medicines 81–6
  Oriental 131–2, 137, 195, 304
  outmoded concepts 20
  professional bodies 55, 67, 195
  registration issues 74
  research issues 21, 137, 193–4
  in Scandinavia 99
  social class and 36
  in South Africa 112
  in Switzerland 48, 99
  therapists 48, 194–5
  UK herbal market 49
  UK organizations 295
  in West Germany 99, 100–1
  in Western Europe 99
Hering, Constantine 200
Hippocrates 11
history of medicine/CM 10–13
  acupuncture 12, 13, 125
  chiropractic 13, 162–3
  herbalism 12, 186–8
  hypnotherapy 13, 80, 210
  legal aspects 70–1
  licensing of medicines 81
  massage 12, 220
  osteopathy 13, 258–9
  radionics 13, 266–7
holistic medicine 9–10
  defined 3–4
  holistic approaches 5–6

Holistic Health Centres 52
patient beliefs and 34
UK organizations 291, 298
Holistic Nurses Association 94
Holland, *see* Netherlands
Homeopathic Medical Association 60, 67
homeopathy 199–209
Bach flower remedies 208
in Belgium 99, 103
in Eastern Europe 107
education/training issues 60–1
equipment needed 51
in France 32, 99, 102
homeopathic hospitals 79, 297–8
in India 117
in Scandinavia 99
in Western Europe 99
legal aspects 86–7
origins of 12, 199
outmoded concepts 20
professional bodies 60, 60–1, 67, 297
research issues 24–5, 202, 204–6
short courses in 57
therapist numbers 48
UK organizations 295–8
Hooper, Baroness 58
Horder, Thomas 267
hospitals
CM in secondary care 94–5
homeopathic 79, 297–8
for natural therapy 52, 53
Huxley, Aldous 240
hydrotherapy 245, 253
oil dispersion baths 151
spas 106, 245, 248
hygienic systems 244, 248
British Natural Hygiene Society 301
hypnotherapy/hypnosis 210–19
advertising claims 72
autogenic therapy and 238
in Bulgaria 107
historical aspects 13, 80, 210
for irritable bowel syndrome 94, 216
legal aspects 79–80
numbers seeking 32
social class and 36
therapist numbers 48
training aspects 61, 65
UK organizations 298
hypoglycaemia 246–7

Illich, Ivan 14
Independent Therapists Examining Council
(ITEC) 48, 66
Indian medicine (Ayurvedic) 5, 115–18, 157–61
UK organizations 294
Industrial Injuries Board 78
infants, *see* children
infections (chronic) 36

Ingham, Eunice 222
INRAT (International Network for Research on
Alternative Therapies) 104
Institute for Complementary Medicine 66,
81, 306
insurance
medical insurance 77
professional indemnity 72–3
International College of Oriental Medicine
59–60
International Network for Research on
Alternative Therapies, *see* INRAT
iridology 8, 245, 247
Society of Iridologists 302
irritable bowel syndrome
acupuncture for 139
hypnotherapy for 94, 216
relaxation for 236
Iscador (mistletoe) 87, 151, 154–5
Italy 99, 103

Japanese medicine
herbalism (Kanpo) 132, 304
shiatzu 131, 225–6, 302
Jersey 99

Kanpo (Japanese herbalism) 132, 304
kinesiology 226–7, 300
Kingston Clinic 53
Kinnoul, Lord 80
Kirlian Institute 306
Kirlian photography 9, 135, 178
Kneipp, Sebastian 100, 244
Kneipp system 100
Kunert, W. 164

La Leche league 306
Lannoye, Paul 105
Laurence, George 271
law, *see* legal and policy aspects
laying on of hands 179, 181
legal and policy aspects 70–96
acupuncture needles 80–1
advertising standards 51, 72, 77
CM within the NHS 87–95
European Union and 76–7
herbs and medicines 81–6
homeopathy 78–9, 86–7
hypnotherapy 79–80
insurance 77
medical incompetence/malpractice 64, 72
registration of therapists 73–6
sickness and death certificates 77–8
Lewisham Complementary Therapy Centre 93
Lindlahr, Henry 245
Littlejohn, John Martin 258–9
Liverpool Clinic 78–9, 91–2, 297

London College of Classical Homeopathy 61
Luxembourg 99

McManaway, Bruce 177
McTimoney Chiropractic School 55, 168–9
magnesium supplements 251
magnetic healing 178
Maharishi Ayur-Veda 160
manipulation, *see* manual therapies
Manning, Matthew 180, 182
manual therapies 220–31
    Alexander technique 143–5, 145–6
    bonesetting 12, 13, 70, 162
    cranial osteopathy 259, 262
    Feldenkrais technique 145
    kinesiology 226–7
    massage 12, 61, 151, 220–2
    polarity therapy 221
    reflexology 55, 61, 67, 222–4
    Rolfing 224–5
    shiatzu 131, 225–6, 302
    spinal touch treatment 227
    therapist numbers 48
    UK organizations 298–300
    see also chiropractic; osteopathy
Mao, Chairman 113
Marylebone Centre Trust 306
Marylebone Health Centre 93–4
massage 220–2
    historical aspects 12, 220
    rhythmical 151
    rolfing 224–5
    shiatzu 131, 225–6, 302
    training issues 61
    UK organizations 299–300
ME (myalgic encephalopathy) 36
medical dowsing 9, 268–70, 305
medical insurance 77
medical litigation 72–3
Medical Research Council 20
medicines
    anthroposophical 151
    historical aspects 11–12, 81, 187
    licensing of herbal medicines 81–6
    licensing of homeopathic remedies 86–7
    move away from 14
    Natural Medicines Society 84, 307
    in Third World 112
Medicines Bill (1971) 82
Medicines Control Agency 87
meditation 235–6
    Transcendental Meditation 160, 235
Mesmer, Franz Anton 210
Middlesex University 60
migraine 37
    acupuncture for 5, 136
    anthroposophical medicines for 151
    biofeedback for 237
    chiropractic for 164, 167

Mikheev, Dr 168
mind-body therapies 232–43
    autogenic therapy 57, 238–40
    bioenergetics 13, 234
    biofeedback 236–8
    eyesight training 240–1
    meditation 160, 235–6
    prayer healing 179
    relaxation techniques 235–6
    UK organizations 300–1
    visualization 179–80
    see also hypnotherapy; hypnosis
mistletoe (Iscador) 87, 151, 154–5
modern medicine, *see* conventional medicine
monodiets 249
MORA system 138
moxibustion 130
Mozambique 112
MRC (Medical Research Council) 20
multiple sclerosis 36
Muntendam, Professor 102
musculoskeletal problems 36–9
    chiropractic for 162–70
music therapy 172–3
    UK organizations 292–3
National Childbirth Trust 306
National Health Service (NHS) 88
    CM within 17, 19, 87–95, 139, 155
    recent reforms 89–90
National Institute of Health (NIH) 98
National Institute of Homeopathy (Calcutta) 117
National Institute of Medical Herbalists 55,
    195, 295
National Poisons Unit 192
National Vocational Qualifications scheme 61
Natural Health Foundation 306–7
Natural Health Network 307
natural medicine 3–4
Natural Medicines Society 84, 307
Nature Cure Clinic 52
naturopathy 4, 8, 38–9, 244–57
    in Australia 107
    hygienic systems 244, 248
    numbers seeking 32
    nutrition therapy 250–4
    therapist numbers 48
    UK organizations 301–2
    UK variations 36
    in the United States 98
    in West Germany 99, 100
    in Western Europe 99
nausea, acupuncture for 134, 137
Netherlands 102–3
    anthroposophical medicine 148
    CM legal position 99, 102–3
    patient surveys 31–2, 34, 41–2
neurological diseases 36
New Zealand 107, 109
NHS, *see* National Health Service
Nogier, Dr 138

Northern College of Acupuncture 56, 60
nurses/nursing care 94–5
  Alexander technique for nurses 145–6
  massage by 221
  reflexology by 224
  therapeutic touch 181
nutrition therapy 12, **250–4**
  fasting 248–9, 254
  monodiets 249
  short courses in 57
  UK organizations 301–2, 307
  vegetarianism 253
NVQ scheme 61

Occupational Standards Councils 61
Office of Alternative Medicine (US) 32
Oriental medicine **125–42**
  diagnostic skills 8
  herbal medicine 131–2
  professional bodies 59–60
  Qi concept 7, 125–6
  UK organizations 302
  see also acupuncture
orthodox medicine, *see* conventional medicine
OSC for Health and Social Care 61
osteoarthritis 159
osteopathy **258–65**
  in Belgium 103
  cranial 259, 262
  education/training issues 55, 57, 67
  historical aspects 13, 258–9
  insurance costs 73
  numbers seeking 32
  patient satisfaction 40–1
  professional bodies 55, 67, 259
  state registration 19, 74–5
  therapist numbers 48, 49
  UK organizations 304–5
  UK variations 36
  in the United States 74, 261, 262, 264
  versus chiropractic 164
Ottery St Mary's Hospital 53
outcome measures 39; *see also* research studies

pain (chronic) 36
pain relief
  acupuncture for 133–4, 136, 215
  hypnotherapy for 214, 215
  massage for 222
  TENS for 138
painting therapy 76, 152, **153**, 171–2, 173
Palmer, D.D. 162–3
Park Attwood Therapeutic Centre 155
Patel, Chandra 236
patients 31–45
  numbers seeking CM 31–3
  patient satisfaction 39–43
  reasons for seeking CM 33–9

who are they? 35–6
pendulum 9, 268, 271
Persian medicine 112
pharmacopoeias 87, 187
  herbal 193
  homeopathic 87
Pharmacy and Poisons Act (1933) 81
physical therapy, *see* manual therapies
phytotherapy
  ESCOP 86
  School of Phytotherapy 60
  see also herbalism
Pierce-Jones, Frank 144
placebo response 233
polarity therapy 221, 300
policy, *see* legal and policy aspects
polyclinics 52
Popp, Fritz 204
Portsmouth University 55
postural therapies
  Alexander technique 57, **143–5**, 145–6
  Feldenkrais technique **145**
  UK organizations 289–90
prayer healing 179
Priessnitz, Vincent 244
private medical insurance 77
professional bodies 66–8
  in acupuncture 56, 58–60, 67, 302–3
  in chiropractic 55
  in herbalism 55
  in homeopathy 60, 60–1, 67, 297
  in osteopathy 55, 67, 259
  registration of therapists 73–6
Professions Supplementary to Medicine 71, 75–6
psionic medicine 271, 305
psychic diagnosis 9
psychic surgery 182–3
psychological therapies, *see* mind-body
  therapies
psychoneuroimmunology 232
psychotherapy
  art therapy and 171–2
  hypnotherapy in 214
  Reichian 234
publicity/advertising restrictions 51, 77

Qigong 132, 137–8
quackery 64–6
questionnaires, *see* surveys

radiesthesia, *see* radionics
radionics **266–71**
  historical aspects 13, 266–7
  medical dowsing 9, 268–70, 305
  therapist numbers 48
  UK organizations 305
Rasayana therapy 159
Raynaud's phenomenon 239

RCCM (Research Council for Complementary
    Medicine) 22
  survey on therapist numbers 47
  survey on use of CM 31
reflexology 222–4
  Therapy Group of Reflexologists 67
  training issues 56, 61
  UK organizations 298–9
registration 73–6
  historical aspects 71
  international aspects 97–118
  see also professional bodies
Reich, William 13
Reichian psychotherapy 234
Reilly, Taylor 63
relaxation techniques 235–6
  meditation 160, 235–6
  UK organizations 300–1
Research Council for Complementary Medicine
    (RCCM) 22, 307
research studies 20–7
  acupuncture 9, 20–2, 25, 133–7
  anthroposophical medicine 154–5
  aromatherapy 228
  autogenic therapy 239
  chiropractic 164, 165–8
  herbalism 21, 137, 193–4
  homeopathy 24–5, 202, 204–6
  hypnotherapy 215–16
  Indian medicine 159
  music therapy 173
  naturopathy 251–3
  osteopathy 262–4
  outcome measures 39
  reflexology 224
  in Russia 106
  shiatzu 226
  spiritual healing 180–3
  therapist training and 57
residential clinics 52–3
  Tyringham 52–3, 307
rheumatic disorders 174, 244
rheumatoid arthritis 191, 206, 248, 253
Rolf, Ida 224
rolfing 224–5
Rosenthal, Marilyn 115
Royal Liverpool Hospital 78–9
Royal London Homeopathic Hospital 79
Rudolf Steiner schools 148
Russia 106–7

St Mary's Hospital 93
scabies 159
Scandinavia 99, 103–4
Schatz, J. 101
School of Phytotherapy 60
School of Spiritual Science 147
Schroth, Johannes 244
Schultz, Johannes 238, 239

Schumacher, E.F. 149
scientific medicine *see* conventional medicine
Selye, Hans 232, 245–6
sense therapies 173–4
  colour therapy 173–4
  sound therapy 174
  UK organizations 293–4
sex distribution of CM users 36
Shackleton, Basil 249
shamanism 12
Sharma, Chandra 158
Sharma, Ursula 33
Shelton, H.M. 248
shiatzu 131, 225–6
  UK organizations 302
Shrubland Hall 53
sickness certificates 77–8
  in Australia 108
Siddha medicine 115–16, 158
sleep disorders 36
social class and CM 35–6
Society of Homeopaths 60, 67, 297
Sofia University 106–7
sound therapy 174
South Africa 107, 109
Spain 99, 103
spas 106, 245, 248
spinal touch treatment 227
spiritual healing 48, 176–85
  radionics and 268
  UK organizations 294, 299
  see also healing therapies
Spiritualist National Union (SNU) 48
Sri Lanka 116, 117
statistics
  CM consultations 50–1
  CM usage 31–43
  GP consultations 32–3, 50–1
Stebbing, Dr 205
Steiner, Rudolf 147–50, 271
Still, Andrew Taylor 258
Stone, Randolph 221
stress-related illnesses 36, 232–3; *see also*
    mind-body therapies
surveys
  CM usage 31–43
  number of UK therapists 47–9
  workload of therapists 49–50
Sutherland, William Garner 262
Sweden 104
Switzerland 99
  anthroposophical medicine 147–8

T'ai-chi 126, 132, 234
  Qigong 132, 137–8
Tamil Nadu 116
Tanzania 109
technical medicine, *see* conventional medicine
TENS 138

Therapeutic Goods Act 108–9
Therapeutic Substances Act (1956) 81–2
therapists 46–69
  competence and quackery 64–6
  consultation statistics 50–1
  herbal 194–5
  numbers in UK 47–9
  professional bodies 66–8
  training/education issues 53–63
  workload 49–50
Therapy Group of Reflexologists 67
Third World countries 109–18; *see also* Chinese
    medicine; Indian medicine
Tibetan medicine
  herbalism 131–2
  in Russia 106
  UK organizations 304
Tinbergen, Nikko 144
traditional medicine 4, 109–12
  bonesetting 12, 13, 70, 162
  in China 113–15
  in India 115–18, 157–61
  in Russia 106
  see also healing therapies; herbalism
training, *see* education/training issues
Transcendental Meditation 160, 235
transcutaneous nerve stimulation (TENS) 138
tryptophan 83
Turkestan 106
turmeric 159
Tyringham Naturopathic Clinic 52–3, 307

Uganda 109
Unani medicine 116, 158, 160
UNESCO 106
United States 97–8
  CM statistics 32, 98
  cost of CM 49

Holistic Health Centres 52
University of Exeter 57
University of Glasgow 64
University of Maryland 98
University of Portsmouth 55
University of Wales 55, 56, 60
University of Westminster 55, 57
USA, *see* United States

vegetarianism/veganism 253
  UK organizations 307
Vietnam 114
village medicine, *see* traditional medicine
visualization 179–80
vitamin supplements 83, 251, 252
Voll, Dr 138
von Peczely, Edmund 245

Wala (pharmaceutical company) 151
Waldorf Schools 148
Wales, Prince of 18
Watson, Lyall 183
Wegman, Ita 147, 151
Weiskrantz, L. 80
Weleda (UK) Ltd 151, 298
Wellbeing Centre 52
West Germany 100–1
  anthroposophical medicine 148
  CM legal position 99
Westminster University 55, 57
World Health Organization (WHO)
  acupuncture guidelines 133
  traditional medicine and 111

yoga therapy 234
  UK organizations 300, 301